Basic and Clinical Applications of Vision Science

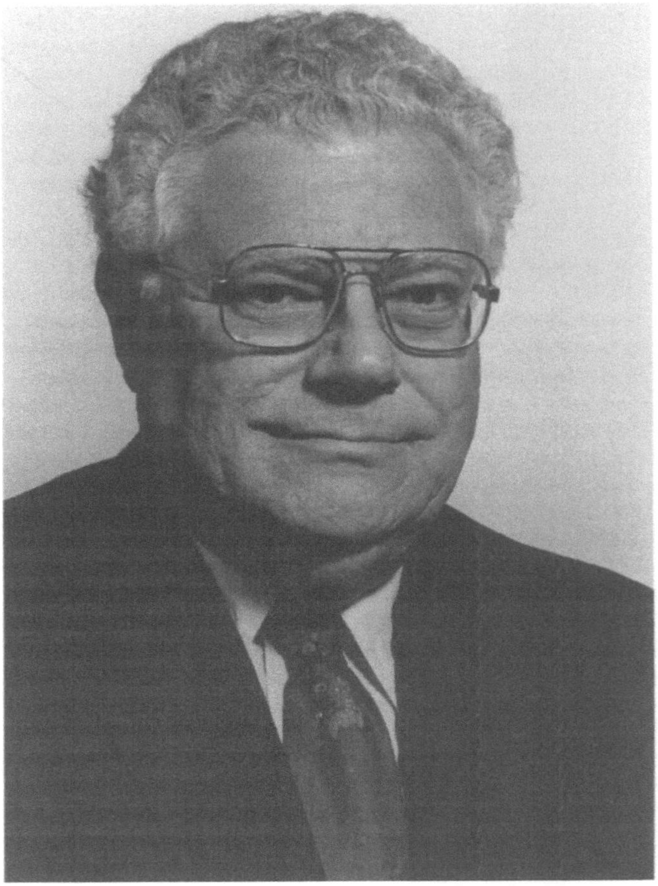

Professor Jay M. Enoch, O.D., Ph.D., D.Sc.(H.C.)

Basic and Clinical Applications of Vision Science

The Professor Jay M. Enoch Festschrift Volume

Edited by

V. LAKSHMINARAYANAN

School of Optometry and
Department of Physics and Astronomy,
St. Louis, Miss., U.S.A.

SPRINGER-SCIENCE+BUSINESS MEDIA, B.V.

A C.I.P. Catalogue record for this book is available from the Library of Congress

ISBN 978-94-010-6403-3 ISBN 978-94-011-5698-1 (eBook)
DOI 10.1007/978-94-011-5698-1

Printed on acid-free paper

Documenta Ophthalmologica Proceedings Series

VOLUME 60

The titles published in this series are listed at the end of this volume.

CONTENTS

PREFACE

I first met Jay Enoch in 1981 at a Christmas party held in Minor Hall at Berkeley. He had recently arrived as Dean and I was a junior graduate student. When he found out that my training was in Physics, he gave me a copy of his recently published book on photoreceptor optics, which I read through that Christmas break. Little did I realize that this was the start of a long relationship in which he played the role of dissertation advisor, mentor, boss, colleague and more importantly, friend, and that 15 years later I would be the chief organizer of the Enoch Vision Science Symposium (EnochFest; April 27-30, 1996) and the editor of this volume celebrating his numerous contributions to Vision Science, Optometry and Ophthalmology.

When Dean Tony Adams first asked me to serve as organizer of the EnochFest, it was with trepidation I accepted. However, my task was lightened by the labor of the Scientific Program Committee (Profs. G. Westheimer, H. Kaufman, and Dr. D. Birch) and the Local Organizing Committee (Profs. I. Bailey, C. Johnson, W. Eng, Mr. C. Campbell, and Mr. R. Knowles). I use this opportunity to acknowledge their advice and considerable work in making this meeting a success. The topics presented at the Fest were representative of the many facets of Jay's career. Fourteen countries from four continents were represented by the participants. A report on the meeting is to be published in an upcoming issue of the journal Optometry and Vision Science (Vol 73, No. 11, 1996).

This book contains many of the papers delivered at the EnochFest, as well as papers by others who could not be present at the Fest. The range and breadth of Jay's interests are truly reflected in the nature of the contributions in this volume. Due to constraints beyond my control, I regret that I could not accommodate the articles of several others who would have gladly contributed to this volume. On behalf of all the contributors, EnochFest participants and all of his colleagues, friends and admirers, this Enoch Festschrift volume is dedicated to Professor Jay M. Enoch.

V. Lakshminarayanan
St. Louis, MO
September 3, 1996

ACKNOWLEDGMENTS

This book and the Enoch Vision Science Symposium would not have been possible without the generous support, financial and otherwise, of many people and organizations. A special thanks goes to the University of California, Berkeley School of Optometry and Dean A. J. Adams. UCBSO not only hosted the meeting, but was also a major symposium and publication sponsor. I also gratefully acknowledge the other corporate and individual sponsors whose financial contribution helped underwrite the Symposium and this Volume (in alphabetical order):

Alcon Laboratories, Inc.
Allergan, Inc.
Dr. Shinobu Awaya
Drs. David and Eileen Birch
The Family of Raymond Eng
Heidelberg Engineering, Inc.
Hoya Corp.
Dr. Donald Korb
Nidek Corp.
Dr. Hitoshi Ohzu
Optische Werke G. Rodenstock
Pentax - Asahi Optical Co.
Retina Foundation of the Southwest
Smith Kettlewell Eye Research Institute
Dr. Shinichi Yamade
Dr. Tetsushi Yasuma
Welch Allyn, Inc.

Financial support for the Symposium was also provided by:

Dr. Irvin M. Borish
Dr. Edward Revelli

Logistical and clerical support at Berkeley was provided by Lois Quick, who also served as the central co-ordinator. She was assisted by Renisa Andrika, Brenda Marshall and Michael Phipps. At St. Louis, invaluable assistance in preparation of this book in the prescribed format was provided by Srinivasa Varadharajan. Thanks also go to Judie Walter and Janice White.

V. Lakshminarayanan
St. Louis, MO
September 3, 1996

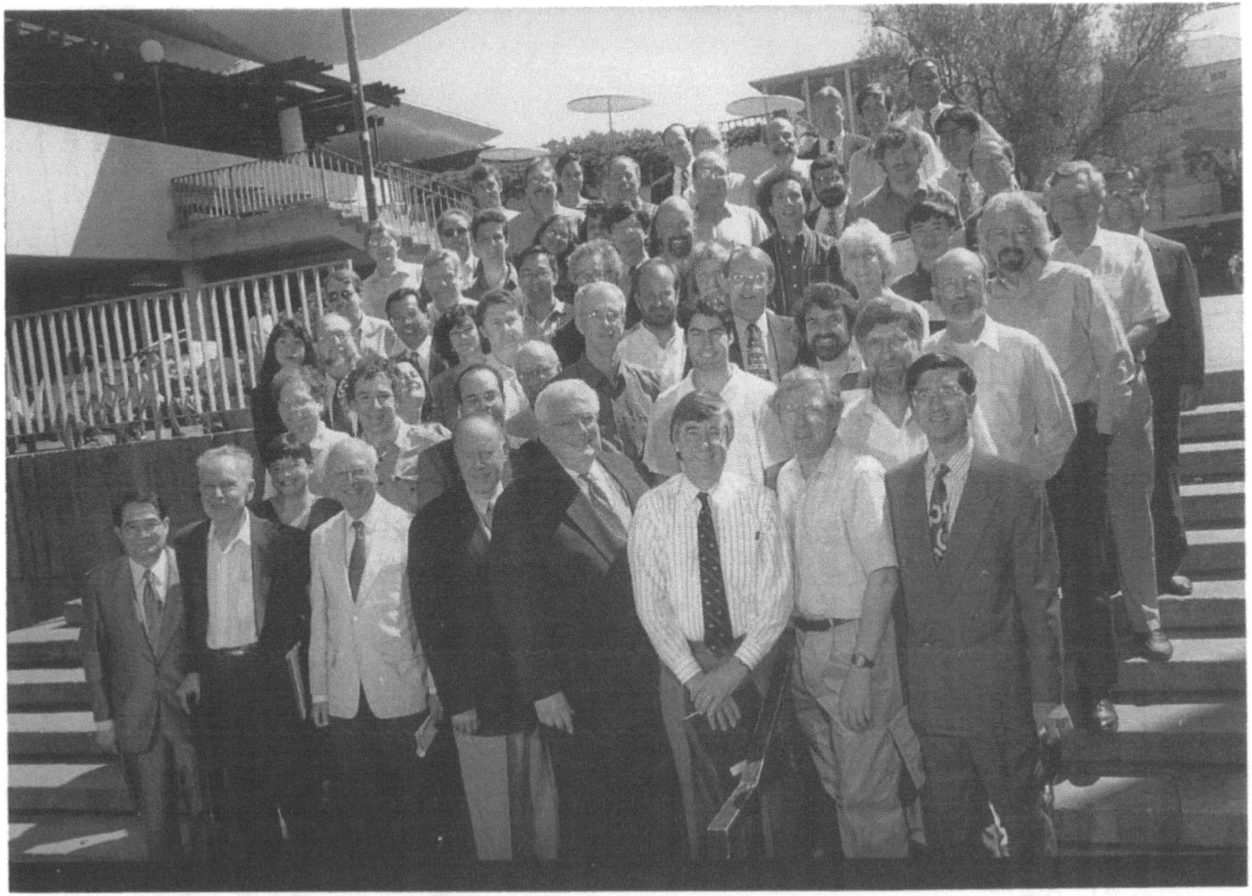

The Enoch Vision Science Symposium, April 27-30, 1996, Berkeley, CA.
Note: Not all participants are in the photograph.

LIST OF CONTRIBUTORS

Note: Only the address of the primary/senior author is given.

Cheryl AINE

Gholamali AMIRKHIABANI
Faculty of Arts, Dept of Psychology
Central Queensland University
Rockhampton, QLD4702, AUSTRALIA

Patricia APKARIAN

Masashi ARAI

Amir AREF

Shinobu AWAYA
Nagoya University, School of Medicine
Department of Ophthalmology
65 Tsurma-cho, Showa-ku
Nagoya 466, JAPAN

Ian L. BAILEY
School of Optometry
University of California - Berkeley
Berkeley, CA 94720

James E. BAILEY
Southern California College of Optometry
2575 Yorba Linda Blvd
Fullerton, CA 92631

Alessandra BALDI

Patrizia BARALDI
Dip. Scienze Biomediche
Universita'di Modena
Via Campi 287, 41100 Modena, ITALY

Michael BARRIS
College of Optometry
Nova Southeastern University
North Miami Beach, FL 33162

Christopher BEAVER

Harold E. BEDELL
College of Optometry
University of Houston
4901 Calhoun Blvd
Houston, TX 77204

Eliot L. BERSON
Berman-Gund Laboratory for the Study of
Retinal Degenerations
Harvard Medical School
Massachusetts Eye and Ear Infirmary
243 Charles Street
Boston, MA 02114

Sanjiv K. BHATIA

David BIRCH
Retina Foundation of the Southwest
9900 North Central Expressway #400
Dallas, TX 75231

Jyothirmay BISWAS
Medical and Vision Research Foundation
18 College Road
Madras 600 006, INDIA

Lo BOUR
Clinical Neurophysiology
Department of Neurology
Academic Medical Center, H2-214
Meibergdreef 9
1105 AZ Amsterdam
THE NETHERLANDS

Renee BOVELLE

Arthur BRADLEY

Maria L. CALVO
Departamento de Optica
Facultad de Ciencias Fisicas
Universidad Complutense
28040 Madrid, SPAIN

Melanie C.W. CAMPBELL
School of Optometry
University of Waterloo
Waterloo, Ontario N2L 3G1
CANADA

Thomas J. CAMPEN

Emilio C. CAMPOS
Clinica Oculistica Ia
Universita di Bologna
via Massarenti 9
40138 Bologna, ITALY

Valentina CETTOLO

Hai-Wen CHEN
Biophysics group, MS D454
Los Alamos National Laboratory
Los Alamos, NM 87545

Margarita CHEVALIER

Yun CHOI

Gerhard CIBIS
Children's Mercy Hospital Department of
Surgery and Pediatrics
24th and Gillham
Kansas City, MO 64112

Alexander I. COGAN
The Smith-Kettlewell Eye Research Institute
2232 Webster Street
San Francisco, CA 94115

Theodore E. COHN
School of Optometry
Univeristy of California - Berkeley
Berkeley, CA 94720

James COMERFORD
The New England College of Optometry
424 Beacon Street
Boston, MA 02115

Joseph M. CORLESS

Melanie CRANDALL

Mary Ann CROFT

Mathew E. DIAMOND

Alvin EISNER
R.S. Dow Neurological Sciences Institute
Good Samaritan Hospital
1120 NW 20th Avenue
Portland, OR 97209

William R. ELLIOT

Nader ENGHETA

Jay M. ENOCH
School of Optometry
Univeristy of California - Berkeley
Berkeley, CA 94720

Edward A. ESSOCK
Departments of Psychology and
Ophthalmology and Visual Sciences
University of Louisville
Louisville, KY 40292

Franz FANKHAUSER
Lindenhofspital Bern
Bremgartenstrasse 117
CH-3012 Bern, SWITZERLAND

Frederick W. FITZKE
Department of Visual Science
Institute of Ophthalmology
University College London
11-43 Bath Street
London EC1V 9EL, UK

Edward FLYNN

Maria P. FRANCESCATO

Gregory GANCARZ

Stephen J. GANGE

Adrian GLASSER

David A. GOSS

Theodore GROSVENOR
Indiana University School of Optometry
800 E Atwater Avenue
Bloomington, IN 47405

Gunther GUILINO
Optische Werke G. Rodenstock
Isartalstrasse 43
D-80469 Munich, GERMANY

Toyohiko HATADA

PUBLICATIONS OF PROFESSOR JAY M ENOCH

This list was prepared from Professor Enoch's Curriculum Vitae. It does not include Technical Reports, Standards documents, Editorials, Book Reviews, etc. This list is current as of August 1996.

BOOKS

[1] Enoch JM, editor. *Perimetric Standards and Perimetric Glossary of the International Council of Ophthalmology*; Concilium Ophthalmologicum Universale; The Hague: Dr. W. Junk bv Publishers, 1979.
[2] Enoch JM, Fitzgerald CR, and Campos EC. *Quantitative Layer-by-Layer Perimetry: an extended analysis*. New York: Grune and Stratton, 1980.
[3] Enoch JM, and Tobey FL Jr. *Vertebrate Photoreceptor Optics*. Springer Series in Optical Sciences. Volume 23. Heidelberg: Springer-Verlag, 1981.
[4] Proenza L, Enoch JM and Jampolsky A, editors. *Clinical Applications of Visual Psychophysics*. Cambridge: Cambridge University Press, 1981.
[5] Dawson W and Enoch JM, editors. *Foundations of Sensory Science*. New York-Heidelberg:Springer-Verlag, 1984.
[6] Enoch JM and Cavanaugh HD, editors. *Contact lenses: Challenges, Controversies and Opportunities*. CORNEA, Vol. 9, Suppl. 1, New York: Raven Press, 1990.

BOOK CHAPTERS

[1] McGraw J and Enoch JM. Summary of Army Medical Research Laboratory, Report No. 99. In: Obrig TE and Salvatori PL,editors. *Contact Lenses*. New York: Obrig Laboratories, 1957: 404-423.
[2] Enoch JM. Physiology: Vision. In: Sorsby A, editor. *Modern Ophthalmology. Vol. 1, Basic Aspects*. Butterworths, London: 1963: 202-289.
[3]. Enoch JM. The retina as a fiber optics bundle. Appendix B In: Kapany NS, editor. *Fiber Optics, Principles and Applications*. New York: Academic Press, 1967: 372-396.
[4] Enoch JM. An attempt to restore binocular stereoscopic vision in selected unilateral aphakic patients. In: Becker B and Burde R, editors. *Current Concepts in Ophthalmology*. St. Louis: CV Mosby, 1969: 236-247.
[5] Enoch JM. The two-color threshold technique of Stiles and derived component color mechanisms.In:Hurvich L, editor. *The Handbook of Sensory Physiology*. Vol. VII/4. Berlin: Springer-Verlag,1972:537-567.
[6] Enoch JM. Vertebrate rod receptors are directionally sensitive. In: Snyder AW and Menzel R, editors. *Photoreceptor Optics*. Berlin: Springer-Verlag, 1975: 17-37.
[7] Enoch JM. Retinal stretch and accommodation. In: Kaufman H and Zimmerman T, editors. *Current Concepts of Ophthalmology*. Vol 4. St. Louis: CV Mosby, 1976: 59-78.
[8] Provine RR and Enoch JM. On voluntary ocular accommodation in biofeedback and self-control. In: *An Aldine Annual on the Regulation of Bodily Processes and Consciousness*. Chicago: Aldine Publishing Company, 1976: 526-528.
[9] Enoch JM. Vertebrate photoreceptor orientation. In: Kaufman H and Zimmerman T, editors. *Current Concepts in Ophthalmology*. Vol 6. St. Louis: CV Mosby, 1979: 69-96.

[10] Enoch JM and Campos EC. New quantitative perimetric tests designed to evaluate receptive-field-like properties in diseases of the retina and the optic nerve. In: Sokol S, editor. *Electrophysiology and Psychophysics: Their Use in Ophthalmic Diagnosis;* International Ophthalmology Clinics. Vol 20(1). Boston: Little, Brown and Co. Inc., 1980: 83-133.
[11] Enoch JM. Vision Problems of the Aging Patient: An Overview. In: Rosenbloom AA and Morgan MW, editors. *Vision and Aging: General and Clinical Perspectives.* 2nd ed. New York: Professional Press Books, Fairchild Publications, 1985: 77-82.
[12] Enoch JM, Williams RA, Essock EA, and Fendick MG. Hyperacuity: A Promising Means of Evaluating Vision Through Cataract. In: Osborne NN and Chader GL, editors. *Progress in Retinal Research.* Vol. 4. Oxford and New York: Pergamon Press, 1985: 67-88.
[13] Adams AJ, Bodis-Wollner I, Enoch JM, Jeannerod M, and Mitchell DE. Normal and Abnormal Mechanisms of Vision: as Revealed by Visual Disorders and Visual Deprivation. In: Spillmann L and Werner JS, editors. *Visual Perception: the Neurophysiological Foundations.* New York: Academic Press, 1990.
[14] Campos E and Enoch JM. The Management of the Aphakic Neonate. In: Rosenbloom AA and Morgan MW, editors.*Pediatric Optometry.* Philadelphia: JB Lippincott, 1990: 420-433.
[15]. Enoch JM and Lakshminarayanan V. Clinical Visual Psychophysics Measurements. In: Masters BR, editor. *New Developments in Noninvasive Studies to Evaluate Ocular Function.* New York: Springer-Verlag, 1990: 454-78.
[16]. Enoch JM and Lakshminarayanan V. Retinal Fibre Optics. In: Charman WN, editor. *Vision and Visual Dysfunction. Vol. 1: Visual Optics and Instrumentation.* London: Macmillan Books, 1991: 280-309.

PAPERS

[1] Enoch, J.M.: Prescribing the prism correction. Optical Journal Review 88:27-31, 1951.
[2] Enoch, J.M. and McGraw, J.L.: Contact lenses: Some aspects of visual acuity and photophobia. Part I. Am. J. Optom. and Arch. Am. Acad. Optom , Visual Acuity. 31:1-27, 1954.
[3] Enoch, J.M. and McGraw, J.L.: Contact lenses: Some aspects of visual acuity and photophobia, Part II. Am. J. Optom. and Arch. Am. Acad. Optom, 31:78-87, 1954.
[4] McGraw, J.L and Enoch, J.M.: Contact lenses - An evaluating study. Trans. Amer. Acad. of Ophth. & Optom., 58:561-575, 1954.
[5] Boynton, R.M., Bush, W.R., and Enoch, J.M.: Rapid changes in foveal sensitivity resulting from direct and indirect adapting stimuli. J. Opt. Soc. Am. 44:56-60, 1954.
[6] Boynton, R.M., Enoch, J.M. and Bush, W.R.: Physical measures of stray light in excised eyes. J. Opt. Soc. Am. 33:879-886, 1954.
[7] Enoch, J.M.: Descartes' contact lens. Am. J. Optom. and Arch. Am. Acad. Optom. 33:77-8, 1956.
[8] Enoch, J.M.: Review of Zigler's work. Intersociety Color Council Newsletter, 126:2-5, 1956.
[9] Enoch, J.M.: Amblyopia and the Stiles-Crawford effect. Am. J. Optom. and Arch. Am. Acad. Optom. 34:298-309, 1957.
[10] Enoch, J.M.: Summated response of the retina to light entering different parts of the pupil. J. Opt. Soc. Am. 48:392-405, 1958. (Ph. D. Dissertation, Ohio State University, 1956.)
[11] Enoch, J.M. and Fry, G.A.: Characteristics of a model retinal receptor studied at microwave frequencies. J. Opt. Soc. Am. 48:899-911, 1958.
[12] Enoch, J.M.: Effect of the size of a complex display upon visual search. J. Opt. Soc. Am. 49:280-286, 1959.
[13] Enoch, J.M.: Further studies on the relationship between amblyopia and the Stiles-Crawford effect. Am. J. Optom. and Arch. Am. Acad. Optom. 36:111-128, 1959.

[14] Enoch, J.M.: Natural Tendencies in Visual Search of a Complex Display. In: *Visual Search Techniques*, Publication #171, National Academy of Sciences, National Research Council, Washington D.C: 92-93; 187-193; 251-252, 1959.
[15] Enoch, J.M.: Environmental stress as related to the visual mechanism. Human Factors 2:76-83, 1960.
[16] Enoch, J.M.: Receptor amblyopia. Am. J. Ophthalmol. 48 Part II:262-273, 1959.
[17] Enoch, J.M.: Optical interaction effects in models of parts of the visualreceptors. Arch. Ophthalmol. 63:548-558, 1960.
[18] Enoch, J.M.: Response of a model retinal receptor as a function of wavelength. J. Opt. Soc. Am. 50:315-320, 1960.
[19] Kalk, M. and Enoch, J.M.: An objective test procedure designed to aid in selecting, training and rating photo interpreters. Photogrammetric Engineering 228-237, 1960.
[20] Constant, M.A. and Enoch, J.M.: A simple optical aid for obtaining calibration curves in tonography. Am. J. Ophthalmol. 49 Part I:1030-1031, 1960.
[21] Enoch, J.M.: Waveguide modes: Are they present, and what is their possible role in the visual mechanism? J. Opt. Soc. Am. 50:1025-1026, 1960.
[22] Enoch, J.M.: Waveguide modes in retinal receptors. Science 133, No. 3461:1353-1354, 1961.
[23] Enoch, J.M.: Visualization of wave-guide modes in retinal receptors, Am. J. Ophthalmol. 51 Part II:1107-1118, 1961.
[24] Fankhauser, F., Enoch, J.M. and Cibis, P.: Receptor orientation in retinal pathology: A first study. Am. J. Ophthalmol. 52 Part II:767-783, 1961.
[25] Enoch, J.M.: Nature of the transmission of energy in the retinal receptors. J. Opt. Soc. Am. 51:1122-1126, 1961.
[26] Enoch, J.M. and Stiles, W.S.: The color change of monochromatic light with retinal angle of incidence. Optica Acta 8:329-358, 1961.
[27] Fankhauser, F. and Enoch, J.M.: The effects of blur upon perimetric thresholds. Arch. Ophthalmol. 68:240-251, 1962.
[28] Enoch, J.M.: Optical properties of retinal receptors. J. Opt. Soc. Am. 53:71-85, 1963.
[29] Enoch, J.M.: The use of tetrazolium to distinguish between retinal receptors exposed and not exposed to light. Invest. Ophthalmol. 2:16-23,1963.
[30] Enoch, J.M.: Some waveguide characteristics of retinal receptors. Giornale di Fisica IV, No. 4:cover, p. 242 and opposite p. 248, October-December 1963.
[31] Enoch, J.M.: Validation of an indicator of mammalian retinal receptor response: Action spectrum. J. Opt. Soc. Am. 54:368-373, 1964.
[32] Enoch, J.M.: Physical properties of the retinal receptors and response of the retinal receptors. Psychol. Bull. 61:242-251, 1964.
[33] Enoch, J.M.: Validation of an indicator of mammalian retinal receptor response: Absolute threshold. J. Opt. Soc. Am. 54:1027-1030, 1964.
[34] Enoch, J.M.: An approach towards the study of retinal receptor optics. Am. J. Optom. & Arch. Am. Acad. Optom 42:63-70, 1965.
[35] Enoch, J.M.: Validation of an indicator of mammalian retinal receptor response: Density of stain as a function of stimulus magnitude. J. Opt. Soc. Am. 56:116-123, 1966 and Erratum J. Opt. Soc. Am. 56:529, 1966.
[36] Enoch, J.M. and Glismann, L.E.: Physical and optical changes in excised retinal tissue: Resolution of retinal receptors as a fiber optics bundle. Invest. Ophthalmol. 5:208-221, 1966.
[37] Enoch, J.M.: Retinal microspectrophotometry. J.Opt. Soc. Am. 56:833-835, 1966.
[38] Enoch, J.M.: The current status of receptor amblyopia. Doc. Ophthalmol. 23:130-148, 1967.
[39] Enoch, J.M.: Comments on "Excitation of waveguide modes in retinal receptors." J. Opt. Soc. Am. 57:548-549, 1967.

[40] Enoch, J.M.: Validation of an indicator of mammalian retinal receptor response: Recovery in the dark following exposure to a luminous stimulus. Invest. Ophthalmol. 6:647-656, 1967.
[41] Enoch, J.M.: A spectacle-contact lens combination used as a reverse Galilean telescope in unilateral aphakia. Am. J. Optom. & Arch. Am. Acad. Optom 45:231-240, 1968.
[42] Enoch, J.M. and Windsor, C.E.: Remission of nystagmus following fitting contact lenses to an infant with aniridia. Am. J. Ophthalmol. 66:333-335, 1968.
[43] Enoch, J.M., Goldmann, H. and Sunga, R.: The ability to distinguish which eye was stimulated by light. Invest. Ophthalmol. 8:317-331, 1969.
[44] Enoch, J.M. and Sunga, R.N.: Hans Goldmann Festschrift article. Development of quantitative perimetric tests. Doc. Ophthalmol. 26:215-229, 1969.
[45] Krill, A., Potts, A., Johanson, C. and Enoch, J.M.: A discrepancy between dark adaptation and the electroretinogram in chloroquine retinopathy. Proc. ISCERG: 317-339, 1969.
[46] Enoch, J.M. and Sunga, R.N.: The development of quantitative perimetric tests. Osterreich Ophthalmologische Gesellshaft, 12 Jahreshauptversammlung, Vienna:69 and enclosures, June 5-7, 1969.
[47] Enoch, J.M.: Photoreceptor orientation following retinal detachment. Am. J. Ophthalmol. 67:603-604, 1969.
[48] Enoch, J.M.: Amblyopia, eccentric fixation and the Stiles-Crawford effect. Am. J. Optom. 47:482-484, 1970.
[49] Enoch, J.M., Sunga, R.N. and Bachmann, E.: Static perimetric technique believed to test receptive field properties. I. Extension of Westheimer's experiments on spatial interaction. Am. J. Ophthalmol. 70:113-126, 1970.
[50] Enoch, J.M., Sunga, R.and Bachmann, E.: Static perimetric technique believed to test receptive field properties. II. Adaptation of the method to the quantitative perimeter. Am. J. Ophthalmol. 70:126-137, 1970.
[51] Sunga, R. N. and Enoch, J.M.: A static perimetric technique believed to test receptive field properties: III. Clinical trials. Am. J. Ophthalmol. 70:244-272, 1970.
[52] Sunga, R.N. and Enoch, J.M.: Further perimetric analysis of patients with lesions of the visual pathways. Am. J. Ophthalmol. 70:403-422, 1970.
[53] Enoch, J.M. and Sunga, R.N.: Neue wege der quantitativen Perimetrie. Albrecht V. Graefes. Arch. klin. exp. Ophthalmol. 179:259-270, 1970.
[54] Brown, R. and Enoch, J.M.: Combined rules of thumb in aniseikonic prescriptions. Am. J. Ophthalmol. 69:118-126, 1970.
[55] Enoch, J.M., Berger, R. and Birns, R.: A static perimetric technique believed to test receptive field properties: Extension and verification of the analysis. Doc. Ophthalmol. 29:127-153, 1970.
[56] Enoch, J.M., Berger, R. and Birns, R.: A static perimetric technique believed to test receptive field properties: Responses near visual field lesions with sharp borders. Doc. Ophthalmol. 29:154-167, 1970.
[57] Enoch, J.M.: Office evaluation of rhodopsin. Am. J. Ophthalmol. 70:995-996, 1970.
[58] Zappia, R., Enoch, J.M., Stamper, R. Winkelman, J. and Gay, A.: The Riddoch phenomenon revealed in non-occipital lobe lesions. Brit. J. Ophthalmol. 55:416-420, 1971.
[59] Enoch, J.M. and Goldberg, M.: Lateral and longitudinal magnification in direct and indirect ophthalmoscopy. Arch. Ophthalmol. 86:536-547, 1971.
[60] Enoch, J.M.: Retinal directional resolution. In: Pierce J and Levene J, editors. *Visual Science*. 1971: Indiana Univ. Press, Bloomington, Indiana: 40-57.
[61] Laties, A. and Enoch, J.M.: An analysis of retinal receptor orientation: I. Angular relationship of neighboring photoreceptors. Invest. Ophthalmol. 10:69-77, 1971.
[62] Enoch, J.M. and Laties, A.: An analysis of retinal receptor orientation: II. Predictions for psychophysical tests. Invest. Ophthalmol. 10:959-970, 1971.

[63] Enoch, J.M. and Scandrett, J.: Human foveal far-field radiation pattern. Invest. Ophthalmol. 10:167-170 and cover picture, 1971.
[64] Winston, R. and Enoch, J.M.: Retinal cone receptor as an ideal light collector. J. Opt. Soc. Am. 61:1120-1121, 1971.
[65] Enoch, J.M.: The needs for standards in tests of vision. Am. J. Ophthalmol. 72:836-837, 1971.
[66] Enoch, J.M.: Comments on "Binocular considerations for the monocular aphakic." J. Am. Optom. Assn. 42:1077, 1971.
[67] Ohzu, H., Enoch, J.M. and O'Hair, J. Optical modulation by the isolated retina and retinal receptors. Vision Res. 12:231-244, 1972.
[68] Ohzu, H. and Enoch, J.M.: Optical modulation by the isolated human fovea. Vis. Res. 12:245-251, 1972.
[69] Ohzu, H. and Enoch, J.M.: Optische Modulation durch isolierte Netzhaute. Optica Acta 19:347-350, 1972.
[70] Enoch, J.M.: Retinal receptor orientation and the role of fiber optics in vision. The First Glenn Fry Lecture. Am. J. of Optom. & Arch. Am. Acad. Optom. 49:455-470, 1972.
[71] Enoch, J.M. and Hope, G.M.: An analysis of retinal receptor orientation: III. Results of initial psychophysical tests. Invest. Ophthalmol. 11:765-782, 1972.
[72] Enoch, J.M. and Hope, G.M.: An analysis of retinal receptor orientation. IV. Center of the entrance pupil and the center of convergence of orientation and directional sensitivity. Investmol. Ophthal. 11:1017-1021, 1972.
[73] Enoch, J.M.: On the presentation of the Friedenwald Award in Ophthalmology to Dr. Alan Laties. Invest. Ophthalmol. 11:550-552, 1972.
[74] Enoch, J.M.: The fitting of hydrophyllic (soft) contact lenses to infants and young children: I. Mensuration data on aphakic eyes of children born with congenital cataracts. Contact Lens Med. Bull. 5:36-47, 1972.
[75] Enoch, J.M.: The fitting of hydrophyllic (soft) contact lenses to infants and young children: II. Fitting techniques and initial results on aphakic children. Contact Lens Med. Bull. 5:48-49, 1972.
[76] Enoch, J.M., Scandrett, J. and Tobey, F.L. Jr.: A study of the effects of bleaching on the width and index of refraction of frog rod outer segments. Vis. Res. 13:171-183, 1973.
[77] Enoch, J.M. and Hope, G.M.: Interferometric resolution determinations in the fovea and parafovea. Doc. Ophthalmol. 34:143-156, 1973.
[78] Honda, Y. and Enoch, J.M.: The appearance of rhythmic wavelets on the ERG of alphachymotryipsin poisoned mammalian retinas. Doc. Ophthalmol. 34:91-103, 1973.
[79] Enoch, J.M. and Tobey, F.L. Jr.: A special microscope microspectrophotometer: Optical design and application to the determination of waveguide properties of frog rods. J. Opt. Soc. Am. 63:1345-1356, 1973.
[80] Daw, N. and Enoch, J.M.: Contrast sensitivity, Westheimer function and Stiles-Crawford effect in the blue cone monochromat. Vis. Res. 13:1669-1681, 1973.
[81] Blank, K. and Enoch, J.M.: Monocular spatial distortions induced by marked accommodation. Science 182:393-395, 1973.
[82] Enoch, J.M.: Effect of substantial accommodation on total retinal area. J. Opt. Soc. Am. 63:899, 1973.
[83] Enoch, J.M. and Hope, G.M.: Directional sensitivity of the foveal and parafoveal retina. The Becker Festschrift. Invest. Ophthalmol. 12:497-503, 1973.
[84] Enoch, J.M., Van Loo, J.A. and Okun, E.: Realignment of photoreceptors disturbed in orientation secondary to retinal detachment. Invest. Ophthalmol. 12:849-853, 1973.
[85] Tobey, F.L., Jr. and Enoch, J.M.: Directionality and waveguide properties of optically isolated rat rods. Invest. Ophthalmol. 12:873-880, 1973.
[86] Enoch, J.M.: Comment on "Morphologic changes in photoreceptor outer segments following photic injury." Ophthalmic Res. 6:372-373, 1974.

[87] Enoch, J.M.: A rapid, accurate technique for retinoscopy of the aphakic infant or child in the operating room. Am. J. Ophthalmol. 78:335-336, 1974.
[88] Enoch, J.M.: International visual field test standards. Annee Ther. Clin. Ophthalmol. 24:371-375, 1974.
[89] Verriest, G., Aulhorn, E., Enoch, J.M. and Israel, A.: An attempt at standardization of the terminology in visual field investigation. Annee Ther. Clin. Ophthalmol. 24:376-390, 1974.
[90] Enoch, J.M.: Directional sensitivity and directional selectivity. Vis. Res. 15:1172, 1975.
[91] Enoch, J.M.: Marked accommodation, retinal stretch, monocular space perception and retinal receptor orientation. Charles F. Prentice Award lecture. Am J. Optom. Physiol. Opt. 52:375-392; 435, 1975.
[92] Blank, K., Provine, R.R. and Enoch, J.M.: Shift in the peak of the photopic Stiles-Crawford function with marked accommodation. Vis. Res. 15:499-507, 1975.
[93] Benson, W.E., Kolker, A.E., Enoch, J.M., Van Loo, J.A. Jr. and Honda, Y.: Best's vitelliform macular dystrophy. Am. J. Ophthalmol. 79:59-66, 1975.
[94] Enoch, J.M. and Lawrence, B.: A perimetric technique believed to test receptive field properties: Sequential evaluation in glaucoma and other conditions. Annee Ther. Clin. Ophthalmol. 25:215-235, 1974. NOTE: With permission of President of the Symposium, Am. J. Ophthalmol. 80:734-758, 1975.
[95] Enoch, J.M. and Horowitz, B.R.: The vertebrate retinal receptor as a waveguide. In: Fox J, editor. *Proc. of the Symposium on Optical and Acoustical Micro Electronics*,Vol XXIII, 1975: Microwave Research Institute Symposia Series, Polytechnic Press, N.Y.:133-159
[96] Tobey, F.L., Jr., Enoch, J.M. and Scandrett, J.M.: Experimentally determined optical properties of goldfish cones and rods. Invest. Ophthalmol. 14:7-21, 1975.
[97] Van Loo, J.A., Jr. and Enoch, J.M.: The scotopic Stiles-Crawford effect. Vis. Res. 15:1005-1009, 1975.
[98] Provine, R. and Enoch, J.M.: On voluntary ocular accommodation. Perception and Psychophysics, 17:209-212, 1975.
[99] Enoch, J.M.: Use of inverted telescopic corrections incorporating soft contact lenses in the (partial) correction of aniseikonia in cases of unilateral aphakia. Adv Opthalmol. 32: 54-66, 1976.
[100] Enoch, J.M., Lazarus, J. and Johnson, C.: Human psychophysical analysis of receptive field-like properties: I. A new transient-like visual response using a moving windmill (Werblin-type) target. Sens. Processes, 1:14-32, 1976.
[101] Bourne, W. and Enoch, J.M.: Some optical principles of the clinical specular microscope. Invest. Ophthalmol. 15:29-32, 1976.
[102] Johnson, C.A. and Enoch, J.M.: Human psychophysical analysis of receptive field-like properties - II. Dichoptic properties of the Westheimer function. Vis. Res. 16:1455-1462, 1976.
[103] Johnson, C.A. and Enoch, J.M.: Human psychophysical analysis of receptive field-like properties - III. Dichoptic properties of a new transient-like psychophysical function. Vis. Res. 16:1463-1470, 1976.
[104] Enoch, J.M. and Johnson, C.A.: Additivity of effects within sectors of the sensitization zone of the Westheimer function. Am. J. Optom. Physiol. Opt. 53:350-358, 1976.
[105] Enoch, J.M.: Vertebrate photoreceptor orientation. Int. J. Quantum Chem. Quantum Biol. 3:65-88, 1976.
[106] Johnson, C.A. and Enoch, J.M.: Human psychophysical analysis of receptive field-like properties - IV. Further examination and specification of the psychophysical transient-like function. Doc. Ophthalmol. 41:329-345, 1976.
[107] Enoch, J.M., Johnson, C.A. and Fitzgerald, C.R.: Human psychophysical analysis of receptive field-like properties: V. Adaptation of stationary and moving windmill target characteristics to clinical populations. Doc. Ophthalmol. 41:347-370, 1976.

[108] Johnson, C.A. and Enoch, J.M.: Human psychophysical analysis of receptive field-like properties. VI. Current summary and analysis of factors affecting the psychophysical transient-like function. Doc. Ophthalmol.Proc. Ser. 14:367-372, 1976.
[109] Enoch, J.M., Johnson, C.A. and Fitzgerald, C.R.: Human psychophysical analysis of receptive field-like properties: VII. Initial clinical trials of the psychophysical transient-like function. Doc. Ophthalmol. Proc. Ser. 14:373-378, 1976.
[110] Enoch, J.M. and Rabinowicz, I.M.: Early surgery and visual correction of an infant born with unilateral eye lens opacity. Doc. Ophthalmol. 41:371-382, 1976.
[111] Enoch, J.M.: Re: "Try this: Equalizing the Images." Contact Lens Forum 1:7, 1976.
[112] Enoch, J.M. and Johnson, C.A.: The Westheimer function as an indicator of fixation locus. Am. J. Ophthalmol. 83:495-498, 1977.
[113] Campos, E.C., Enoch, J.M. and Rabinowicz, I.M.: Tentativi di rieducazione in un paziente di sei mesi con afachia monolaterale dovuta a cataratta congenita. Giorn. It. Ortott. 5:65-68, 1977.
[114] Enoch, J.M. and Campos, E.C.: Analisi di pazienti con glaucoma ad angolo aperto mediante tecniche perimetriche che riflettono proprieta' del tipo di quelle dei campi recettivi retinici. Atti della Societa Oftalmologica Italiana, 1-14, 1977.
[115] Enoch, J.M.: Histochemical psychophysics, or would you believe psychophysical histochemistry. Invest. Ophthalmol. Vis Sci. 16:1-4, 1977.
[116] Campos, E.C., Bedell, H.E., Enoch, J.M. and Fitzgerald, C.R.: Retinal receptive field-like properties and Stiles-Crawford effect in a patient with a traumatic choroidal rupture. Doc. Ophthalmol. 45:381-395, 1978.
[117] Enoch, J.M. and Tobey, F.L. Jr.: Use of the waveguide parameter V to determine the difference in the index of refraction between the rat rod outer segment and the interstitial matrix. J. Opt. Soc. Am. 68:1130-1134,1978.
[118] Enoch, J.M.: The relationship between retinal receptor orientation and photoreceptor optics. Int. Ophthalmol. Clin. 18:41-80, 1978.
[119] Enoch, J.M.: Restoration of binocularity in unilateral aphakia by non surgical means. Int. Ophthalmol. Clin. 18:273-282, 1978.
[120] Enoch, J.M., Bedell, H.E. and Campos, E.C.: Local variations in rod receptor orientation. Vis. Res. 18:123-124, 1978.
[121] Enoch, J.M.: Quantitative layer-by-layer perimetry. The Francis I. Proctor Lecture (1977). Invest. Ophthal. Vis. Sci. 17:208-257, 1978.
[122] Campos, E.C., Enoch, J.M. and Rabinowicz, I.M.: Prismatic therapy in aphakia due to congenital cataract. In: Reinecke RD, editor. *Strabismus*. 1978: Grune and Stratton, Inc., New York: 319-325.
[123] Sloan, L. and Enoch, J.M.: Considerations related to "going metric": The best metric distances for measuring visual acuity and the correct use of the Snellen fraction. Arch. Ophthalmol. 96:1567, 1978.
[124] Enoch, J.M.: The receptor fiber optics bundle and retinoscopy. Am. J. Optom. Physiol. Opt. 56:661-662, 1979.
[125] Enoch, J.M., Rabinowicz, I.M. and Campos, E.C.: Visual correction of infant sensory deprivation amblyopia: Post-surgical management in unilateral aphakia. In: Gernet H, editor. *Diagnosstica Ultrasonica in Ophthalmologica.* SIDUO VII. 1979: R.A. Remy, Verlag, Munster: 209-220.
[126] Enoch, J.M., Campos, E.C. and Bedell, H.E.: Visual resolution in a patient exhibiting a visual fatigue or saturation-like effect: Probably multiple sclerosis. Arch. Ophthalmol. 97:76-78, 1979.
[127] Bedell, H.E. and Enoch, J.M.: A study of the Stiles-Crawford (S-C) function at 35° in the temporal field and the stability of the foveal S-C function peak over time. J. Opt. Soc. Am. 69:435-442, 1979.

[128] Enoch, J.M. and Bedell, H.E.: Specification of the directionality of the Stiles-Crawford function. Am. J. Optom. Physiol. Opt. 56:341-344, 1979.
[129] Enoch, J.M., Rabinowicz, I.M. and Campos, E.C.: Post surgical contact lens correction of infants with sensory deprivation amblyopia associated with unilateral congenital cataract. J. Jpn. Contact Lens Soc. 21:95-104, 1979.
[130] Enoch, J.M.: Fitting parameters which need to be considered when designing soft contact lenses for the neonate. Contact and Intraocular Lens Med. J. 5:31-37, 1979.
[131] Fitzgerald, C.R., Enoch, J.M., Campos, E.C. and Bedell, H.E.: Comparison of visual function studies in two cases of senile macular degeneration. Albrecht v. Graefe's Arch. klin. exp. Ophthalmol. 210:79-91, 1979.
[132] Enoch, J.M., Campos, E.C., Greer, M. and Trobe, J.: Measurement of visual resolution at high luminance levels in patients with possible demyelinating disease. Ophthalmol. 1:99-104, 1979.
[133] Enoch, J.M., Fitzgerald, C.R. and Campos, E.C.: The relationship between fundus lesions and areas of functional change. Doc. Ophthalmol. Proc. Series. 19:381-393, 1979.
[134] Enoch, J.M. and Campos, E.C.: Analysis of patients with open-angle glaucoma using perimetric techniques reflecting receptive field-like properties. Doc. Ophthalmol. Proc. Series 19:137-149, 1979.
[135] Enoch, J.M.: Physiology of monocular aphakia. Ophthalmol. 86:391-398, 1979.
[136] Enoch, J.M., Bedell, H.E. and Kaufman, H.E.: Interferometric visual acuity in anterior segment pathology. Arch. Ophthalmol. 97:1916-1919, 1979.
[137] Enoch, J.M.: Techniques for evaluating scleral curvature and corneal vault. Die Contactlinse 13:19-25, 1979 (German). Contact Lens J., UK 8:5, 19-31, 1979.
[138] Enoch, J.M., Ohzu, H. and Itoi, M.: Contrast (modulation) sensitivity functions measured in patients with high refractive error with emphasis on aphakia: I. Theoretical considerations. Doc. Ophthalmol. 47:139-145, 1979.
[139] Enoch, J.M., Yamade, S. and Namba, A.: Contrast (modulation) sensitivity functions measured in patients with high refractive errors with emphasis on aphakia: II. Determinations on patients. Doc. Ophthalmol. 47:147-162, 1979.
[140] Karlan, M.S. and Enoch, J.M.: Virtual image of the incus from a saline lens: An aid to safe dissection of the mastoid antrum. Otolaryngol. Head Neck Surg. 87:904-910, 1979.
[141] Enoch, J.M., Birch, D.G. and Birch, E.E.: Monocular light exclusion for a period of days reduces directional sensitivity of the human retina. Science. 206:705-707, 1979.
[142] Enoch, J.M.: The Stiles-Crawford Effect and Vertebrate Photoreceptor Optics. Adv. Ophthalmol. 41:206-211, 1980.
[143] Enoch, J.M.: Need for standard test techniques in order to enhance interchangeability of test results. Adv. Ophthalmol. 41:170-171, 1980.
[144] Enoch, J.M.: Keynote Presentation by Chairman, Proceedings of NEI Workshop on the Role of Psychophysics and Physiological Optics in Ophthalmic Diagnosis and Patient Evaluation, Bethesda, Maryland, September 9-10, 1976. Adv. Ophthalmol. 41:149-216, 1980.
[145] Enoch, J.M.: Research directed towards improved localization of lesions at various loci along the visual pathways. Adv. Ophthalmol. 41:206-211, 1980.
[146] Enoch, J.M.: Techniques for treating and optimizing performance in children born with sensory deprivation anomalies. Adv. Ophthalmol. 41:181-182, 1980.
[147] Enoch, J.M.: Vertebrate receptor optics and orientation. Doc. Ophthalmol. 48:373-388, 1980.
[148] Bedell, H.E. and Enoch, J.M.: An apparent failure of the photoreceptor alignment mechanism in a human observer. Arch. Ophthalmol. 98:2023-2026, 1980.
[149] Fitzgerald, C.R., Enoch, J.M., Birch, D.G., Benedetto, M.D., Temme, L.A. and Dawson, W.W.: Anomalous pigment epithelial/photoreceptor relationships and receptor orientation. Invest. Ophthal. Vis. Sci. 19:956-966, 1980. Erratum, Invest. Ophthal. Visual Sci. 90:1052, 1980.

[150] Temme, L.A., Enoch, J.M., Fitzgerald, C.R. and Merimee, T.J.: Transient-like function and associated retinal capillary anomalies: Analysis of a patient with early retinopathy secondary to juvenile onset diabetes mellitus. Invest. Ophthal. Vis. Sci. 19:991-1008, 1980.
[151] Fitzgerald, C.R., Birch, D.G. and Enoch, J.M.: Functional analysis of vision in patients following retinal detachment repair. Arch. Ophthalmol. 98:1237-1244, 1980.
[152] Enoch, J.M., Birch, D.G. Birch, E.E. and Benedetto, M.D.: The effect of uniocular occlusion on selected visual functions. Trans. Ophthalmol. Soc. U.K. 99:407-412, 1980.
[153] Birch, D.G., Birch, E.E. and Enoch, J.M.: Visual sensitivity, resolution, and Rayleigh matches following monocular occlusion for one week. J. Opt. Soc. Am. 70:954-958, 1980.
[154] Enoch, J.M. and Birch, D.G.: Evidence for alteration in photoreceptor orientation. Ophthalmology 87:821-833, 1980.
[155] Campos, E.C., Enoch, J.M., Fitzgerald, C.R. and Benedetto, M.D.: A simple psychophysical technique provides early diagnosis in optic neuritis. Doc. Ophthalmol. 49:325-335, 1980.
[156] Enoch, J.M., Birch, D.G., Birch, E.E. and Benedetto, M.D.: Alteration in directional sensitivity of the retina by monocular occlusion. Vis. Res. 20:1185-1189, 1980.
[157] Enoch, J.M., Fitzgerald, C.R., Campos, E.C. and Temme, L.A.: Different functional changes recorded in open angle glaucoma and anterior ischemic optic neuropathy. Doc. Ophthalmol. 50:169-184, 1980.
[158] Campos, E.C. and Enoch, J.M.: Amount of aniseikonia compatible with fine binocular vision: Some old and new concepts. J. Pediatr. Ophthalmol. Strabismus 17:44-47, 1980.
[159] Enoch, J.M. and Campos, E.C.: New quantitative perimetric tests designed to evaluate receptive-field-like properties in diseases of the retina and the optic nerve. Int. Ophthalmol. Clin. 20:83-133, 1980.
[160] Enoch, J.M., Fitzgerald, C.R. and Temme, L.A.: Remission of anomalies: An important aid to analysis. In:Proenza LM, Enoch JM, Jampolsky A, editors. *Clinical applications of visual psychophysics*. 1981: Cambridge University Press, Cambridge:198-233.
[161] Fitzgerald, C.R., Enoch, J.M. and Temme, L.A.: Kinetic perimetry (in the plateau region of the field) as a sensitive indicator of visual fatigue or saturation-like defects in retrobulbar anomalies. Doc. Ophthalmol. Proc. Ser. 26:293-303, 1981.
[162] Enoch, J.M. and Birch, D.G.: Inferred positive phototropic activity in human photoreceptors. Philos. Trans. R. Soc. Lond. (Biol) 291:323-351 1981.
[163] Fitzgerald, C.R., Enoch, J.M. and Temme, L.A.: Radiation therapy in and about the retina, optic nerve, and anterior visual pathway: Psychophysical assessment. Arch. Ophthalmol. 99:611-623, 1981.
[164] Bedell, H.E., Enoch, J.M. and Fitzgerald, C.R.: Photoreceptor orientation. A graded disturbance bordering a region of choroidal atrophy. Arch. Ophthalmol. 99:1841-1844, 1981.
[165] Enoch, J.M., Binder, P.S. and Bourne, W.M.: The need to measure added parameters in order to properly specify hydrogel lenses in the treatment of corneal pathology. Contact and Intraocular Lens Med. J. 7:331-336, 1981.
[166] Baron, W.S. and Enoch, J.M.: Calculating photopic illuminance. Am. J. Optom. Physiol. Opt. 59:338-341, 1982.
[167] Enoch, J.M., Eisner, A. and Bedell, H.E.: Further evaluation of an apparent failure of the photoreceptor alignment mechanism in a human observer. Arch. Ophthalmol. 100:1280-1281, 1982.
[168] Eisner, A. and Enoch, J.M.: Some effects of 1 week's monocular exposure to long-wavelength stimuli. Perception and Psychophysics 31:169-174, 1982.
[169] Enoch, J.M.: Quantitative layer-by-layer perimetry: an update. Am. J. Optom. Physiol. Opt. 59:952-53, 1982.
[170] Enoch, J.M.: To woo a Helmholtz.Am. J.Optom.Physiol.Opt.59:843, 1982.
[171] Enoch, J.M.: Historical Vignette: "Joseph Le Conte." Am. J. Optom. Physiol. Opt. 60:1003, 1983.

[172] Enoch, J.M. and Williams, R.A.: Development of clinical tests of vision: Initial data on two hyperacuity paradigms. Perception and Psychophysics 33: 314-322, 1983.
[173] Enoch, J.M. and Hamer, R.D.: Image size correction of the unilateral aphakic infant. Ophthalmic Pediatrics and Genetics 2:153-165, 1983.
[174] Hudson, D.K., Enoch, J.M., Scandrett, J.H. and Bernstein, M.: A study of the effects of bleaching on the width and index of refraction of goldfish cone outer segments. In: Breinin GM and Seigel IM, editors. *Advances in Diagnostic Visual Science*. 1983: Springer-Verlag, Heidelberg: 30-34.
[175] Enoch, J.M., Moses, R.A., Nygaard, R.W. and Allen, D.: Perimetric techniques used to assess retinal strain during accommodation. Doc. Ophthalmol. Proc. Ser. 35:413-420, 1983.
[176] Enoch, J.M.: Automation of perimetry and modern methods of subjective eye examination. In: Henkind P, editor. *Acta: XXIV International Congress of Ophthalmology*. 1983: J.B. Lippincott Co. 1:136-146.
[177] Enoch, J.M.: Perimetry, today and tomorrow. Doc. Ophthalmol. 55:307-22, 1983.
[178] Williams, R.A., Essock, E.A. and Enoch, J.M.: Influence of variable-sized backgrounds on a hyperacuity threshold. In: Breinen GM and Seigel IM, editors. *Advances in Diagnostic Visual Science*. Springer Series in Optical Sciences, 41. 1983: Springer-Verlag, Heidelberg: 232-238, .
[179] Marmor, M.F., Aguirre, G., Arden, G., Berson, E., Birch, D.G., Boughman, J.A., Carr, R., Chatrian, G.E., Del Monte, M., Dowling, J., Enoch, J.M. et al.: Retinitis pigmentosa: A symposium on terminology and methods of examination. Ophthalmol. 90:126-131, 1983.
[180] Enoch, J.M.: Fool's gold, the alchemist's pot, psychophysics and glaucoma. Invest. Ophthalmol. Vis. Sci. 24:1440-1442, 1983.
[181] Williams, R.A., Enoch, J.M. and Essock, E.A.: The resistance of selected hyperacuity configurations to retinal image degradation. Invest. Ophthal. Vis. Sci. 25:389-399, 1984.
[182] Essock, E.A., Williams, R.A., Enoch, J.M. and Raphael, S.: The effects of image degradation by cataract on vernier acuity. Invest. Ophthalmol. Vis. Sci. 25:1043-1050, 1984.
[183] Enoch, J.M., Williams, R.A., Essock. E.A. and Barricks, M.: Hyperacuity perimetry: Assessment of macular function through ocular opacities. Arch. Ophthalmol. 102:1164-1168, 1984.
[184] Campbell, S.R. and Enoch, J.M.: Clinical comparison of the Coopervision Dicon Auto Perimeter 2000 to Goldmann Hagg-Streit Perimetry. Optometric Monthly. 75:274-279, 1984.
[185] Enoch, J.M., Essock, E.A. and Williams, R.A.: Relating vernier acuity and Snellen acuity in specific clinical populations. Doc. Ophthalmol. 58:71-77, 1984.
[186] Williams, R.A., Enoch, J.M. and Raphael, S.: Retinal image noise and vernier acuity. Vis. Res. 24:1735-38, 1984.
[187] Enoch, J.M., Williams, R.A., Essock, E.A. and Raphael, S.: Application of hyperacuity to assess vision through media and retinal opacities: methodology. Doc. Ophthalmol. Proc. Ser. 42:569-575, 1985.
[188] O'Donnell, J.J., Fendick, M.G. and Enoch, J.M.: Abnormal inner retinal function in gyrate atrophy. Doc. Ophthalmol. Proc. Ser. 42:473-479, 1985.
[189] Webb, R.H., Essock, E.A., Enoch, J.M. and Williams, R.A.: Measurement of layer-by-layer perimetry responses using direct retinal projection by the scanning laser ophthalmoscope. Doc. Ophthalmol. Proc. Ser. 42:481-486, 1985.
[190] Centaro, A., Savage, G.L., Enoch, J.M. and Newman, N.: Studies of drusen of the optic nerve head. Doc. Ophthalmol. Proc. Ser. 42:467-472, 1985.
[191] Williams, R.A., Enoch, J.M., Essock, E.A. and Barricks, M.A.: Application of hyperacuity to assess vision through media and retinal opacities: clinical trials. Doc. Ophthalmol. Proc. Ser. 42:577-584, 1985.
[192] Essock, E.A., Lehmkuhle, S., Frascella, J. and Enoch, J.M.: Temporal modulation of the background affects the sensitization response of x- and y-cells in the dLGN of cat. Vis. Res. 25:8:1007-1019, 1985.

[193] Enoch, J.M. and Campos, E.C.: Helping the aphakic neonate to see. Ophthalmol., 8:237-248, 1985.

[194] Essock, E.A., Enoch, J.M., Williams, R.A., Barricks, M. and Raphael, S.: Joint application of hyperacuity perimetry and gap test in assessment of visual function behind cataracts: initial trials. Doc. Ophthalmol. 60:293-312, 1985.

[195] Enoch, J.M., Essock, E.A., Williams, R.A. and Barricks, M.: Functional visual effects of lesions located near the optic nerve head. Doc. Ophthalmol. 61:137-156, 1985.

[196] Lakshminarayanan, V. and Enoch, J.M.: Shape of the Stiles-Crawford function for traverses of the entrance pupil not passing through the peak of sensitivity. Am. J. Optom. Phys. Opt. 62:127-28, 1985.

[197] Enoch, J.M., O'Donnell, J., Williams, R.A. and Essock, E.A.: Retinal boundaries and visual function in gyrate atrophy. Arch. Ophthalmol. 102:1314-1316, 1984. Erratum, 103:1284, 1985.

[198] Savage, G.L., Centaro, A., Enoch, J.M. and Newman, N.: Drusen of the optic nerve head: an important model. Ophthalmology 92:793-799, 1985.

[199] Enoch, J.M. and Birch, D.G.: Comment on inferred positive phototropic activity in human photoreceptors. Phil. Trans. R. Soc. Lond. B309:611-613, 1985.

[200] Verriest, G. (ed.), Bailey, I.L., Calabria, G., Campos, E.C., Crick, R.P. Enoch, J.M., et al.: The occupational visual field: II. Practical aspects: the functional visual field in abnormal conditions and its relationship to visual ergonomics, visual impairment and job fitness. Doc. Ophthalmol. Proc. Ser. 42:281-326, 1985.

[201] Enoch, J.M., Birch, D.G. and Birch, E.E.: Photoreceptor alignment. Science 229:4715: 708, 1985.

[202] Lakshminarayanan, V., Enoch, J.M., Raasch, T., Nygaard, R. and Crawford, B.: Effects of intraocular lens (IOL) tilt and displacement. In: Technical Digest. Noninvasive Assessment of the Visual Function, Optical Society of America. Washington D.C., 1985.

[203] Hamer, R.D., Lakshminarayanan, V., Enoch, J.M., Yasuma, T., Birch, D.G. and Birch, E.E.: Stiles-Crawford functions are not broader after one week of total light exclusion.In: Technical Digest. Noninvasive Assessment of the Visual Function, Optical Society of America. Washington D.C., 1985.

[204] Williams, R.W., and Enoch, J.M.: Hyperacuity: Assessing visual function behind ocular opacities. In: Technical Digest. Noninvasive Assessment of the Visual Function, Optical Society of America. Washington D.C., 1985.

[205] Fausset, T.M. and Enoch, J.M.: A rapid, simple means of testing kinetic visual fields in young children.In: Technical Digest. Noninvasive Assessment of the Visual System, Optical Society of America,Washington D.C., 1986.

[206] Lakshminarayanan, V., Enoch, J.M. and Yamade, S.: The Stiles-Crawford effect (SCE) of the first kind: studies of the SCE in an aniridic observer.In: Technical Digest. Noninvasive Assessment of the Visual System, Optical Society of America, Washington D.C., 1986.

[207] Baraldi, P., Enoch, J.M., Savage, G., Lakshminarayanan, V. and Fendick, M.: Evaluating metamorphopsia in the presence of ocular opacities. In: Technical Digest. Noninvasive Assessment of the Visual System, Optical Society of America, Washington D.C., 1986.

[208] Lakshminarayanan, V., Enoch, J.M., Raasch, T., Crawford, B. and Nygaard, R.W.: Refractive changes induced by intraocular lens tilt and longitudinal displacement. Arch. Ophthalmol. 104:90-92, 1986.

[209] Enoch, J.M., Lakshminarayanan, V. and Yamade, S.: The Stiles-Crawford effect (SCE) of the first kind: studies of the SCE in an aniridic observer. W.S Stiles Memorial Issue. Perception, 15:777-784, 1986.

[210] Baraldi, P., Enoch, J.M. and Raphael, S.: Vision through nuclear and posterior subcapsular cataract. Int. Ophthalmol. 9:173-178, 1986.

[211] Yasuma, T., Hamer, R.D., Lakshminarayanan, V., Enoch, J.M. and O'Donnell, J.J.: Retinal receptor alignment and directional sensitivity in a gyrate atrophy patient. Clin. Vis. Sci. 1:93-102, 1986.
[212] Hamer, R.D., Lakshminarayanan, V., Yasuma, T., Enoch, J.M. and O'Donnell, J.J.: Selective adaptation of the Stiles-Crawford function in patient with gyrate atrophy. Clin. Vis. Sci. 1:103-106, 1986.
[213] Yamade, S., Lakshminarayanan, V. and Enoch, J.M.: A comparison of two fast quantitative methods for evaluating the Stiles-Crawford function. Am. J. Optom. Physiol. Opt., 64:621-626, 1987.
[214] Enoch, J.M., Hamer, R.D.,Lakshminarayanan, V., Yasuma, T., Birch, D.G. and Yamade, S.: Effect of monocular light exclusion on the Stiles-Crawford function. Vis. Res. 27:507-510, 1987.
[215] Enoch, J.M. and Nygaard, R.W.: Retinal strain induced by accommodation: an overview. In: Stark L and Obrecht G, editors. *Presbyopia: Recent Research and Reviews*. 1987: Professional Press Books, Fairchild Publications, New York: 142-146.
[216] Heitz, R.F. and Enoch, J.M.: Leonardo da Vinci: an assessment of his discourse on image formation in the eye. In: Fiorentini A, Guyton DL, Siegel IM, editors. *Advances in Diagnostic Visual Optics*. 1987: Springer-Verlag, 19-26.
[217] Baraldi, P. and Enoch, J.M.: Hyperacuity: successful evaluation of visual function through ocular opacities.In: Fiorentini A, Guyton DL, Siegel IM, editors. *Advances in Diagnostic Visual Optics*. 1987: Springer-Verlag: 82-87.
[218] Lakshminarayanan, V., Enoch, J.M. and Yamade, S.: Human photoreceptor orientation: normals and exceptions. In: Fiorentini A, Guyton DL, Siegel IM, editors. *Advances in Diagnostic Visual Optics*. 1987: Springer-Verlag: 28-32.
[219] Enoch, J.M. and Baraldi, P.: Design for a field model of a hyperacuity apparatus suitable for application in developing countries. In: Fiorentini A, Guyton DL, Siegel IM, editors. *Advances in Diagnostic Visual Optics*. 1987: Springer-Verlag: 88-92.
[220] Enoch, J.M.: It is proposed that the cornea of the eye of the bull's head rhyton from the Little Palace of Knossos (artifact dated 1550-1500 B.C.) is a true lens. In: Fiorentini A, Guyton DL, Siegel IM, editors. *Advances in Diagnostic Visual Optics*. 1987: Springer-Verlag: 15-18.
[221] Enoch, J.M., Savage, G. and Lakshminarayanan, V.: Anomalous visual response in Tourette's syndrome. Doc. Ophthalmol. Proc. Series, 49:667-672, 1987.
[222] Fausset, T.M. and Enoch, J.M.: A rapid technique for kinetic visual field determination in young children and adults with central retinal lesions. Doc. Ophthalmol. Proc. Series, 49:495-501, 1987.
[223] Baraldi, P., Enoch, J.M. and Raphael, S.: A comparison of visual impairment caused by nuclear (NC) and posterior subcapsular (PSC) cataracts. Doc. Ophthalmol. Proc. Series, 49:43-50, 1987.
[224] Enoch, J.M.: A Note on the Late W.S. Stiles and Directional Sensitivity of the Retina. Ophthalmic. and Physiol. Optics, 7:509-510, 1987.
[225] Enoch, J.M., Lakshminarayanan, V., Savage, G. and Knowles, R.: Fundus photoperimetric analysis of pigmented chorioretinal lesions. In: Technical Digest. Noninvasive Assessment of the Visual System, Optical Society of America, Washington D.C., 174-178, 1987.
[226] Enoch, J.M., Savage, G. and Lakshminarayanan, V.: Psychophysical tests of dopamine anomalies in the retina. In: Technical Digest. Noninvasive Assessment of the Visual System, Optical Society of America, Washington D.C., 162-166, 1987.
[227] Enoch, J.M.: Life Span Planning for Human Needs: An International Perspective. J. Am. Optom. Assn., 59:282-284, 1988.
[228] Bailey, J.E., Lakshminarayanan, V., and Enoch, J.M.: Stiles-Crawford functions in an aphakic subject with retinitis pigmentosa. In Technical Digest. Noninvasive Assessment of the Visual System, Optical Society of America, Washington D.C., 58-61, 1988.

[229] Peters, H.B., Enoch, J.M., and Sarver, M.D.: Meredith Walter Morgan - A Salute. Am. J. Opt. Physiol. Optics, 65:322-324, 1988.
[230] Enoch, J.M., Baraldi, P., Lakshminarayanan, V. Savage, G. and Fendick, M.: The measurement of metamorphopsia in the presence of ocular media opacities. Morgan Festschrift. Am. J. Optom. Physiol. Optics, 65:349-353, 1988.
[231] Enoch, J.M., Lakshminarayanan, V., Itzhaki, A., Shechter, G. and Marmor, M.: Layer-by-layer perimetry and haloperidol: Implications for schizophrenia and other diseases. In Belmaker RH, Sandler M and Dahlstrom A, editors. *Progress in Catecholamine Research, Part C: Clinical Aspects. 1988:* Alan R. Liss, Inc. New York, 131-136.
[232] Enoch, J.M., Heitz, R., Lakshminarayanan, V.: John Frederick William Herschel on testing for astigmatism in 1845. Ophthal. Physiol. Optics, 8:349-350, 1988.
[233] Enoch, J.M., Lakshminarayanan, V., Itzhaki, A.: Psychophysical studies of neuropsychiatric patients on and off haloperidol. In: Bodis-Wollner I and Piccolino M, editors. *Dopaminergic Mechanisms in Vision*, IBRO Roundtable Conference 1988: Alan R. Liss, Inc., New York: 227-237.
[234] Lakshminarayanan, V., Enoch, J.M.: The MacLeod selective adaptation paradigm in cases with modest cataracts. Clin. Vis. Sci., 3:155-156, 1988.
[235] Enoch, J.M., Itzhaki, A., Lakshminarayanan, V., Comerford, J.P. Lieberman, M. and Lowe, T.: Gilles de la Tourette syndrome: visual effects. Neuro-Ophthalmol. 8:251-257, 1988.
[236] Enoch, J.M., Itzhaki, A., Lakshminarayanan, V., Comerford, J.P., M. Lieberman, M. and Lowe, T.: Gilles de la Tourette syndrome: genetic marker. Neuro-Ophthalmol. 8:259-265, 1988.
[237] Enoch, J.M., Itzhaki, A., Lakshminarayanan, V., Comerford, J.P., Lieberman, M. and Lowe, T.: Anomalous kinetic visual fields in Gilles de la Tourette syndrome patients and family members. In: Heijl A, editor. *Proceedings of the VIII International Perimetric Society Meeting, Perimetry Update 1988/89*. 1989: Kugler & Ghedini; Amsterdam: 77-84.
[238] Enoch, J.M., Itzhaki, A., Lakshminarayanan, V., Comerford, J.P. and Lieberman, M.: Visual field defects in patients with Gilles de la Tourette syndrome: Preliminary report. Int. Ophthalmol. 13:331-344, 1989.
[239] Khamar, B.M., Enoch, J.M., Lowe, T.L., Schreier, H.: Temporal Steps in the Visual Field in Neuropsychiatric Disorders. Lancet, 2(8674):1283-1284, 1989.
[240] Enoch, J.M., Lakshminarayanan, V.: Biological light guides. Nature, 340:6230, p. 194, 1989.
[241] Enoch, J.M., Itzhaki A., Lakshminarayanan, V.: Visual field anomalies in Tourette syndrome patients and family members. In: Technical Digest. Noninvasive Assessment of the Visual System, Optical Society of America. Washington D.C.,7:132-139, 1989.
[242] Enoch, J.M.: Glenn Ansel Fry: An 80th Birthday Celebration. Optom. Vis. Sci., 67:57, 1990.
[243] Aziz, S., Lakshminarayanan, V., Enoch, J.M.: PC-based hyperacuity tests. In: Technical Digest. Noninvasive Assessment of the Visual System, Optical Society of America. Washington D.C. 3:191-194, 1990.
[244] Enoch, J.M., Hudson, D.K., Lakshminarayanan, V., Scandrett, J., Bernstein, M.: Effect of bleaching on the width and index of refraction of goldfish rod and cone outer segment fragment. Optom. Vis. Sci., 67:600-605, 1990.
[245] Khamar, B.M., Enoch, J.M., Lakshminarayanan, V., Chader, G.J.: Dopamine and Myopia. Optom. Vis. Sci. 67:908-910, 1990.
[246] Enoch, J.M., Khamar, B.M., Lakshminarayanan, V.: Fluctuating field defects - A preliminary report. Neuro-Ophthalmol., 10:311-314, 1990.
[247] Enoch, J.M., Khamar, B.M., Lakshminarayanan, V.: An analysis of step-like Field Defects in Gilles de la Tourette syndrome. Neuro-Ophthalmol., 10:299-309, 1990.
[248] Khamar, B.M., Enoch, J.M., Lakshminarayanan, V.: Step manifestations and sensitivity changes in Gilles de la Tourette syndrome. Neuro-Ophthalmol., 10:293-298, 1990.

[249] Enoch, J.M, Khamar, B.M., and Lakshminarayanan, V.: Static and kinetic perimetric field defects in Gilles de la Tourette syndrome: Quantifying step-like field defects. Clin. Vis. Sci., 6:361-369, 1991.

[250] Enoch, J.M., Khamar, B.M., Lakshminarayanan V.: Changes in step-like effects in Gilles de la Tourette syndrome measured after a period of one year. Clin. Vis. Sci. 6:371-377, 1991.

[251] Enoch, J.M., Lakshminarayanan, V., and Khamar, B.M.: Time variation of step-like field defects in Gilles de la Tourette syndrome.In: Mills RP and Heijl A, editors. *Proceedings of the IXth International Perimetric Society Meeting, Perimetry Update, 1990/91.* 1991: Kugler Publishers, Amsterdam: 137-141.

[252] Lakshminarayanan, V., Aziz, S., Enoch, J.M.: Quantification of metamorphopsia using hyperacuity techniques.: Optom. Vis. Sci., 68:940-945, 1991.

[253] Enoch, J.M., Khamar, B.M., Lakshminarayanan, V.: Step-like field defects in Gilles de la Tourette syndrome: Changes during a day, Neuro-Ophthalmol., 11:307-317, 1991.

[254] Enoch, J.M.: The design of an instrument for evaluation of vision, before, during and after refractive surgery, Lasers and Light in Ophthalmol. 4:111-119, 1991.

[255] Enoch, J.M., Itzhaki, A., Lakshminarayanan, V., Surendran, T., Comerford, J.: Anomalous kinetic visual fields found in family members of patients with a confirmed diagnosis of Gilles de la Tourette syndrome. Optom. Vis. Sci., 68:807-812, 1991.

[256] Reich, L., Lakshminarayanan, V. and Enoch, J.M.: Analysis of the method of adjustment for testing potential acuity with the hyperacuity gap - A preliminary report. Clin. Vis. Sci., 6:451-456, 1991.

[257] Bailey, J.E., Lakshminarayanan, V. and Enoch, J.M.: The Stiles-Crawford function in an aphakic subject with retinitis pigmentosa. Clin. Vis. Sci., 6:165-170, 1991.

[258] Lakshminarayanan, V., Aziz, S., Enoch, J.M.: Gap function trends in different age groups.In: Technical Digest. Noninvasive Assessment of the Visual System, Optical Society of America, Washington D.C., 1:133-135, 1991.

[259] Enoch, J.M., Campos, E.C.: Visual Correction of Unilateral Aphakic Neonates, Binocular Vision Quarterly, 6:7, 1991.

[260] Enoch, J.M.: Extended comments with figures. In: McNicol A, editor. *Workshop on Corneal Biophysics II, Optics, Measurement, and Modeling of the Cornea.* 1992: National Eye Institute, National Institutes of Health, Bethesda, MD: 215-240.

[261] Enoch, J.M., Knowles, R.A.: The instrument design and hyperacuity tasks used for precision alignment of optics and evaluating vision before, during, and after refractive surgery. Ophthalmic Technologies II, Proceedings of SPIE, 1644:145-154, 1992.

[262] Enoch, J.M.: Hans Goldmann, M.D. Obituary. Optom. Vis. Sci., 69:168-169, 1992.

[263] Enoch, J.M.: Hyperacuity, an extremely sensitive technique for evaluation of vision, may be of value in the assessment of results of refractive surgery, CLAO Journal, 18:64-71, 1992.

[264] Lakshminarayanan, V., Knowles, R.A., Enoch, J.M., Vasudevan, R.: Measurement of Fixational Stability While Performing a Hyperacuity Task Using the Scanning Laser Ophthalmoscope: Preliminary Studies, Clin. Vis. Sci., 7:557-563, 1992.

[265] Lakshminarayanan, V., Aziz, S., Enoch, J.M.: Variation of the hyperacuity gap function with age. Optom. Vis Sci., 69:423-426, 1992.

[266] Lakshminarayanan, V., Bailey, J.E., Enoch, J.M.: The Optics of Phakic, Pseudophakic, and Aphakic Eyes: effects on the Stiles-Crawford (SCE I) function. Optom. Vis. Sci., 70:404-408, 1993.

[267] Lakshminarayanan, V., Enoch, J.M., Knowles, R.A.: Residual aniseikonia among patients fitted with one or two intraocular lenses (pseudophakic corrections). Optom. Vis. Sci., 70:107-110, 1993.

[268] Enoch, J.M., Barroso, L., Huang, D.: Cataract: a critical problem in the developing world. Optom. Vis. Sci. 70:986-989, 1993.

[269] Enoch, J.M., Lakshminarayanan, V., Knowles, R.A.: Aniseikonia with Intraocular Lenses - Reply. Optom. Vis. Sci. 70:608-610, 1993.

[270] Enoch, J.M.: Aniseikonia with Intraocular Lenses: A continuing saga.: Optom. Vis. Sci. 71:67-68, 1993.

[271] Lakshminarayanan, V.. Bailey, J.E., Enoch, J.M.: Aniseikonia in intraocular lens (IOL) implants: An optical analysis.: Eur. J. Implant and Refract Surg. 6:22-29, 1994.

[272] Bailey, J.E., Lakshminarayanan, V., Enoch, J.M.: Photoreceptor orientation in iris coloboma. Optom. Vis. Sci. 71:120-124, 1994.

[273] Enoch, J.M.: Tribute: Hans Goldmann (1899-1991). Ophthal. Physiol. Opt. 14:330-332, 1994.

[274] Enoch, J.M.: Paul Boeder, Ph.D., the years after 1947. In Bisno D, editor. *Eyes in the Storm. President Hopkins's Dilemma: The Dartmouth Eye Institute.*1994: Norwich Press Books, Norwich VT: 203-207.

[275] Bailey, J.E., Lakshminarayanan, V., Enoch, J.M., Brookman, K.E.: Aniseikonia in Pseudophakia: General trends. In: Technical Digest. Vision Science and Its Applications, Optical Society of America, Washington D.C., 2:43-46, 1994.

[276] Lakshminarayanan, V., Lang, A., Bailey, J.E., Enoch, J.M.: Aniseikonia in Bilateral Pseudophakia. In: Technical Digest. Vision Science and Its Applications, Optical Society of America, Washington D.C., 2:192-195, 1994.

[277] Enoch, J.M.: The Anniversary of the National Eye Institute. Optometric Education 19: 104-105, 1994.

[278] Enoch, J.M.: Vision science in the developing world: Challenges, problems and opportunities, and example. In: Technical Digest. Vision Science and Its Applications, Optical Society of America, Washington D.C., 1: 50-53, 1995.

[279] Bolzani, R., Campos, E.C., Dickmann, A., and Enoch, J.M.: Stability of target fixation. In: Technical Digest. Vision Science and Its Applications, Optical Society of America, Washington D.C., 1: 187-189, 1995.

[280] Enoch, J.M., Schwartz, A., Chang, D., and Hirose, H.: Aniseikonia, metamorphopsia, and perceived entoptic pattern: Some effects of a macular epiretinal membrane, and the subsequent spontaneous separation of the membrane (A case study). Ophthal. Physiol. Opt. 15:339-343, 1995.

[281] Enoch, J.M., Giraldez-Fernandez, M.J., Huang, D., Hirosi, H., Knowles, R., Namperumalsamy, P., LaBree, L., and Azen, S.P.: Vision assessment behind dense cataracts in developing nations. In: Mills RP and Wall M, editors. *Proceedings of the XII International Perimetric Society Meeting Perimetry Update, 1994/95.* 1995: Kugler Publications, Amsterdam: 319-327.

[282] Enoch, J.M., Giraldez-Fernandez, M.J., Knowles, R., Huang, D., Hunter, A., LaBree, L., and Azen, S.P.: Hyperacuity test to evaluate vision through dense cataracts: Research preliminary to a clinical study: I. Studies conducted at the University of California at Berkeley prior to travel to India. Optom. Vis. Sci. 72: 619-629, 1995.

[283] Enoch, J.M., and Knowles, R.: Hyperacuity test to evaluate vision through dense cataracts: Research preliminary to a clinical study: II. Initial trials of the India instrument and HASP protocol at Aravind Eye Hospital, Madurai, India. Optom. Vis. Sci. 72: 630-642, 1995.

[284] Enoch, J.M., Lakshminarayanan, V., Azen, S.P.,and Barroso, L.: Vision assessment behind dense cataracts in developing nations: Implications for quality of life. In: Sridhar R, Srinivasa Rao K and Lakshminarayanan V, editors. *Selected Topics in Mathematical Physics.* 1995: Allied Publishers Ltd., New Delhi: 462-473.

[285] Lakshminarayanan, V., Enoch, J.M.: Vernier acuity and aging. Ophthalmol. 19: 109-115, 1995.

[286] Enoch, J.M., Giraldez-Fernandez, M.J., Huang, D., Hirose, H., Knowles, R., Namperumalsamy, P., LaBree, L., and Azen, S.P.: Hyperacuity test to evaluate vision through dense cataracts: Research Preliminary to a clinical study in India.: Optical Engineering 34: 765-771, 1995.

[287] Rynders, M., Grosvenor, T., and Enoch, J.M.: Stability of the Stiles-Crawford function in a unilateral amblyopic subject over a 38 year period: A case study. Optom. Vis. Sci. 72: 177-185, 1995.
[288] Enoch, J.M.: What if images in the two eyes are of different sizes? Part I: Aniseikonia, then and now. In: Bisno D, editor. *Proceedings of the Dartmouth Eye Institute Commemorative Symposium.* 1995: Norwich Press Books, Norwich, Vermont: 50-69.
[289] Enoch, J.M.: What if the images in the two eyes are of different sizes? Part II: Aniseikonia, new and important dimensions of the problem. In: Bisno D, editor. *Proceedings of the Dartmouth Eye Institute Commemorative Symposium.* In: 1995: Norwich Press Books, Norwich, Vermont: 70-106.
[290] Vilar, E. Yebra-Pimentel, Giraldez-Fernandez, M.J., Enoch, J.M., Lakshminarayanan, V., Knowles, R, Srinivasan, R: Performance on three point Vernier acuity targets as a function of age. J. Opt. Soc. Am. A. 12: 2293-2304, 1995.
[291] Enoch, J.M.: Vision care in the developing world. In: Sridhar R, Srinivasa Rao K and Lakshminarayanan V, editors. *Selected Topics in Mathematical Physics:* 1995: Allied Publishers Ltd., New Delhi: 457-461.
[292] Enoch, J. M.: India: With a population of nearly 1 billion and one-third of the world blind population, currently provides low vision treatment (*per se*) to only a few thousand patients per annum. J. Vis. Rehab. 9: 9-11, 1995. An erratum appears in 9(4), 1995
[293] Enoch, J.M., Rynders, M., Lakshminarayanan, V., Vilar, Eva Y.-P., Giraldez-Fernandez, M.J., Grosvenor, T., Knowles, R., Srinivasan, R.: Two vision response functions which vary little with age. In: Adrian W, editor. *International Symposium on Lighting for Aging Vision and Health.* 1995: Lighting Research Institute, New York: 39-51.
[294] Enoch, J.M., Schreier H.A., and Barroso, L.H.: Visual field defects in psychiatric disorders: possible genetic implications. Biol. Psych. 37:275-277, 1995.
[295] Enoch, J.M.: U.S.-Russian Intrigue. Archaeology 48: 10, 1995.
[296] Enoch J.M., Barroso L., Landau K., Schreier H., and Scorolli, L.: Visual field defects in neuropsychiatric disorders. Neuro-ophthalmol. 16: 77-84, 1996.
[297] Singh, S., Aravind, S., Hirose, H., and Enoch, J.M.: Hyperacuity test to evaluate vision through dense cataracts; research preliminary to a clinical study: III. Data on normal subjects obtained with and without a pseudo-nuclear cataract 6/60 (20/200) at the Aravind Eye Hospital, Madurai, India. Optom. Vis. Sci. 73: 62-64, 1996.
[298] Singh, S., Aravind, S., Hirose, H., Enoch, J.M., Azen, S.P.: Hyperacuity test to evaluate vision through dense cataracts; research preliminary to a clinical study: IV. Data on patients with macular degenerations and minimal media disorders obtained with and without a pseudo-nuclear cataract 6/60 (20/200) at the Aravind Eye Hospital, Madurai, India. Optom. Vis. Sci. 73: 125-126, 1996.
[299] Enoch, J.M.: Aniseikonia, important dimensions of the problem in modern ophthalmology. Implant (J. Intraocular Implant Society, India.) 1:48-60, 1996.
[300] Enoch, J.M.: Comment on "Cataract surgery in one eye or both: A billion dollar per year issue." Ophthalmol. 103:863-864, 1996.
[301] Enoch, J.M. (with assistance from Profs. Westheimer G, Kaiser P and Smith-Pokorney V). Glenn A. Fry Obituary. Color Research and Application. 21:249-251, 1996.

PAPERS SUBMITTED OR IN PRESS AS OF JULY 1996

[1] Hirose, H., Enoch, J.M., Tuan, K-M. Quantification of prism induced metamorphopsia as a model for clinical retinal (and other) distortions. Ophthal. Physiol. Opt.
[2] Lakshminarayanan, V., Bailey, J.E., and Enoch, J.M.: Photoreceptor orientation in nasal fundus ectasia. Optom. Vis. Sci.

[3] Enoch, J.M.: Early lens use: Lens found in context with their original objects. Optom. Vis. Sci.
[4] Enoch, J.M., Vilar, E. Yebra-Pimentel, Giraldez-Fernandez, M.J.: Development of low vision care and rehabilitation services in a developing world country: India as an example Proc. International Low Vision Congress, Madrid, July 7-12, 1996.
[5] Enoch, J.M.: Management of aniseikonia in patients with binocular vision and receiving one or two iols or treated with refractive surgery:A practical approach. J. Refract. Surg.
[6] Enoch, J.M.: Refractive aniseikonia: A source of binocular vision stress and asthenopia. J. Refract. Surg. 12: 1996.
[7] Enoch, J.M.: Lentil beans, early lenses, and when were lenses first used: Lenses found in context with their original objects. Technology and Culture.
[8] Dickmann, A., Bolzani, R., Scorolli, L., Enoch, J.M.: Relations between monocular and binocular gaze stability during fixation. Proceedings of European Strabismological Association Meeting. Cambridge, UK, 1995.

PATENTS ISSUED

[1] Methods for Evaluating Metamorphopsia. Inventor: Enoch, J.M. and Knowles, R. U.S. Patent No. 4,798,456. Issued: January 17, 1989.
[2] Hyperacuity Testing Instrument for Evaluating Visual Function. Inventor: Enoch, J.M. U.S. Patent No. 4,765,732. Issued: August 23, 1988.

PART II

PHOTORECEPTOR WAVEGUIDES - A SIMPLE APPROACH

STANLEY A. KLEIN
School of Optometry, University of California-Berkeley, Berkeley, CA 94720

Abstract

Jay Enoch made important contributions to our understanding of how the waveguide nature of photoreceptors leads to the Stiles-Crawford effect. One of the issues that has been controversial in the past is the dependence of the Stiles-Crawford effect on wavelength. This issue has been difficult to analyze because the mode structure of waveguides involves complex mathematics. The present paper describes a simple approach for understanding aspects of the problem. A numerical approach is advocated.

Introduction

The generations of vision scientists who entered the field less than twenty-five years ago missed out on an exciting set of issues having to do with the Stiles-Crawford effect and the waveguide nature of photoreceptors [1-3]. In a series of papers mainly in the 1960s [4-15 give a sampling of his papers] Jay Enoch made definitive contributions to our understanding of the optical properties of photoreceptors. In particular, he gave experimental evidence for the presence of multiple modes of propagation of light down the photoreceptors. The mode structure of photoreceptors is important for understanding the angular breadth of the Stiles-Crawford effect and its dependence on wavelength.

As part of this Enoch Festschrift I thought it would be appropriate to bring some of those beautiful waveguide computations and issues to those of us vision scientists who missed the action thirty years ago. I rapidly discovered, however, that the computations of the waveguide nature of cones are not simple. The mathematical literature on waveguides requires an understanding of analytic solutions of partial differential equations, a field that requires expertise well beyond that of typical vision scientists. I wanted to develop methods that made analysis of waveguides easier to handle. As will be seen, so far this quest has been only partially successful since I haven't yet developed a general purpose computer program to calculate the antenna pattern of general cones.

This short article covers four points. First, diffraction patterns and Stiles-Crawford patterns are compared while avoiding Bessel functions. Our results are compared to a theoretical calculation by Snyder & Pask [16]. Second, new data on the Stiles-Crawford effect strengthens the relevance of the diffraction approach. Third, a computer program is provided for calculating the general modes of cylindrical waveguides of constant cross section. The program has no "hidden machinery" such as eigenfunction routines. This approach simplifies and demystifies the modes of waveguides. Finally, I comment on extending this approach to the case of non-constant cross section photoreceptors.

Diffraction and the Stiles-Crawford angular tuning

Suppose the cone has a square aperture. The angular dependence of the diffraction pattern is standardly found by summing over the phasors from the top to the bottom of the aperture. This gives the integral:

$$\text{amplitude} = \int \exp(i\phi(y))\, dy \,/ \int 1\, dy \;= \sin(\phi_o/2)/(\phi_o/2) \qquad (1)$$

$$\approx 1 - (\phi_o/2)^2/\, 6. \qquad (2)$$

Standard single slit diffraction theory gives

and $\phi_o/2 = \pi\, d \sin(\theta)/\, \lambda$ (3)

with $\theta = y/24$ mm (4)

where λ is the wavelength in the ocular medium and d is the slit width. Note that θ does not use a reduced eye length (we use 24 rather than 17 mm) since the diffraction pattern takes place entirely in the ocular medium.

For a cone with a circular aperture the only change to Eq. 1 is that there is a weighting function controlling the length of each phasor due to the circular shape. Eq. 1 becomes:

$$\text{amplitude} = \int((d/2)^2 - y^2)^{.5} \exp(i\phi(y))\, dy \,/ \int((d/2)^2 - y^2)^{.5}\, dy \qquad (5)$$

$$\approx 1 - (\phi_o/2)^2/\, 8. \text{ (where 8 is an exact integer)} \qquad (6)$$

The intensity of light is the amplitude squared. For small angles the intensity is:

$$\text{intensity} = 1 - k\, (\phi_o/2)^2 \qquad (7)$$

where k = 1/3 or 1/4 for a rectangular or circular aperture, respectively. Eq. 7 can now be related to the Stiles-Crawford aperture function given by:

$$\text{aperture function} = 10^{\wedge}(-ry^2) \approx 1 - 2.3\, ry^2 \qquad (8)$$

where 2.3 is the natural log of 10. Comparing Eqs. 2, 3, 4, 7 and 8 gives:

$$r = k/2.3\, (\pi d/(24\, \lambda))^2 \qquad (9)$$

This derivation of the Stiles-Crawford parameter r in terms of cone diffraction avoided introduction of Bessel functions. Instead of the Airy factor of 1.22 associated with the first zero of the lowest Bessel function, we have the simpler factor of 1/4 due to the circular aperture. This simplification was possible because for the Stiles-Crawford function we are interested in small values of y, where keeping the leading terms of the Taylor's expansion in Eqs. 2 and 6 is an excellent approximation.

A primary inspiration for writing this article occurred when I compared Eq. 9 to theoretical waveguide calculations by Snyder & Pask [16]. For example, for λ= .7/1.33 μ and an inner segment diameter of 3.2μ, Eq. 9 gives r=.688. This value is about 4% lower than the Snyder & Pask [16] calculation for the lowest mode. Eq. 9 also has the same dependence on d and l as their calculation (Fig. 9, of [16]). One difference is that in our approach (Eq. 9) there is no dependence on the refractive index of the inner segment. In their Fig. 10, Snyder & Pask show that the dependence on inner segment refractive index is very small. Thus the simple diffraction approach is instructive.

New Data

One problem with the previous waveguide approaches is that the Stiles-Crawford tuning tended to be too broad to be compatible with the lowest waveguide mode. That situation may have changed recently. Burns, Wu & Elsner [17] have made objective retinal densitometry measurements that indicate the Stiles-Crawford function may be narrower than previously thought. They find $\rho \approx .07$ in the fovea and $\rho \approx .13$ at an eccentricity of about 1 deg. These values are about double those previously found, indicating narrower angular tuning from previous estimates. The narrower tuning brings one closer to the regime where diffraction is the limiting factor. This is the regime where the lowest mode is dominant. One's intuition is that the lowest waveguide mode should be dominant since it is the only mode that doesn't have a zero intensity node within the cone. The zero intensity node produces reduced absorption by the photopigment.

Calculating the mode structure of constant cross-section waveguides

In order to determine the waveguide modes one starts with the Maxwell's Equations and derives the wave equation for each component of the electric or magnetic field. For monochromatic light whose vacuum wavelength is λ_0 the wave equation becomes:

$$\nabla^2 U + k^2 U = 0 \qquad (10)$$

where ∇^2 is the three-dimensional second derivative, $k = 2\pi n/\lambda_0$ and n is the index of refraction. Inside the cone outer segment n is fixed at $n_o = 1.405$ and the index of the surrounding medium is taken as $n_s = 1.34$. If the waveguide has axial symmetry and a constant cross section then the solution, U, must have the following structure in z (the location along the waveguide) and ϕ the azimuthal angle.

$$U(r, \phi, z) = u(r) \exp(i(m\phi + bz)) \qquad (11)$$

where $b= 2\pi/\lambda_z$ and λ_z is the wavelength of the light inside the fiber in the z direction. In cylindrical coordinates Eq. 10 becomes:

$$d^2u/dr^2 + r^{-1}\, du/dr + (k^2 - b^2 - m^2/r^2)\, u = 0 \qquad (12)$$

For a region of constant index, the solution to Eq. 12 is an mth order Bessel function. For most values of b the solution u(r) diverges at infinity. There are a finite number of b values for which a well behaved solution can be found. These solutions are called eigenfunctions or modes. The modes are difficult to calculate analytically because of the need to smoothly join the inner and outer Bessel function solutions at the photoreceptor boundary. The following annotated Matlab program simplifies the process of calculating the mode shapes and the allowable values of b for m=0 and arbitrary values for the wavelength, indices of refraction and outer segment diameter.

```
lambda=.6;              % the vacuum wavelength in microns
del=.1;                 % the integration interval in the r direction
rmax=6; nr=rmax/del; % nr is number of r intervals, rmax is region of solution)
bndy=floor(.5/del);    % the cone outer segment has radius of .5 microns)
ns=1.34; no=1.405;    % the indices of refraction for surround and outer segment
k=2*pi/lambda*[ones(1,bndy)*no  ones(1,nr-bndy)*ns];% the reciprocal
wavelength
b=[14.271744:.000001:14.2717461]'; %for 1st mode and del=.1)
u(:,1:2)= [b.^0 b.^0]; % initialize the first two r values at r=-.5 and +.5
for ir=3:nr;            % this is the loop that solves the differential equation
 temp= 2*u(:,ir-1)- u(:,ir-2)*(1-1/(2*ir-5)); % where r=(ir-1-1.5)*del
 u(:,ir)= (temp - u(:,ir-1).*del^2.*(k(ir-1)^2-b.^2))/(1+1/(2*ir-5));
end
plot([del/2:del:rmax-del]',u(:,2:nr)');  % plot the curves for each b value
for ib=1:length(b);text(4.5,u(ib,nr-2),sprintf('b=%f', b(ib))); end
xlabel('r (microns)');ylabel('amplitude of electric field')
```

The program's output is shown in figure 1. The three values of b that are used bracket the correct value that converges to zero as r goes to infinity. This correct value (related to the eigenvalue) was obtained in about two minutes of trial and error hunting by hand, with an extra decimal point obtained on each iteration. If the sample size is reduced (del=.1 in above program) then the value of b must be adjusted slightly. The value of b was increased to look for additional modes but none were found given the tiny 1 μ outer segment. If the outer segment diameter is increased (such as is the case for the inner segment) then a second mode is found.

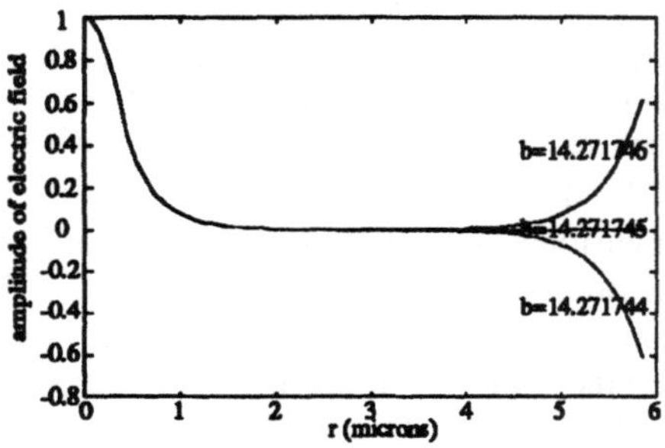

Figure 1: Program Output

Calculating the antenna pattern for general waveguides

The Matlab program shown above was for the special case of rotation symmetry in *f* and translation symmetry in *z* so that Eq. 11 could be used to convert the partial differential equation (Eq. 10) to an ordinary differential equation in *r*. It is my goal to write a Matlab program, somewhat similar to the one above, that assumes axial symmetry, but that allows the cone diameter to change as a function of z. One would work the problem backwards: start with a single mode propagating down the outer segment and solve the differential equation for the antenna pattern entering the inner segment. I have devoted some effort to this task, but so far the solution is not well behaved when the light hits the tapered section of the waveguide. One way to proceed is to use a package such as the Matlab Partial Differential Equation toolbox. By that means one can calculate the Stiles-Crawford effect for cones of any shape without needing to be an expert in mathematics.

References

1. Stiles, WS and Crawford, JB. The luminous efficiency of rays entering the eye pupil at different points. Proc R Soc B 1933;112:428-50.
2. Stiles, WS. The luminous efficiency of monochromatic rays entering the eye pupil at different points and a new colour effect. Proc R Soc B 1937;123:90-118.
3. O'Brien, B. Vision and resolution in the central retina. J Opt Soc Am 1951;41:882-94.
4. Enoch, JM. Response of a modal retinal receptor as a function of wavelength. J Opt Soc Am 1960;50:315-20.
5. Enoch, JM. Wave-guide modes in retinal receptors. Science 1961;133:1353-54.
6. Enoch, JM. Nature of the transmission of energy in the retinal receptors. J Opt Soc Am 1961; 51:1122-26.
7. Enoch, JM. Visualization of waveguide modes in retinal receptors. Am J Ophth 1961;51:1107-18.
8. Enoch, JM. Optical properties of the retinal receptors. J Opt Soc Am 1963;53:71-85.
9. Enoch, JM. The retina as a fiber optics bundle. In: Kapany NS, editor. Fiber Optics. New York: Academic Press; 1967.
10. Enoch, JM. & Tobey, FL eds. Vertebrate Photoreceptor Optics, Berlin: Springer-Verlag, 1981. This book contains several chapters by Enoch providing an excellent summary of his work.
11 Enoch, JM. Commets on "Excitation of waveguide modes in retinal receptors". J Opt Soc Am '67;57:548-49.
12 Enoch, JM & Glissman, LE. Physical and optical changes in excised retinal tissue. Invest. Ophth. 1966; 5:208-21.

13 Enoch, JM & Laties, AM. An analysis of retinal receptor orientation II. Predictions for psychophysical tests. Invesst. Ophth. 1971;10:95.
14. Enoch, JM. & Stiles, WS. The colour change of monochromatic light with retinal angle of incidence. Optica Acta 1961;8:329-58.
15. Enoch, JM, Bedell, HE & Campos, EC. Local variations in rod receptror orientation Vision Res. 1978; 18: 123-24.
16. Snyder, AW & Pask, C. The Stiles-Crawford effect-Explanation and consequences. Vision Res. 1973; 13:1115-37.
17. Burns, SA, Wu, S & Elsner, AE. Variation in photoreceptor directionality across the fovea. ARVO 1996 abstract, 2044.

IMAGING PHOTORECEPTORS IN THE LIVING EYE WITH ADAPTIVE OPTICS

JUNZHONG LIANG, DAVID R. WILLIAMS, DONALD T. MILLER
Center for Visual Science, University of Rochester
Rochester, NY 14627

Abstract

High-resolution images of the living retina are obtained by adaptively compensating for the wave aberration of the human eye. Adaptive optics allows correction for not only defocus and astigmatism, but also coma, spherical aberration, and higher order aberrations in the human eye.

Introduction

Aberrations limit the optical quality of normal human eyes. These aberrations include defocus, astigmatism, coma, spherical aberration, and more complicated higher order aberrations. For small pupil sizes (<2.5 mm), the optics of the eye can be made diffraction-limited using spectacles to correct for both defocus and astigmatism. For a larger dilated pupil, however, the optical quality is often worse due to the uncorrected spherical aberration, coma, and higher order aberrations [1,2]. These aberrations blur images that form on the retina thereby reducing the eye's contrast sensitivity. In addition, they reduce the resolution of fundus cameras that are designed to image retinal structures as small as single photoreceptors[3].

To remove these aberrations for large pupils, we have chosen an approach based on adaptive optics. Adaptive optics is an emerging technology that has been primarily developed in the astronomical and military communities for imaging through the earth's atmosphere [4]. It has been successful in compensating for the phase error induced by atmospheric turbulence for ground-based telescopes. Adaptive compensation requires two main components: a wavefront sensor, which measures the phase error in real time, and a deformable mirror or a liquid crystal device, which compensates for the measured phase error. The use of a deformable mirror in a confocal scanning laser ophthalmoscope has been successful for the correction of astigmatism of the human eye [5], though correction of other aberrations in the eye has not been reported previously. Adaptive compensation for these other aberrations such as spherical aberration, coma, and higher order aberrations requires a wavefront sensor which can provide quick and accurate measurements of the wave aberration in any particular eye.

Method and Results

We have constructed an adaptive optics system that measures the wave aberration of the eye using a Hartmann-Shack wavefront sensor (HSWS) [2,6] and compensates for it with a deformable mirror. An image of a point source is produced on the retina by the optics of the eye that focuses an incoming laser beam of 1.5 mm in diameter. The HSWS consists of an array of 217 lenslets and a CCD camera at the focal plane of the lenslets. It measures the local slopes of the wavefront emerging from a dilated pupil over a diameter of 6.7 mm. The wave aberration of the eye is then reconstructed from the wavefront slopes with a least squares fit, using a sum of 65 Zernike modes as the basis functions. The measured wavefront error across the pupil is then compensated using a PZT deformable mirror (Xinetics, Inc.). The deformable mirror has 37 actuators each with a stroke of 3 μm. After a number of (typically 10-15) closed-loop iterations, each consisting of a wavefront measurement followed by an adaptive correction, the compensated wave aberration of the eye is significantly reduced. In the four eyes tested so far, the peak to valley wavefront error was reduced on average by a factor of four.

Adaptive compensation provides the eye with unprecedented optical quality. Our preliminary psychophysical measurements have shown that the contrast sensitivity function was significantly improved for both tested eyes with adaptive compensation. For example, both subjects easily resolved a high frequency grating at 55 cycles/degree with adaptive compensation, while they could not resolve the same grating even at 100% contrast without adaptive compensation. This improvement is also reflected in the eye's MTF (measured with the HSWS) before and after adaptive compensation. The eye's point spread function with adaptive compensation has a comparable size to that of a single foveal photoreceptor. Both tested observers reported that a monochromatic point source viewed through the deformable mirror produced stunning changes in color over time, which are likely caused by drifts in the retinal image across different cone classes.

High-resolution retinal images were obtained by incorporating a Krypton flash lamp into our adaptive optics system. The flash lamp delivers a brief (4 msec) exposure that uniformly illuminates a patch of retina, often one degree in diameter. The Krypton lamp provides light of a broad spectrum from 100 to 1100 nm. Narrow band illumination of the retina is obtained by a filter with a spectral bandwidth typically 10 to 30 nm. A scientific grade CCD camera, conjugate with the retina, was used to collect images of the living retina. Our experimental results on two eyes so far have shown that adaptive compensation for the wave aberration of the eye provides a significant improvement in image resolution and image contrast from the foveal center to 4 degrees eccentricity. As an example, we show in Figure 1 a high-resolution image of living photoreceptors for one subject over a field of 0.707 x 0.707 degrees. Further details will be reported in a separate paper currently in preparation.

Acknowledgments

The authors are thankful to Houman Tamaddon, Alan Russell, and William Vaughn for their technical assistance. This research is supported by NIH Grants EY04367, EY01319 and a RE&HPB Fellowship.

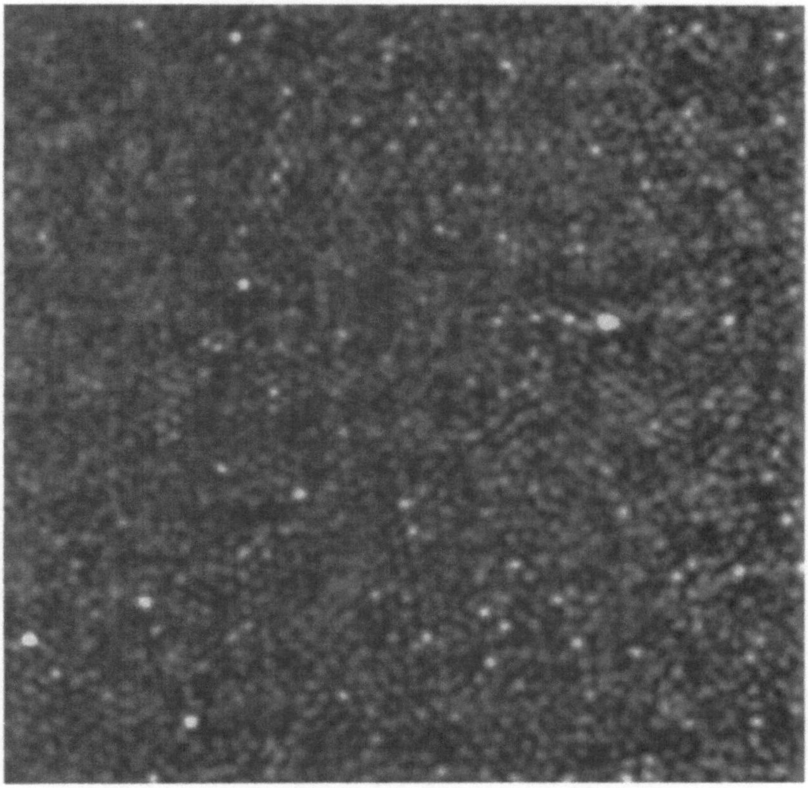

Figure 1. High resolution image of living photoreceptors for subject JL's eye over a field of 0.707 x 0.707 degrees (206 x 206μm^2). The image was taken under adaptive compensation for the wave aberration of the eye for a 6 mm pupil. The retinal illumination is spatially incoherent with a spectral bandwidth of 10 nm centered at 630 nm. The image shown is bandpass filtered to remove low frequencies below 10 cycles/degree, which enhances contrast, and high frequencies beyond 100 cycles/degree, which reduces noise. The center of the field is 0.9 degrees from the foveal center.

References

1. Campbell FW and Green DG. Optical and retinal factors affecting visual resolution. J Physiol Lond 1965; 181: 576-593.
2. Liang J and Williams DR. Effect of higher order aberrations on image quality in the human eye. Vision Science and its Applications, Vol.1, 1995 OSA Technical Digest Series, 70-73, Optical Society of America, Washington, D.C., 1995.
3. Miller DT, Williams DR, Morris GM, and Liang J. Images of the cone mosaic in the living human eye. Vis Res 1995; 36: 1067-1079.
4. Hardy J. Adaptive optics. Sci Amer 1994; 270:60-65.
5. Dreher AW, Bille JF, and Weinreb RN. Active optical depth resolution improvement of the laser tomographic scanner. Appl Opt 1989; 28:804-808.
6. Liang J, Grimm B, Goelz S, and Bille JF. Objective measurement of wave aberrations of the human eye with the use of a Hartmann-Shack wavefront sensor. J Opt Soc Am 1994; A11: 1949-1957.

PHOTOPIGMENT ABSORPTANCE AND DIRECTIONAL SENSITIVITY IN PERIPHERAL PRIMATE RETINA

ORIN S. PACKER & DAVID R. WILLIAMS
Center for Visual Science, University of Rochester, Rochester, NY 14627

Abstract

We simultaneously measured the light being absorbed at every location across a patch of fresh excised primate retina. Rod and cone axial absorptances were 0.5 and 0.3 respectively, consistent with the specific density of photopigment and outer segment length. The photometric quantum efficiency of patches of peripheral retina was 0.12. There was little evidence for directional sensitivity in patches of rods. Great care must be taken when interpreting bright spots in images of excised retina.

Introduction

We have developed an improved version of axial microspectrophotometry (MSP) [1], photopigment transmittance imaging [2], and used it to simultaneously measure the light being absorbed at every location across a patch of fresh primate retina. We used this technique to 1) measure the axial absorptance of each photoreceptor in the mosaic in order to classify it by photopigment type, 2) measure the photometric quantum efficiency of patches of retina [3], and 3) extend Enoch's measurements [4] of photoreceptor directional sensitivity to include measurements of absorbed light.

Methods

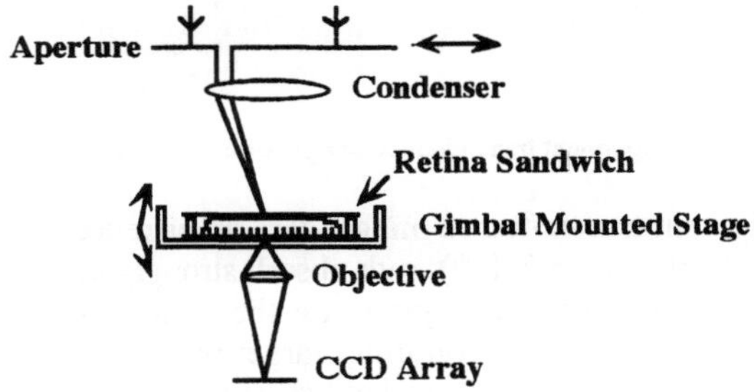

Figure 1. The apparatus.

Under infrared illumination, we superfused macaque monkey eyecups in oxygenated Ames medium, then sandwiched a disk of fresh excised retina between two coverglasses. The optical system (Figure 1) illuminated this disk under conditions comparable to those used in psychophysical experiments. The microscope condenser took the place of the eye lens, while a moveable aperture of variable diameter took the place of the pupil, providing precise control of the angle of incidence and the angular extent of the illuminating beam. The retinal sandwich was mounted on a microscope stage and illuminated from the same direction as retina would be in vivo. The gimbal mounted stage allowed the retina to be tilted to align the optical axis of the microscope with the optical axes of the photoreceptors. The photoreceptor outer segments were imaged with a microscope objective onto a CCD array, which provided precise radiometric measurements at each pixel location in the image, letting us measure not just absorbed light, but also light that fell between or leaked out of photoreceptors.

Results

Photopigment absorptance in individual photoreceptors: To measure the amount of absorbed light, an image of retina collected before bleaching the photopigment was divided by an image taken after a white light bleach.

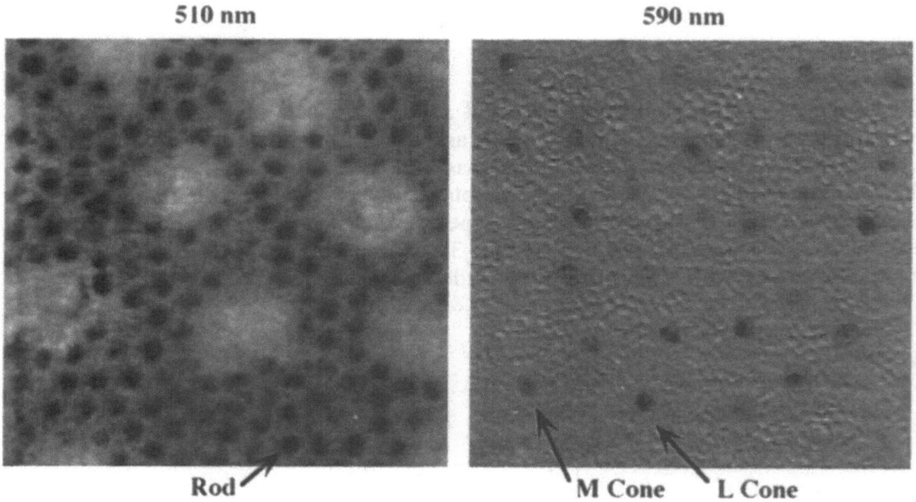

Figure 2. Photopigment transmittance images of peripheral macaque retina.

In a photopigment transmittance image, dark areas represent high photopigment absorptance. At 510 nm (Figure 2, left), rods absorb strongly and the dark spots are rod outer segments. The lighter circular regions are the locations of cones, whose inner segments at this eccentricity are several times larger in diameter than rods. The cone outer segments are shorter than the rods and out of focus.

The mean absorptance of 270 rods was 0.51 ± 0.04, consistent with the specific density of rhodopsin and rod outer segment length. Apparently, the majority of the photons passed through the photopigment-filled outer segments of intact, well-aligned rods.

We also measured the axial absorptances of cones. Changes in wavelength affect which photoreceptors absorb strongly. In Figure 2 (right), taken with 590 nm light, L cones show the highest photopigment absorptance, M cones less, and rods almost none. The mean absorptance of 116 cones corrected for the λ_{max} of the photopigment they contain was 0.3 ± 0.04, consistent with the specific density of photopigment and cone outer segment length. It is also approximately 6 times the value typically reported by axial MSP.

We have imaged patches of peripheral retina with well aligned cones at wavelengths (440, 510, & 590 nm) that produce the highest contrast between the photopigments. We combined the three photopigment transmittance images to show the retina as it would look if it were possible to view it under white light without bleaching the photopigment. In such an image, L cones appear blue, M cones appear purple, and rods appear red. We found approximately equal numbers of L and M cones, and in the largest patch of retina, there was a statistically reliable tendency for L cones to clump with other L cones and M cones with other M cones.

Absorptance across patches of retina: We also measured the average absorptance of whole patches of photoreceptors by averaging all the pixels in the image. The average absorptance in 4 patches of retina that each contained more than 100 rods, like Figure 2 (left), was 0.23 ± 0.08. If we assume that in vivo, 0.8 of a 500 nm stimulus is transmitted by the optics and that 2/3 of the absorbed photons lead to photoisomerizations, then the quantum efficiency or the fraction of quanta incident at the cornea that produced photoisomerizations in rods would be 0.12. Measuring quantum efficiency directly eliminates the need to make separate measurements of the absorptance of individual photoreceptors and the fraction of light that falls between or leaks out of photoreceptors.

The directional sensitivity of patches of rods: In addition to axial measurements of absorptance, we measured the directional sensitivity of photon absorptance in whole patches of retina, by varying the angle of incidence of the illuminating beam. Since measurements of directional sensitivity require comparisons of the numbers of absorbed photons rather than just the fraction absorbed, the images collected before and after bleaching were subtracted rather than divided. The total number of photons absorbed in a patch of retina was calculated by summing the pixels in the difference image.

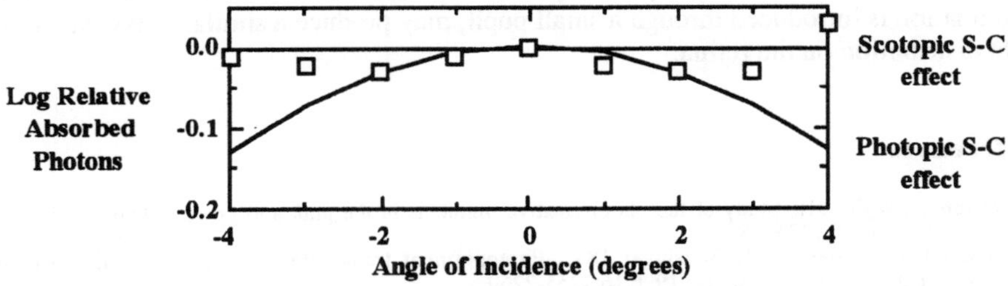

Figure 3. Directional sensitivity for absorbed photons.

The squares in Figure 3 shows the numbers of photons absorbed in a patch of rods as a function of the angle of incidence of the illuminating beam. This patch of rods absorbed similar numbers of photons regardless of angle of incidence, a result that is consistent with the scotopic Stiles-Crawford (S-C) effect (horizontal line). A typical photopic S-C function for these conditions is also plotted. Three of four patches of retina were similar.

Directional sensitivity of individual photoreceptors: The images used to calculate directional sensitivity were made using an aperture equivalent to a 1 mm pupil in the living eye, to more closely match conditions used in Stiles-Crawford experiments. Measured in this way, the directional sensitivity of individual rods and cones was highly variable. Although, on average, there was little evidence of directional sensitivity, several photoreceptors were too narrowly tuned to be consistent with diffraction from an aperture the diameter of a photoreceptor. This led us to discover that the illuminating light was coherent and was interfering with itself, rendering light measurements at single pixels in the image unreliable estimates of light transmittance through the retina. Thus, narrow apertures and filter bandwidths are not appropriate for directional sensitivity measurements in individual photoreceptors. We are modifying the technique to reduce the speckle so that we can compare the directional sensitivity of the photoreceptors in a patch of retina both as individuals and as members of a group.

Conclusions

Photopigment transmittance imaging lets us simultaneously measure the light being absorbed at every location across a patch of fresh excised primate retina. We have 1) made the first axial absorptance measurements in individual primate rods and cones that are consistent with the specific density of photopigment and outer segment length, 2) classified individual photoreceptors simultaneously in large patches of retina, based on the spectral properties of their photopigment, 3) calculated the quantum efficiency of patches of peripheral retina, and 4) found little evidence for directional sensitivity in patches of rods, consistent with the rod Stiles-Crawford effect.

We imaged many cones that appeared to funnel light efficiently, but which had little photopigment absorptance. These bright spots probably represent light leaking from inner segments, and can easily be misinterpreted as outer segment tips unless their absorptances are measured. In addition, it can be difficult to distinguish photoreceptor outer segments from speckle. Care must be taken when interpreting bright spots in images of excised retina. Psychophysical experiments in which monochromatic illumination is introduced through a small pupil, may produce a similar noisy pattern of light distribution on the retina.

References

1. Denton EJ, Wyllie JH. Study of the photosensitive pigments in the pink and green rods of the frog. J Physiol Lond 1955;127:81-89.
2. Packer OS, Williams DR, Bensinger DG. Photopigment transmittance imaging of the primate photoreceptor mosaic. J Neurosci 1996;16:2251-2260.
3. Pelli DG. The quantum efficiency of vision. In: Blakemore C, editor. Vision: coding and efficiency. Cambridge: Cambridge University Press, 1990:3-24.
4. Enoch JM, Lakshminarayanan V. Retinal fibre optics. In: Cronly-Dillon J, editor. Vision and Visual Dysfunction, Vol I. Boca Raton: CRC Press, 1991:280-309.

REFRACTIVE INDEX GRADIENTS IN SUNFISH CONES

MICKEY P. ROWE[1], NADER ENGHETA[1], JOSEPH M. CORLESS[2], and EDWARD N. PUGH, JR.[3]
[1]*Moore School of Electrical Engineering* [3]*Department of Psychology and Institute of Neurological Sciences, University of Pennsylvania, Philadelphia, PA.*
[2]*Departments of Cell Biology, Neurobiology and Ophthalmology, Duke University Medical Center, Durham, NC.*

Abstract

Jay Enoch's pioneering work with whole-mounted retinas established that vertebrate photoreceptors behave as dielectric waveguides. Theoretical analyses lead to the expectation that the distribution of refractive index in the photoreceptor inner segment will affect its waveguiding behavior. To determine the distribution of refractive indices in isolated photoreceptors, we examined them with a scanning microinterferometer. Our measurements of cones from green sunfish (*Lepomis cyanellus*) reveal systematic gradients of refractive index within the inner segments. For example, the refractive index of single cones (averaged over transverse cross-sections) increases from ca. 1.38 to ca. 1.42 along the inner segment longitudinal axis. Such gradients are large enough to affect waveguiding properties. Interferometric measurements and analysis of sub-cellular variations in refractive index will allow us to address a variety of unresolved issues in photoreceptor optics.

Introduction

Following various reports that some vertebrates are sensitive to optical polarization [*e.g.* 1] and knowing that photoreceptor inner segments act as optical waveguides[2], we have pursued the hypothesis that birefringent waveguiding through double cone inner segments provides a basis for vertebrate polarization sensitivity[3]. To test this hypothesis, we used electron microscopy (EM) to determine ultrastructural properties relevant to photoreceptor waveguiding. While examining electron micrographs of a sectioned sunfish retina, we noted systematic variations in the electron density of mitochondria in all cone inner segments[3]. In order to determine if these electron density gradients correspond to relevant variations in refractive index, we examined cone inner segment-outer segments (CIS-COSs) with a scanning microinterferometer.

Methods

Much of this work has been previously reported[3,4], so we will only briefly describe the scanning methods here. CIS-COSs were isolated from sunfish retinas and mounted on the stage of a modified Vickers M86 microscope. Optical components in the microscope split a He-Ne laser beam into two parallel beams which project through the specimen plane as diagrammed in Fig. 1. The positions of the two beams are controlled via a Macintosh computer, and the relative phases of the two beams are compared by optical and electronic elements in the base of the microscope. Ideally the optical path lengths (OPLs) through which the two beams travel are identical except at the specimen plane where one of the beams may be directed through a CIS-COS (or other object of interest). The beams are focused down to 0.3 μm spots at the specimen plane, and can be moved laterally in steps of approximately 0.2 μm. Thus, we can use the instrument to systematically examine variations in OPL with high spatial resolution.

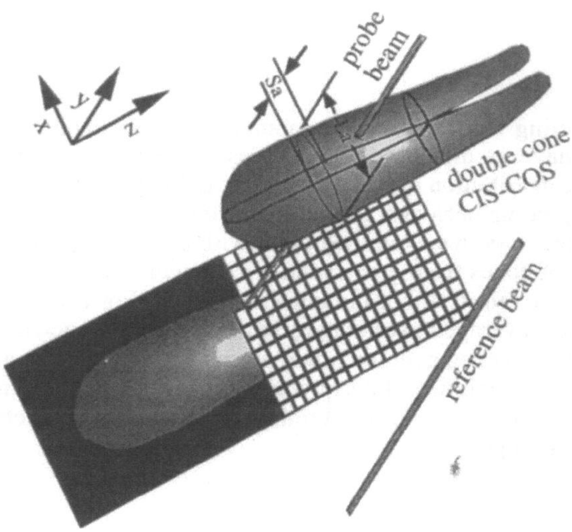

Figure 1. Schematic representation of scanning microinterferometry and aspect ratio determinations. The probe beam and reference beam are moved in a raster pattern over the specimen and the phases of the two beams are compared at each location generating data matrices of OPL(x,z). A partial data set is schematically depicted as an intensity image underneath the double cone that is being scanned here. Complete images are depicted in Figs. 2 and 4. The cross-section outlined in the middle of the inner segments indicates what measurements were made on the EMs to establish the aspect ratios plotted in Fig. 3. Aspect ratios were defined as **La/Sa.**

The OPL measured by the interferometer is the integral of refractive index over the distance the laser beam travels through the object of interest. It is not possible to directly measure refractive index; even if the refractive index is constant along a given physical path, the distance along that path must be known in order to extract refractive index from OPL. Thus to use OPL measurements for inferring underlying refractive index distributions, we need information about the CIS-COS's cross-sections in the planes through which the microinterferometer's beam passes. In our previous report[4] we focused on the single cones because their cross-sections are nominally circular. In this report we will also address refractive index gradients in double cones. To do so, we measured the aspect ratios of double cones in tangential (relative to the retina) EM sections. The measurements made are schematically depicted in Fig. 1.

Results and Discussion

In the coordinate system depicted in Fig. 1, OPL(x, z) is the integral of refractive index along y. If we integrate our OPL's over x and divide the result by the cross-sectional area of the cell as a function of z, we can determine an average refractive index along z ($\bar{n}(z)$). Since the area of a circle can be determined from its radius, it is relatively easy to obtain from OPL(x, z) estimates of the cross-sectional areas of single cones. Fig. 2 depicts a scan of a representative single cone CIS-COS and its $\bar{n}(z)$. Note how $\bar{n}(z)$ increases as a function of z through the inner segment.

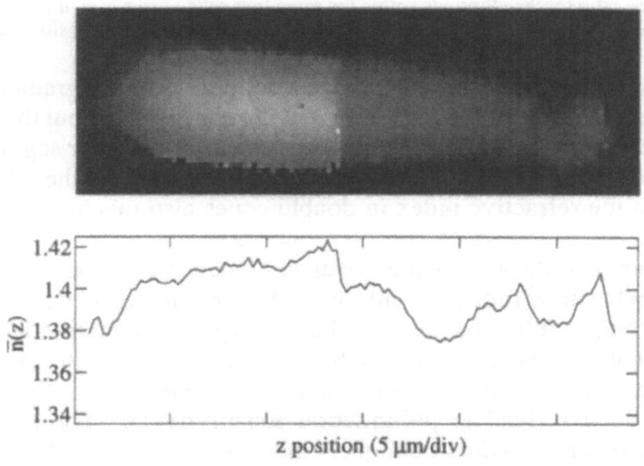

Figure 2. Longitudinal variations in single cone refractive index. The top panel depicts OPL(x,z) - image intensity is proportional to the measured value of OPL each position. The lower panel represents the average refractive index determined as described in the text. Refractive index rises in the inner segment. Refractive index in the outer segment is lower and generally more uniform thatn that in the inner segment, but frequently other objects (such as the accessory outer segment) cause the refractive to appear to fluctuate as here. The principal features of $\bar{n}(z)$ are representative our data from single cone inner setment.

Fig. 3 presents the results of the aspect ratio calculations from EMs of double cones. The origin of the longitudinal axis is arbitrary; the sections analyzed extended from just above the nuclei to the bases of the outer segments. The diamonds represent the aspect ratios of the ellipsoids within the cells; the squares represent the aspect ratios of the cones as diagrammed in Fig. 1 (**La**/**Sa**). Note that the aspect ratios remain relatively constant along most of the length of the inner segment. This indicates that changes in **Sa** are well correlated with changes in **La** -- hence variations in the apparent width of a cell in our OPL(x, z) measurements should correspond to variations in thickness in the perpendicular direction (*i.e.* the direction along which our probe beam travels).

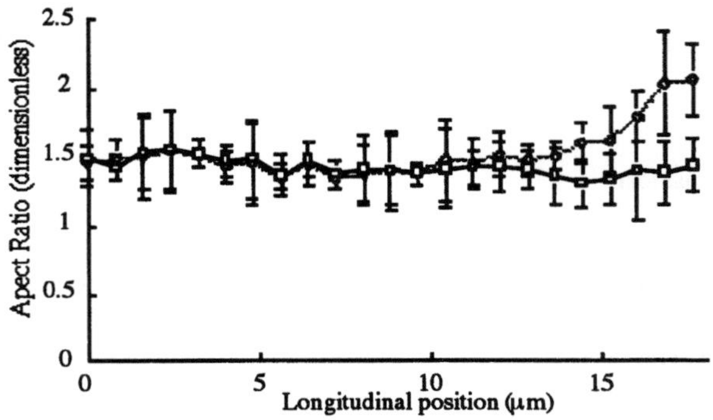

Figure 3. Double cone aspect ratios. The distance across both the long and short axes were measured across four double cones in 23 EM sections. Squares correspond to **La/Sa** as diagrammed in Fig. 1. Diamonds represent the same ratio for the ellipsoids within the same four cells. Error bars indicate one standard deviation. (Editor's note: Ordinate label should be Aspect Ratio (dimensionless)).

Fig. 4 shows evidence for longitudinal refractive index gradients through a double cone. Near the base of the inner segment the cone is wide, but the OPL near the center is relatively low (dotted line). In sections closer to the outer segment, the cell's apparent width is the same (solid line) or smaller (dashed line) but the OPL is larger. It is thus clear that the refractive index in double cones also increases along the inner segment.

These results suggest that the electron density variations evident in EM's correspond to refractive index variations in living sunfish cones. Modeling of waveguiding through sunfish cones must thus incorporate refractive index gradients. Refractive index gradients may act to better concentrate light into the center of the cones' inner segments. Given the non-circular cross-sections of sunfish double cones, this concentration may lead to polarization sensitivity[3]. The refractive index gradients may also help to redirect obliquely incident light such that it travels straight down the axes of the outer segments and enhances the animal's sensitivity both spatially (by preventing cross-talk between photoreceptors) and overall (by aligning the light for maximal absorption by the pigments in the outer segment disks).

Acknowledgements

This work was supported by the U. S. Department of Navy, Office of Naval Research, under grant N00014-93-1-0935.

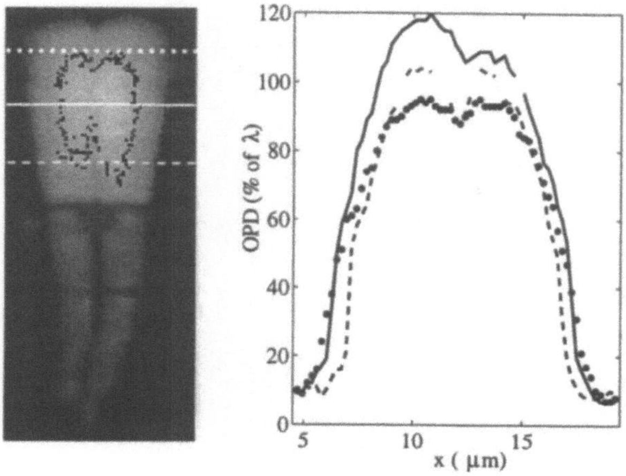

Figure 4. OPL variations in a sunfish cone. The left panel depicts OPL(x, z) for a sunfish double cone CIS-COS. The dark points within the inner segment are places where the data were suppressed because the instrument does not reliably report OPLs when the probe and reference beams are nearly in phase. The right panel redisplays OPL(x) for three positions along the z axis. The dotted, solid and dashed lines come from the positions marked by the corresponding lines marked in the left panel. Comparison of the height of the three curves with the CIS's width (as determined from the positions at which OPL first begins to rise on each side) indicate that refractive index must increase along the orthodromal direction.

References

1. Waterman TH. Polarization Sensitivity. In:Autrum H, editor. Handbook of sensory physiology VII/6B. Invertebrate visual centers and behavior I. Berlin: Springer-Verlag, 1981:281-469.
2. Enoch JM, Lakshminaryanan V. Retinal Fiber Optics. In: Charman WN, editor. Vision and Visual Dysfunction Vol. 1. Visual Optics and Instrumentation. Boca Raton: CRC Press, 1991:280-309.
3. Rowe MP, Engheta N, Easter SS Jr, Pugh EN Jr. Graded-index model of a fish double cone exhibits differential polarization sensitivity. J Opt Soc Am A 1994;11:55-70.
4. Rowe MP, Corless JM, Engheta N, and Pugh EN Jr. Scanning interferometry of sunfish cones I: Longitudinal variation in single cone refractive index. J Opt Soc Am A; in press.

APODIZATION NEUTRALIZATION:

A NEW TECHNIQUE FOR INVESTIGATING THE IMPACT OF THE STILES-CRAWFORD EFFECT ON VISUAL FUNCTION

M. C. RYNDERS[1], L.N. THIBOS[1], A. BRADLEY[1], N. LÓPEZ-GIL [2]
[1]Visual Science Group, Indiana University School of Optometry, 800 Atwater Avenue, Bloomington, IN 47405, [2]Departamento de Física, Universidad de Murcia, 30071 Murcia, SPAIN.

Abstract.

Although the Stiles-Crawford effect (SCE) is of retinal origin, many of its roles in vision have been modeled successfully with an optical apodization of the pupil plane. By neutralizing the postulated apodization of the pupil, and thereby effectively canceling the SCE, we can examine the optical and visual impact of the SCE experimentally. We created reversely apodized filters, which were aligned with the subject's own SCE to create a uniformly transmitting pupil. To demonstrate the new technique, we measured the effect of pupil diameter on ocular transverse chromatic aberration (TCA) under normal conditions and again with the SCE neutralized. Results confirm earlier suggestions that SCE apodization modulates the effect of pupil diameter and location on perceived TCA, monocular chromatic diplopia, and chromostereopsis.

Introduction.

Since the 1930's the SCE has been known to exist and its causes and many of its aspects have since been investigated [1], but what is its effect on visual performance? Campbell has proposed an increased depth of field [2]. Legge, et al suggested that it reduces the effects of blur [3] and Vos suggested that the SCE has a role in chromostereopsis [4]. The latter was later described more in depth by Ye, et al [5], who also considered decentration of the pupil, which is known to induce TCA at the fovea. In agreement with Vos' hypothesis they proposed that the SCE reduces the effects of pupil decentration on perceived or subjective TCA (sTCA).

Of all suggested impacts of the SCE on visual functions, only Ye, et al tested their proposal by measuring sTCA both under photopic conditions (normal SCE present) and scotopic conditions (SCE much reduced), and, as predicted, pupil decentrations from the visual axis produced greater sTCA and chromostereopsis under scotopic conditions.

When Ye, et al. measured under scotopic conditions, the SCE was much reduced, but not fully absent [6]. In addition, foveal visual functions cannot be tested scotopically and the retinal illumination clearly is much reduced.

The currently proposed technique yields a more direct way of canceling the SCE induced apodization of the pupil, thus allowing us to verify the proposed impact of the SCE on the various aspects of visual performance mentioned above, since they all were based on the pupil apodization hypothesis. It does so by placing a filter with a reverse apodization (rSCE filter) conjugate to the eye's entrance pupil plane. With this filter all rays are rendered equally efficient. The filter thus creates a uniform pupil function. (See Fig.1) Differences revealed when taking a set of measurements twice, once under normal viewing conditions and once while looking through the rSCE filter, then yield information on the impact the apodization has on a certain visual function.

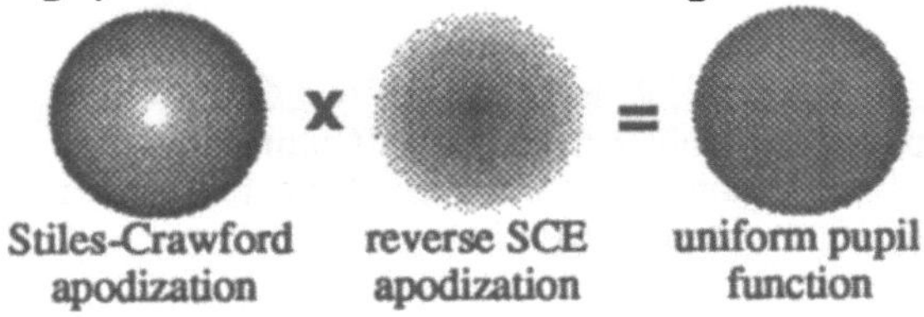

Figure 1. The basic principle: Aligning a reversely apodized filter with the Stiles-Crawford function of the eye in a plane conjugate to the eye's entrance pupil, removes the optical effects of the SCE-induced pupil apodization. This produces a uniform pupil function.

It is expected that in this way one can determine the impact of the SCE on a series of visual aspects, including those mentioned above.

To illustrate the currently proposed technique and to further verify/confirm the ideas of Vos and Ye, et al., we have used this method to determine the impact the SCE has on the psychophysically measured TCA. As predicted, removal of the apodization increased the sTCA, observed with decentered pupils.

Methods.

We first produced a set of rSCE filters with diameters of 5, 6 and 7 mm and with ρ-values ranging from -0.025 to -0.075, so that later any filter from this set could be chosen during experimental sessions. The minus sign indicates that the filter has a reverse apodization and the range of ρ-values was based on distributions of ρ-values found by Applegate and Lakshminarayanan in a large group of normals [7]. The variable ρ is defined as usual. An example can be found in Ref.[7]. In Fig. 2 four different types of filters are presented, each within a black mask. Note how the center of the filter is darker for larger filters and for filters with larger ρ-values, since larger differences in light efficiency have to be compensated. The thin lines within the black masks were used for alignment purposes.

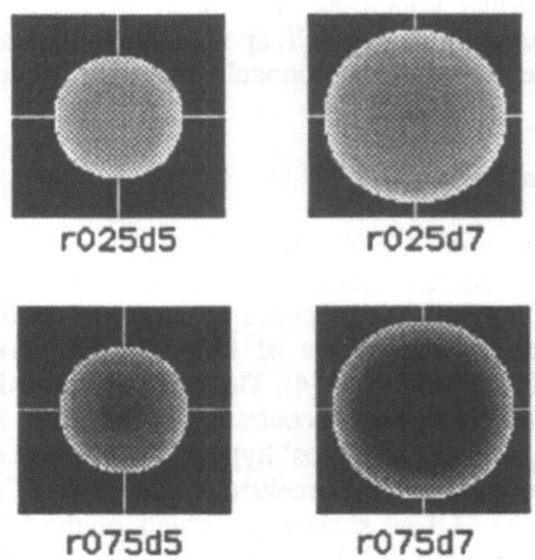

Figure 2. Four of the rSCE filters with radii of 5 mm (left column) and 7 mm (right column) and ρ-values of -0.025 (upper row) and -0.075 (lower row).

For each of the filters and masks the mathematical description was determined and pict-files for the filters were made using the software packet "Spyglas". The resulting pict-files were then "drawn" on slide film with a Montage slidemaker. Transmission of the developed filters was then determined and a Γ-correction function was determined, with which a next set of pict-files was made. After 3 such iterations a full set of rSCE filters was obtained, of which calibration showed remarkable matches with design specifications for the smaller filters and those with smaller ρ-values, while deviations were rarely more than 5% off and always well within 10% of the desired density values for filters with the largest diameters and ρ-values.

The next step was to determine the SC functions (SCF) of the subjects' eyes. The apparatus used has been described elswhere [8]. All alignments were done with the visual axis. Next, SCFs were again determined, but with rSCE filters in place.

Results.

For 2 subjects the SCFs were determined along the horizontal meridian at 0.5 mm intervals, with and without filters. Results are presented in Figures 3a and b. Individual data points represent the averages of 3 measurements. ρ-Values under normal conditions were 0.054 for LT and 0.058 for AB. rSCE- filters with ρ-values of -0.045 and -0.065 respectively were used, resulting in remaining ρ-values of 0.005 and -0.009 respectively.

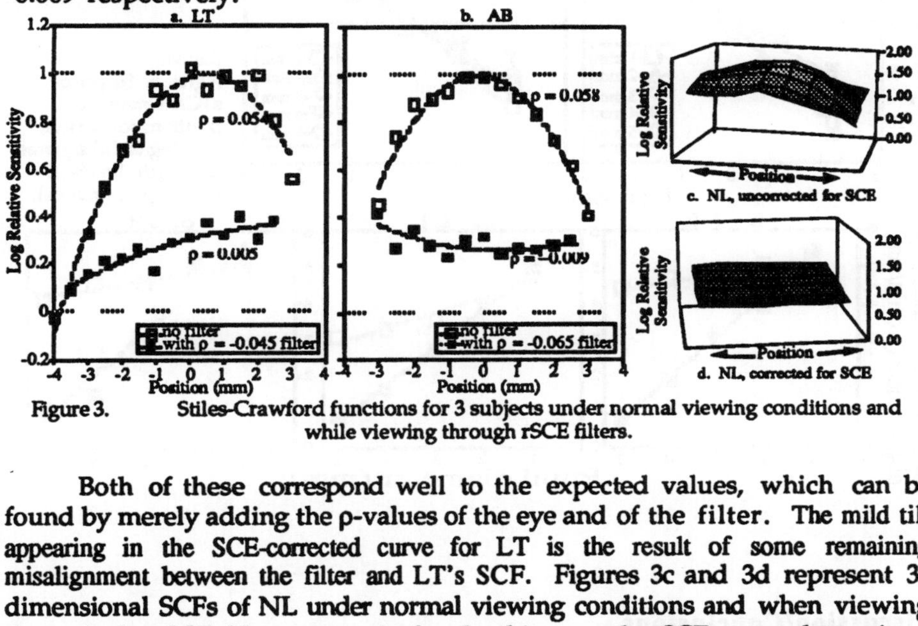

Figure 3. Stiles-Crawford functions for 3 subjects under normal viewing conditions and while viewing through rSCE filters.

Both of these correspond well to the expected values, which can be found by merely adding the ρ-values of the eye and of the filter. The mild tilt appearing in the SCE-corrected curve for LT is the result of some remaining misalignment between the filter and LT's SCF. Figures 3c and 3d represent 3-dimensional SCFs of NL under normal viewing conditions and when viewing through the rSCE filter, respectively. In this case the SCFs were determined by samplng 3x at the points of a 7x7 grid within the pupil plane. Distances between the sampling points were 1mm. The ρ-values along the horizontal meridia are 0.052 (Fig. 3c) and 0.002 (Fig. 3d.), while the rSCE filter had a ρ-value of -0.050.

A first application.

We tested the proposed technique to find the strength of the predicted impact that the SCE-induced pupil apodization has on the perceived TCA (sTCA). The theory has been described in detail in Ref.[4]. Fig. 4 shows the amount of sTCA measured for pupil diameters from 1 through 5 mm and for pupil displacements from the visual axis (x=0) of up to 2 mm. To keep retinal illuminance constant, an ND-filter with value equivalent to the mean of the rSCE filter was used whenever the rSCE filter was not inserted (i.e. under normal viewing conditions). Figure 5 shows the slopes of such graphs as in Fig. 4 for 3 subjects. From Figs. 4 and 5 one can clearly see how, for large pupils, the removal of the apodization (open squares) increases the sTCA's sensitivity to pupil displacement from the visual axis. On the other hand one might also state that under normal conditions (filled squares) the sTCA is clearly reduced by the SCE, particularly for larger pupils.

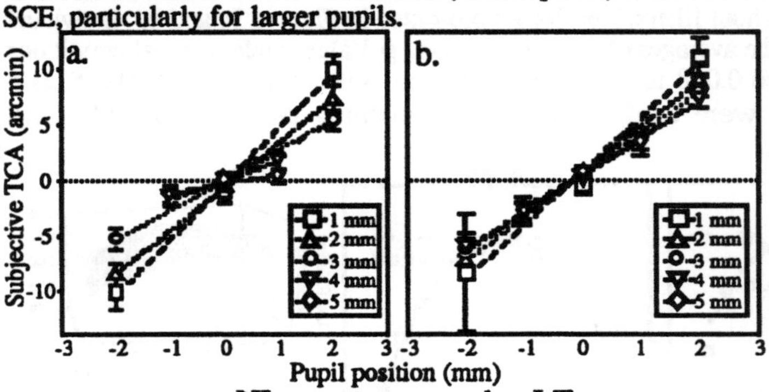

Left:
Figure 4. sTCA for LT under normal viewing conditions (a) and with SCE canceled (b).

Below:
Figure 5. Slopes of sTCA versus pupil positions for normal viewing (solid squares) and with the rSCE filter (open squares).

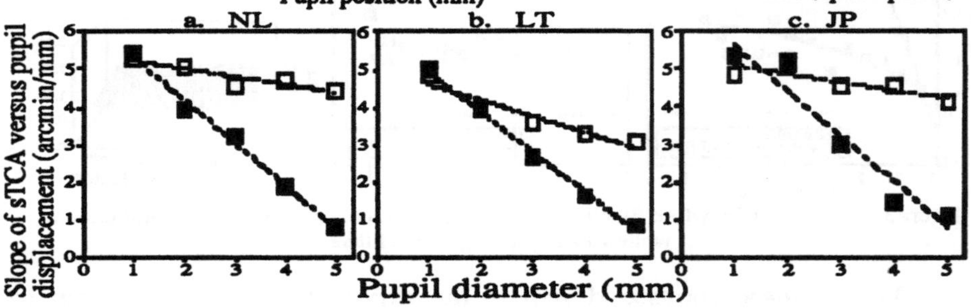

Discussion/Conclusions.

From Fig. 3 we conclude that using appropriate rSCE filters effectively cancels SCE-induced apodization of the eye's pupil. From Figs. 4 and 5 we can see what impact the apodization has on the s TCA: We conclude that for all 3 subjects the SCE reduces the sTCA, with a greater reduction for larger pupil sizes. This also implies that the SCE reduces monocular chromatic diplopia and the chromostereopsis of these subjects [4].

Fig. 5 also shows that our method even allows us to quantify the impact of the SCE on certain visual functions. Although the new method is likely to enable us to determine the impact of the SCE various visual functions, such as those mentioned in the introduction, we do not expect it to be possible to find the SCE's impact on disabililty glare, since some of this type of glare may result from trans-scleral and trans-iral light.

References.

1. Enoch JM, Lakshminarayanan V. Retinal Fiber Optics. In: Charman WN, ed. Visual Optics and Instrumentation. 1 ed. London, U.K.: MacMillan Press, 1991: 280-308. Vision and Visual Dysfunction; vol Vol.1).
2. Campbell FW. The depth of field of the human eye. Optica Acta 1957;4(4):157-164.
3. Legge GE, Mullen KT, Woo GC, Campbell FW. Tolerance to visual defocus. J. Opt. Soc. Am. - A 1987;4(5):851-863.
4. Vos JJ. Some new aspects of color stereoscopy. J. Opt. Soc. Am. 1960;50:785-790.
5. Ye M, Bradley A, Thibos LN, Zhang XX. The Effect of Pupil Size on Chromostereopsis and Chromatic Diplopia: Interaction between the Stiles-Crawford Effect and Chromatic Aberrations. Vision Research 1992;32(11):2121-2128.
6. Van Loo JA, Enoch JM. The scotopic Stiles-Crawford effect. Vision Research 1975;15:1005-1009.
7. Applegate RA, Lakshminarayanan V. Parametric representation of Stiles-Crawford functions: normal variation of peak location and directionality. J. Opt. Soc. Am. - A 1993;10(7):1611-1623.
8. Rynders MC, Grosvenor TP, Enoch JM. Stability of the Stiles-Crawford Function in a Unilateral Amblyopic Subject over a 38-Year Period: A Case Study. Optometry & Vision Science. 1995;71(3):177-185.

ANALYSIS OF HUMAN RECEPTOR DENSITY

CHRISTOPHER W. TYLER
Smith-Kettlewell Eye Research Institute,
2232 Webster St., San Francisco CA 94115

Abstract

Data for densities and sizes of human cones were analyzed as a function of retinal eccentricity. Density of cones followed a decreasing power of about -2/3 over much of the eccentricity range. This decrease, and the subsequent increase in cone density toward the ora serrata, were predictable on the basis of a hypothetical density-control mechanism to equate the integrated luminous flux at the photoreceptors per unit retinal area, together with the empirical rule that cone diameter increases with a power of about 1/3 with eccentricity beyond the foveola. The analysis implies that cones aggregate in inverse proportion to the light impinging on them, and provides an explanation for the pronounced increase to 100% cone density at the ora serrata.

Introduction

Knowledge of the density of receptors as a function of retinal eccentricity is important in studies of spatial resolution, visual sensitivity and the dissection of neural contributions to the visual response. Until recently, the only extensive investigation of overall receptor density in human was by Oesterberg [1], and it has yielded a much-reproduced graph of rod and cone densities as a function of eccentricity. Oesterberg's data, which still cover the widest range of any data available on human retina, are fully validated by studies using more modern techniques [2], but there have been few attempts to characterize the data analytically or determine what principles may be operating to control the receptor distributions.

Cone distribution as a function of eccentricity: Oesterberg's complete data for cone densities in each measured location in the horizontal meridian and four retinal sectors are plotted as a function of eccentricity in double logarithmic coordinates in Fig.1. This type of plot reveals two salient characteristics of the cone distribution. First, the density falls approximately on a straight line with a slope of about -2/3 between 0.2 and 20° eccentricity, most clearly for the horizontal temporal meridian (0°) in Fig. 1 but also supported by the sparse data for the other quadrants. Over this range, a regression analysis of the temporal data indicates a density exponent of z=-0.63 with 99% confidence limits of ±0.022 (eq. 1).

$$d_c \propto \theta^z \qquad (1)$$

where θ is eccentricity in terms of visual angle from the fovea.

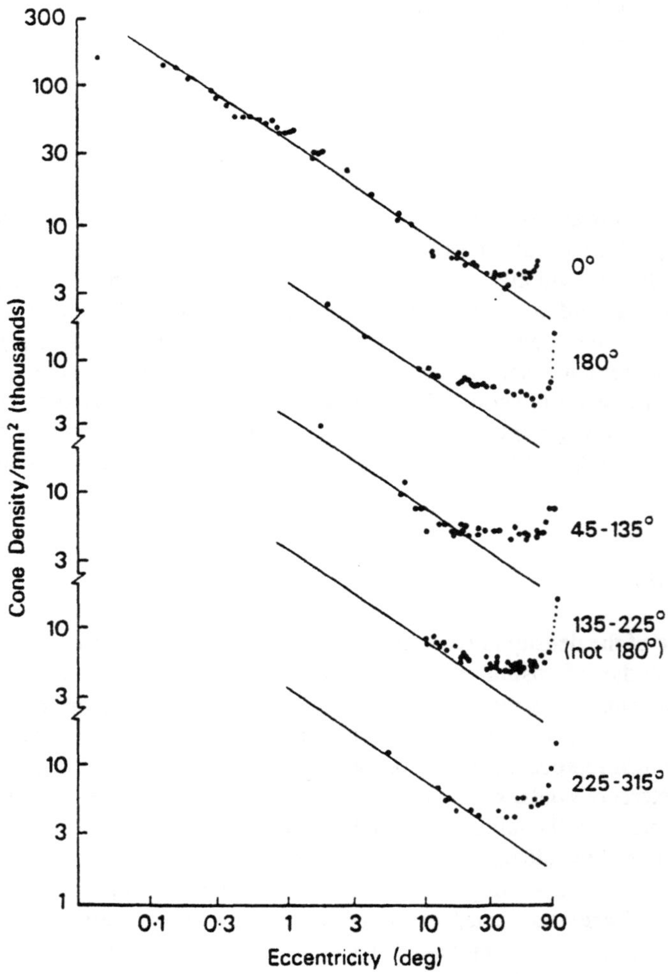

Fig. 1. Log-log plot of cone densities as a function of eccentricity for 5 retinal sectors, with successive plots displaced by 1 log unit, for a narrow sector close to the temporal (0°) meridian and nasal (180°) meridians, and for the upper, temporal and lower quadrants, respectively. Straight lines have slopes of -2/3 for comparison. Note departure of data from these functions beyond about 20° and steep rise in cone density near the ora serrata emphasized by the dotted connecting lines in two cases. From Oesterberg [1].

This confidence range strongly excludes a hyperbola with a density exponent of -1 (reciprocity between cone density and eccentricity) and also excludes a density exponent of -0.5 (reciprocity between linear cone spacing and eccentricity). For one female macaque retina, Schein [3] has similarly shown exponents with a value of -0.768 for the mean data of the four cardinal meridians and -0.771 for the temporal meridian alone, based on data out to 2.5 mm eccentricity (about 10° in visual angle).

A second point about the data of Fig. 1 is that, both in the central fovea and beyond about 20°, cone density deviates from the power function of eq. 1 and stabilizes for a large range of peripheral retina between about 20 and 60° (compressed to a small region on this logarithmic plot). In all five data sets there is, then, an increase in cone density of up to a factor of 3 as the oraserrata is reached, as noted by Oesterberg and as recently validated quantitatively by direct anatomical studies [4].

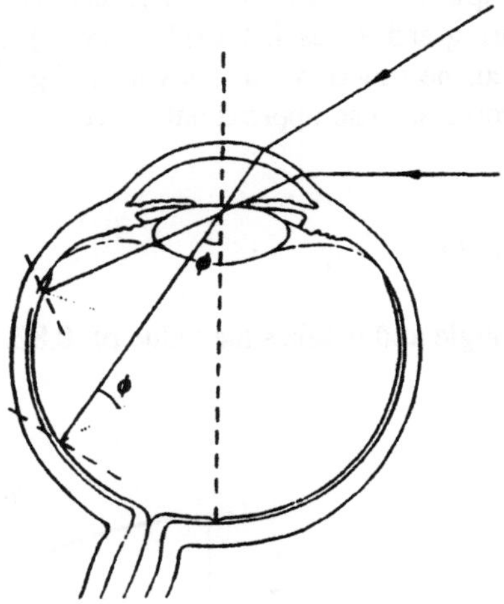

Fig. 2. Anatomic and projective geometry of the eyeball, showing oblique pupil entry for peripheral rays, projective distance to the retina, and angle of the retina relative to incident rays increasing towards the ora serrata.

Estimation of the luminous flux incident on the cones: In this section, the projective geometry for the luminous flux received by each cone with retinal eccentricity is developed as a guiding principle to explain the changes in cone density toward the ora serrata. The resulting function will be shown to be descriptive of the data in several respects, although whether this is a true functional relationship between the two will have to be determined by further comparative studies. With this proviso, it is hypothesized that the decrease in cone density with eccentricity is such as to compensate for the variation in luminous flux received by each cone. The luminous flux, F, is given simply by the product of the light-catching aperture of each cone and the retinal illuminance, L, reaching that aperture. If the aperture of the cone corresponds to the area of the inner segment, then the incident luminous flux will be

$$F = 2 \cdot \pi \cdot r_c^2 \cdot L \tag{2}$$

where r_c is the inner segment radius.

If the cone density is inversely proportional to luminous flux, then all that is required for a quantitative prediction is to determine the variation of the two variables, L and r_c, as a function of eccentricity. Major factors affecting the illuminance falling on the receptor as eccentricity is increased (see Fig. 2) are: (i) reduction of effective pupil area as its angle to the incident ray reduces the pupil aperture to an ellipse, and (ii) decrease in the path length to the retina causing an increase in the flux per unit retinal area.

The effective pupil area with eccentricity, and hence the incident flux, has been quantified by Spring and Stiles [5] and by Jay [6] and can be well approximated by an adjusted cosine function, as shown in Fig. 3 for Jay's data for the normal pupils of 8 observers. The approximating curve for pupil area A_p has the equation:

$$A_p = \cos(\nu \cdot \theta) \tag{3}$$

where θ is the incident angle and ν takes the value of 0.82.

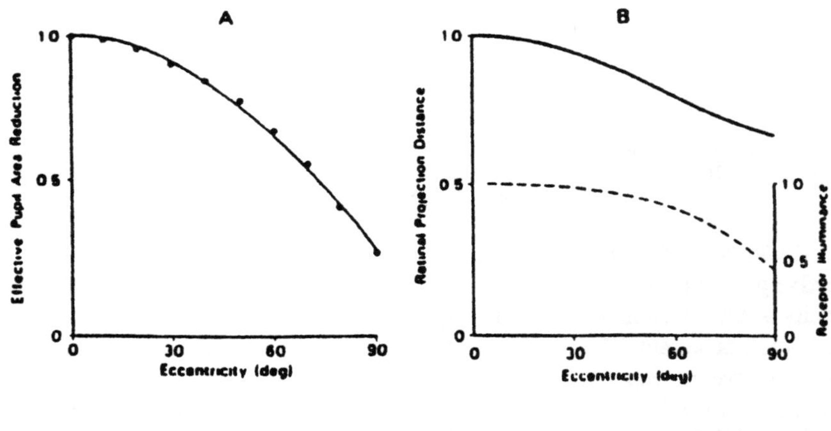

Fig 3. A. Retinal illuminance reduction as a function of eccentricity produced by oblique pupil entry. Data from Jay [6] are fitted by the cosine function of eq. 2. B. Projective distance (left ordinate; thick line) of internal rays as a function of eccentricity. Data from the wide-angle schematic model [7] are fitted by eq. 3. Dashed line and right ordinate show the reduction in receptor illuminance implied by the combination of the pupil size and projection distance functions.

The distance that the light rays have to travel to reach the retina at various eccentricities has been derived with the use of a wide-angle schematic model of the eye [7]. As the distance becomes shorter the retinal area of incident rays from a unit visual angle is reduced, with a reciprocal increase in the luminous flux per unit retinal area. The resulting estimates of the flux are shown in Fig. 3B, based on the assumption that the receptors are oriented towards the axis of the incident light [8,9]. Thus, the normalized data for optical path length, x, are fitted by the arbitrary function:

$$x = 1 - w \cdot (1 - \cos(u \cdot \theta)) \tag{4}$$

with $w = 0.19$ and $u = \pi / 2$, as shown by the solid line in Fig. 3B. The implied receptor illuminance, L, varies with the square of this path length and with the pupil aperture from eq. 3 as given by:

$$L = A_p / x^2 \tag{5}$$

The dashed line in Fig. 3B plots the resultant receptor illuminance function, L, which shows that the decrease in distance of the retina from the lens does not increase the illuminance sufficiently to compensate for the decreased luminous flux with pupil angle. A similar conclusion was reached by Charman [10].

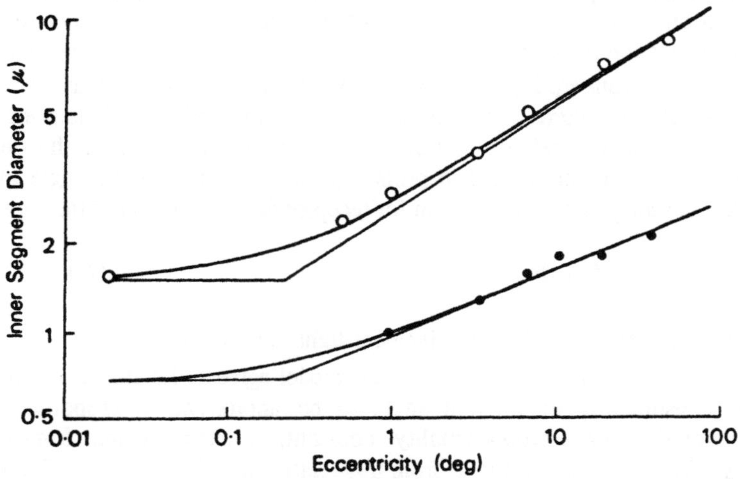

Fig. 4. Fit of function in eq. 5 to data for cone (filled circles) and rod (open circles) inner segment diameters from Polyak [8], as a function of eccentricity on double logarithmic coordinates.

The final aspect of receptor anatomy which pertains to the luminous flux impinging on each receptor is the variation in area of the inner segments with eccentricity. The most complete data available [8] for the diameter of the cone inner segments at a range of eccentricities are shown in Fig. 4 in double logarithmic coordinates. The cone inner segments show a large increase in diameter with eccentricity (a total factor of 6), which must be taken into account for any process based on the quantum catch of each cone.

Using a similar approach to a previous analysis of these data [11], the data for cone diameters r_c are well fit by the function:

$$r_c = m_c \cdot (B+\theta)^{0.33} \tag{6}$$

where m_c= 1.25 μ/deg and B = 0.2 deg. This function is shown as the full line in Fig. 4, and provides a good description of the data. The thin lines show the asymptotic limits of the function when θ = 0 and when θ >> B. The functions are assumed for the present purpose to continue out to the far periphery, although the increased cone density near the ora serrata suggests that the sizes in this region need detailed verification for a complete analysis.

Mathematical description of the cone density variation: Sufficient information is now available to provide a mathematical description of the variation in cone density with eccentricity. The basic equation that prevails for two log units over the mid range of eccentricities from 0.2 to 20° (eq. 1) will now be replaced by the assumption of the previous section that the cone density is inversely proportional to the luminous flux impinging on each receptor. It should be noted that the density will be expressed in terms of retinal area, and must therefore take account of the angle of the retina with respect to the incident rays (see Fig. 2). The final function for cone density, d_c, is therefore inversely proportional to luminous flux, F, (from eq. 2), with compensation for the angle of the receptors to the retina. In other words, if the receptor density projected to a plane normal to the incident light is inversely proportional to the luminous flux, then the density on the retina itself will be reduced in proportion to the cosine of the angle of the retina to that normal plane. The equation for receptor density then takes the form

$$d_c \approx \cos(\phi)/F \tag{7a}$$

where ϕ is the internal angle of the incident light on the retina.

Drasdo and Fowler [7] show that their model agrees with the data of Lotmar [12] in estimating the internal angle to be approximately proportional to the external angle, with a proportionality constant, v, close to that from eq. 3, which was 0.82. Substitution for ϕ from this relation and for F from eq. 2, and the substitution of expressions for cone radius from eq. 6 and receptor illuminance from eqs. 3,4 and 5, results in the full expression for cone density:

$$d_c = \frac{A\cdot\left[1-w\cdot(1-\cos(u\cdot\theta))\right]^2}{m_c\cdot(B+\theta)^{0.33}} \tag{7b}$$

where A is an areal constant of proportionality which includes the 2π term from eq. 2.

This equation represents the final form of the mathematical description of the cone density function, and it has only the density scaling constant, A, as a free parameter. Fig. 5 shows the fit of this function (full line) to the most complete set of data, close to the horizontal temporal (0°) meridian from Fig. 1. The value of the scaling constant, A, was 30,000 cones/mm^2.

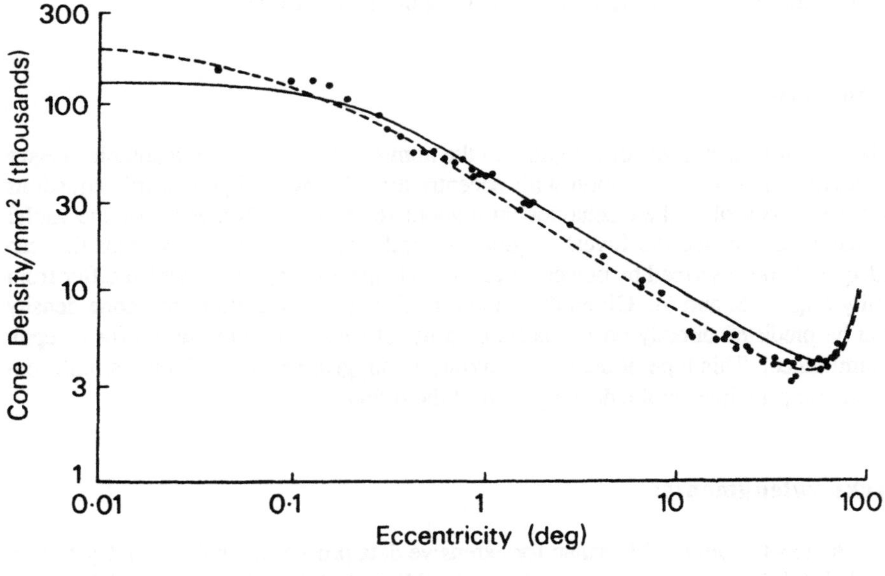

Fig. 5. Fit of function in eq. 6 (full line) to cone densities near the horizontal temporal (0°) meridian, based on the principle of compensation for integrated luminous flux at the receptors, with no free parameters other than a vertical scaling constant. Dashed line shows improved fit obtained by assuming an eccentricity constant of 5' for the foveolar singularity.

Equation 6 provides a good fit to the cone density data across the full range of eccentricities, although it is slightly low in the foveola and somewhat high in the mid periphery for the temporal data.

In the midrange of eccentricities, where $\theta >> B$, the cone density is governed by the power law of the cone inner segment areas with a slope of -0.33 x 2 or -0.66, close to the empirical value of -0.63 found from eq. 1. A slight reduction is to be expected from the asymptotic behavior at the two extremes. Note also that the deviation from the basic power law provided by the cosine terms gives an excellent description of the upturn in the far periphery, again with no free parameters. The steep portion beyond the range of the temporal data shows the increase of up to a factor of 3 above the mid-peripheral densities required to fit the other data sets in Fig. 1.

To show that the present approach is capable of completely fitting the data with a little extra freedom in the parameters, the dashed line in Fig. 5 gives a second solution to eq. 6 assuming a different eccentricity constant of 0.080 (5') for Polyak's data [8] (which are not well determined in the foveola), smaller by a factor of 2.5 than the best fitting value. The function was then rescaled to a density of 36,500 at the center but all other parameters relating to the receptor illuminance hypothesis were the same. With this small adjustment the function now fits the cone density data within the error of estimation of 0.1 log units for each point.

Conclusion

The densities and sizes of receptors in the human retina show a remarkable degree of regularity in their variation with eccentricity. A few straightforward equations suffice to describe their behavior throughout the retina. Over most of the useful visual range outside the foveal singularity, both cone sizes and cone densities can adequately be described by power functions with specific exponents which differ from unity (eqs. 1, 5, and 6). Given the function of cone size variation, the cone density can be predicted directly on the basis of a hypothesis of compensation for receptor illuminance. This type of analytic anatomy is suggestive of relatively simple ontogenetic principles in the development of the retina.

Acknowledgments:

My thanks to Gerald Silverman for extensive data processing and to Stanley Schein for helpful discussion. Supported by NSF BNS 8711217 and NIH grant RR 5566.

References

1. Oesterberg GA. Topography of the layer of rods and cones in the human retina. Acta Ophthal Suppl VI 1935.
2. Curcio CA, Sloan KR, Packer O, Hendrickson AE, Kalina RE. Distribution of cones in human and monkey retina: Individual variability and radial asymmetry. Science 1987;236:579-582.
3. Schein S.J. Anatomy of macaque fovea and spatial densities of neurons in foveal representation. J Comp Neurol 1988;269:479-505.
4. Williams RW. The human retina has a cone-enriched rim. Vis Neurosci 1991;6:403-406.
5. Spring KH, Stiles WS. Apparent shape and size of the pupil viewed obliquely. Br J Ophth 1948;32:347-354.
6. Jay BS. Effective pupillary area at varying perimetric angles. Vision Res 1962;1:418-24.
7. Drasdo N, Fowler CW. Non-linear projection of the retinal image in a wide-angle schematic

eye. Br J Ophth 1974; 58:709-714.
8. Polyak S. The retina. Chicago: University of Chicago Press 1941.
9. Laties AM, Liebmann PA, Campbell CEM. Photoreceptor orientation in the primate eye. Nature 1968;218: 172-173.
10. Charman WN. The retinal image in the human eye. In: Osborne NN, Chader GJ, editors. Progress in retinal research. Oxford: Pergamon Press, 1983: 1-50.
11. Tyler CW. Analysis of visual modulation sensitivity II. Peripheral retina and the role of photoreceptor dimensions. J Opt Soc Am A 1985;2:393-398.
12. Lotmar W. Theoretical eye model with aspherics. J Opt Soc Am 1971;61:1522-1529.

DIRECTIONAL SENSITIVITY OF THE CONE SYSTEMS IN NORMAL AND ANOMALOUS COLOR VISION

PIETER L. WALRAVEN
Em. TNO Human Factors Research Institute
P.O.Box 23, 3769 ZG Soesterberg
THE NETHERLANDS

Abstract

Stiles published in 1937 that the hue of a monochromatic beam of light depends upon its angle of incidence on the retina. In the early 60's the effect has been remeasured by Enoch and Stiles, including saturation-shifts.Walraven and Bouman proposed in 1960 an explanation of the chromatic SC-effect by considering selfscreening of the photopic visual pigments, and by attributing a difference between the directional sensitivity of the S-cone system with respect to the L- and M-cone systems. It is now suggested that this larger directional sensitivity of the S-system might be attributed to the larger cross-sectional diameter of the S-cones with respect to L- and M-cones.Huge hue shifts might occur in anomalous colour vision. These hue shifts can be explained in the same way as for normal colour vision, provided the appropriate pigment densities are chosen, together with a shift of the absorption curve of the M-pigment along the wavelength axis in the case of deuteranomaly.

Introduction

Stiles and Crawford [1] showed that the sensitivity of the retina varies with the place of entry of the light in the pupil, and thus with the direction of incidence of light upon the retina. Sensitivity is generally greatest near the centre of the pupil and progressively decreases for more eccentric entry points. This phenomenon is known in the literature as the Stiles-Crawford effect of the first kind (SCE I). The hue shift associated with the SC-effect was discovered [2] in a further study of the retinal direction effect. This effect is called the chromatic Stiles-Crawford effect, often also referred to as the Stiles-Crawford effect of the second kind (SCE II).

Walraven and Bouman [3] explained this directional effect by assuming a. that the S-system has a larger directional effect than the L- and M-systems, and b. that due to selfscreening the decrease of the pathlength of the light through the pigment results in narrowing of the absorption curves for oblique incident light. The explanation of this character of the S-system, and the application of the theory to anomalous color vision are the goals of this paper.

The Stiles-Crawford effect I

If η is the luminous efficiency of the light for peripheral entry in the pupil at radius r, the efficiency at the radius of maximum efficiency r_0 being 1, the relationship between η and r along the horizontal traverse of the pupil is expressed by

$$\log_{10} \eta = - p\ (r-r_0)^2$$

p being in the fovea about 0.05 (r in mm). The center of maximum efficiency is usually located near the centre of the pupil with a slight nasal bias.

Stiles and Crawford [1] indicated that the effect must be a property of the receptors themselves, because the effect is dependent on luminance. Starting from this finding, Wright and Nelson [4] gave an explanation which is based on the fact that the refractive index of the cone is somewhat higher than that of the surrounding tissue. Rays entering the receptor only slightly obliquely are caught by total reflection, whereas more slanting rays partially pass to the tissue outside. So only the perpendicularly incident light is totally gathered into the outer segment, thus being more effective than oblique light. Toraldo di Francia [5] described this in terms of cones as dielectric antennas or as we would say presently in terms of cones as waveguides.

The p-value increases, according to Enoch and Hope [6], as one moves to the retinal periphery, from 0.05 in the fovea to 0.08 at 5°. The magnitude is supposed by Westheimer [7] to be associated with the shape of the receptors: directional sensitivity is most pronounced for the squat parafoveal cones, slightly smaller for the elongated (rodlike) cones in the central fovea.

The value of p is also dependent on wavelength. After correcting the available data with a factor for the differences in absorption of the center and the periphery of the lens, Vos and van Os [8] derived the data for the p-values at retinal level as shown in Figure 1.

The Stiles-Crawford effect II in normal and anomalous color vision

Stiles [2] noted a change in hue and saturation accompanying the change in luminous efficiency. These measurements were confirmed by Walraven and Bouman [3] and Stiles and Enoch [9], and described by Walraven and Bouman [3] by applying the selfscreening hypothesis to the L- and M-cones, and attributing a larger directional sensitivity of the S-cones with respect to the L- and M-cones.

The selfscreening hypothesis connects the SC-effect II with the SC-effect I because it predicts that the dip in the p-value versus wavelength curve as displayed in Figure 1 would disappear when the pigments are bleached. This is, according to Walraven [10], indeed the case.

The selfscreening hypothesis can also be applied to the SC-effect II in anomalous vision. The data of protanomalous vision [11,12] are described by a low density of the L-pigment. In deuteranomalous vision there is a large variation, from almost normal up to huge hue shifts [11,12]. Assuming that the deuteranomalous M-absorption curve (M'-absorption curve) is a normal M-absorption curve shifted about 10 nm to longer wavelengths on a $1/\lambda$ scale [13,14], a variation in density of the M'-pigment

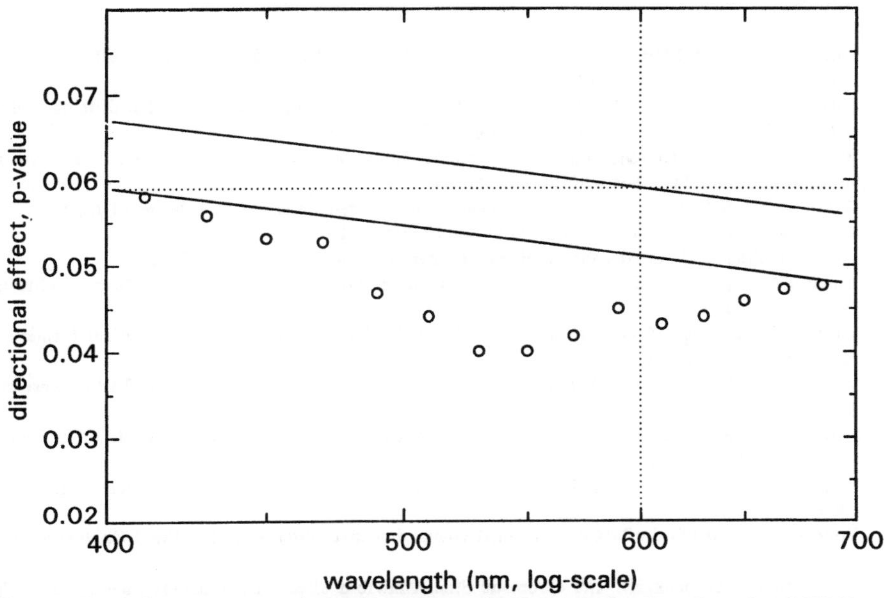

Figure 1. The circles represent experimental p-values at retinal level as a function of wavelength [8]. Drawn lines are supposed to be the relationship between p-value and wavelength for low pigment concentration, the upper curve belonging to 1.5 times larger cone diameter than the lower curve.

describes the variation in hue shifts in deuteranomalous vision. Space does not permit to go now into more detail about this hypothesis.

The directional sensitivity of the S-cones.

The theory on the Stiles-Crawford effect II requires a p-value of the S-cones about 30 % larger than the p-values of the L- and M-cones. These values are confirmed by Stiles [15], Alpern and Kitahara [16] and Geri et al [17] by measuring the p-values of the π-1 mechanism. The same value is obtained in blue cone monochromasy by Daw and Enoch [18]. This high value of directional sensitivity is never explained.

I suggest that it is due to the larger diameter of the S-cones. In the fovea, according to Curcio et al [19], the diameters of blue cone ellipsoids are larger than neighbouring R/G cones: 3.2 +/- .4 μm vs 2.2 +/- .4 μm. This difference in diameter is reflected in the p-value in the same way Westheimer [7] explained the difference between the directional sensitivity of the fovea and the parafovea.

Assuming that the relationship op p and wavelength is described in Figure 1 by the lower straight line, the line for low pigment density all over the spectrum, the values for a 50% larger diameter can be derived by shifting the straight line horizontally by a factor of 1.5. This results indeed in an about 30% larger p-value.

Waveguide theory [20] should be used to check the soundness of this hypothesis.

References

1. Stiles WS, Crawford BH. The luminous efficiency of rays entering the eye pupil at different points. Proc Roy Soc London 1933;B112:428-50.
2. Stiles WS. The luminous efficiency of monochromatic rays entering the eye pupil at different points and a new colour effect. Proc Roy Soc London 1937;B123:90-118.
3. Walraven PL, Bouman MA. Relation between directional sensitivity and spectral response curves in human cone vision. J Opt Soc Am 1960;50:780-84.
4. Wright WD, Nelson JH. The relation between the apparent intensity of a beam of light and the angle at which it strikes the retina. Proc Phys Soc 1936;48:401-05.
5. Toraldo da Francia G. Retina cones as dielectric antennas. J Opt Soc Am 1947;39:324.
6. Enoch JM, Hope GM. Directional sensitivity of the foveal and parafoveal retina. Invest Ophthalm 1973;12:497-503.
7. Westheimer G. Dependence of the magnitude of the Stiles-Crawford effect on retinal location. J Physiol Lond 1967;192:309-15.
8. Vos JJ, van Os FJ. The effect of lens density on the Stiles-Crawford effect. Vision Research 1975;15:749-51.
9. Stiles WS, Enoch JM. The colour change of monochromatic light with retinal angle of incidence. Opt Acta 1961;8:329-58.
10. Walraven PL. Recovery from the increase of the Stiles-Crawford effect after bleaching. Nature 1966;206:311-12.
11. Voke J. Stiles-Crawford effect in congenital colour defective observers. Mod Probl Ophthalm 1974; 13:140-44.
12. Walraven PL, Leebeek HJ. The chromatic Stiles-Crawford effect of anomalous trichromats. J Opt Soc Am 1962;52:836-37.
13. Walraven PL, Leebeek HJ, Fundamental response curves of a normal and a deuteranomalous observer derived from chromatic adaptation data. J Opt Soc Am 1966;56:125-27.
14. DeMarco P, Pokorny J, Smith VC. Full-spectrum cone sensitivity functions for X-chromosome-linked anomalous trichromats, J Opt Soc Am A 1992;9:1465-76.
15. Stiles WS. The directional sensitivity of the retina and the spectral sensitivities of the rods and cones. Proc Roy Soc Lond 1939;B127:64-105.
16. Alpern M, Kitahara K. The directional sensitivities of the Stiles' colour mechanisms. J Physiol 1983;338:627-49.
17. Geri GA, Kandel GL, Roy Genter II C, Breed HE. Meridional differences in the directional sensit ivity of human color mechanisms. Am J Optom Physiol Opt 1988;65:880-89.
18. Daw NW, Enoch JM. Contrast sensitivity, Westheimer function and Stiles-Crawford effect in a blue cone monochromat. Vision Research 1973 13 1669-1680
19. Curcio CA, Allen KA, Sloan KR, Lerea CL, Hurley JB, Klock IB, Milam AH. Distribution and morphology of human cone photoreceptors stained with anti-blue opsin. J Comp Neurology 1991;3 12:610-24.
20. Lakshminarayanan V, Calvo ML. Incoherent spatial impulse response in variable-cross-section photoreceptors and frequency-domain analysis, J Opt Soc Am A 1995;12:2339-47.

A FORMALISM FOR ANALYZING DEGRADED EDGES USING MODIFIED HEAVISIDE FUNCTIONS

M.L. CALVO[1], A. MANZANARES[1], M. CHEVALIER[1] and V. LAKSHMINARAYANAN[2]
[1]*Universidad Complutense, 28040 Madrid, SPAIN.*
[2]*University of Missouri-St. Louis, MO 63121.*

Abstract.

We present a mathemathical formalism to analyze saturated edge imaging using various modified Heaviside functions.

Introduction.

For the past few decades an enormous amount of work has been done in the field of the theory of edge detection. This area of optical, hybrid and digital image processing interrelates different aspects of image formation, visual optics and robotic vision. It is well established that edge detection is a primary mechanism in visual object recognition [1]. These have been studied as a major application for pattern recognition. Studying the established models and formalisms one is concerned with the specific phenomena related to blurred edge detection. From the literature, we find that only approximate calculations have been done in the sense of explaining the different contributions to the total image intensity distribution of a blurred or degraded edge. Our main goal in our current studies is to establish well-defined blurred (or degraded) edge functions to interpret different pattern and object recognition in a two dimensional scene. The idea is illustrated in the scheme shown in Fig.1. These edge functions depend on a variable parameter which accounts for the degree of degradation or edge blurring. We are interested in defining a unique edge generator as a general function to be applied to represent different features of edge image processing. The calculation of a first derivative defines a line object. From these two functions one can either represent Edge Spread Function(ESF), Line Spread Function (LSF) and the associated Modulation Transfer Function (MTF), through the well established reciprocity for perfect optical systems. On the other hand, one could obtain a larger class of degraded (or blurred) edges and the corresponding class of thick lines. Calculating second derivatives from the first function, one is able to define a class of differential operators to be applied for edge detection mechanism, namely, zero-crossing location. This aspect has been also largely discussed and our main interest is to achieve a generalization of this procedure.

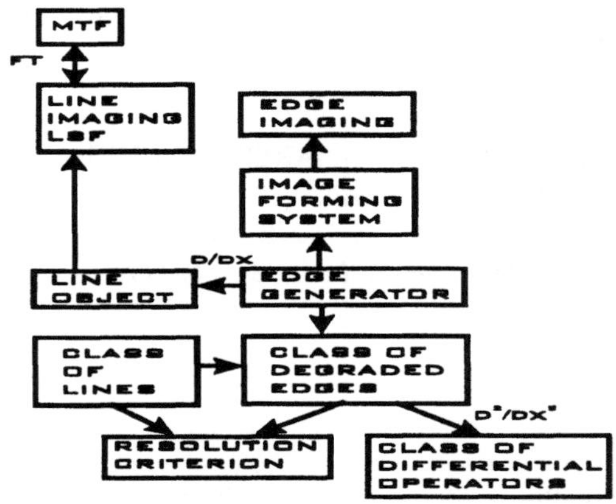

Fig. 1: Scheme of the proposed processes

As for resolution criterion applied to blurred edges very little information is available in the literature, in part because it is not easy to design a simple experiment from which one could infer objective criteria, and partially also because there is an inadequate formalism. Recently, Marshall et al. [2] have shown that identification of two identical images except for the nature of boundaries between different regions of the picture (sharp edge and blurred edge) is related to the so-called *occlusion edge blur* on the relative depth seen on a scene, which is related to depth perception. To interpret their experiment, they define an approximate model in which the total intensity (stimuli) is given as a sum of two contributions [3]. 1) A convolution of a gaussian blur kernel and the intensity image of the blurred object. 2) A vignetting function defined as the convolution of the gaussian kernel and a perfect edge, multiplied by the intensity image of the sharp object.

We propose a more rigorous formalism as an alternative approach to those in that the gaussian kernel is substituted by the exact LSF of an incoherent and diffraction-limited system. This formalism is also consistent with the definition of resolution criteria and a large class of second order differential operators to be applied to various blurred edge detection processes.

Proposed Formalism: LSF Definition and Blurred Edge Representation.

Fig.2 displays various representations for different analytical formulations of the LSF availables in the literature. The LSF in terms of the Struve function can be represented as a polynomial expansion or represented in terms of a Bessel functions series (dashed line), as proposed earlier by Steel [4]. Here we have found a major error. Approximate formulations are also given by Barakat-Houston [5] (dots) and Gaskill-Hufnagel [6] (solid line). We have applied the exact representation obtained by us as a Bessel functions expansion, showing the appropiate high speed of convergence of the series.

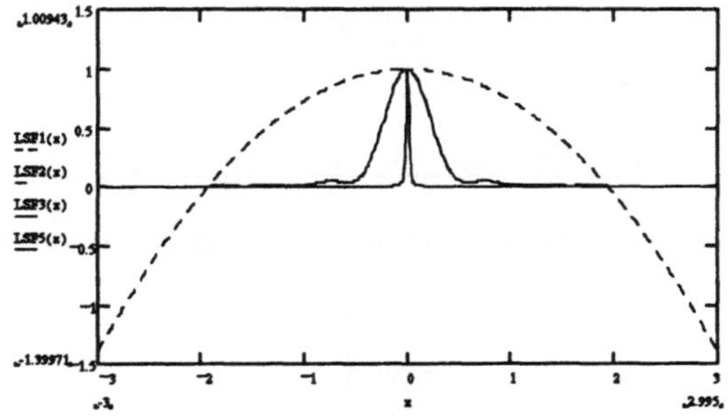

Fig. 2: Comparison of different definitions for the LSF.

The representation of blurred edges has been defined as in the earlier work of Shanmugen et al. [7] in terms of a sigmoid where the blurring parameter gives the *degree of blur*. We have introduced an alternative representation called *saturated degraded edges* (Fig.3) in terms of the so-called *degradation parameter*.

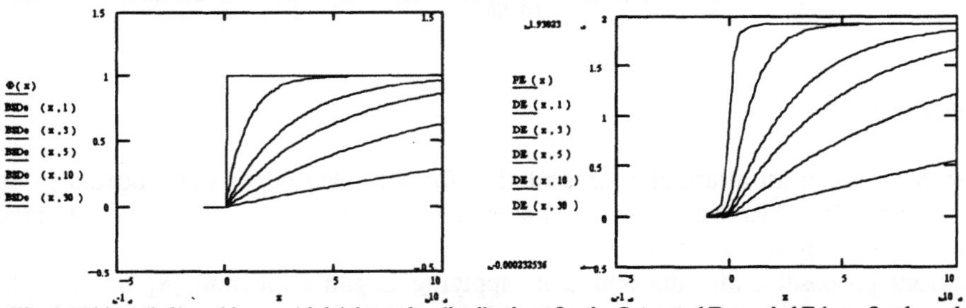

Fig. 3: Object (left) and image (right) intensity distributions for the Saturated Degraded Edges, for degradation parameters 0, 1, 3, 5, 10, 30.

They fit the type of experimental edge distribution recorded by a detector (e.g., CCD camera), since the white zone is more saturated than the black one . The degradation parameter is related to the degree of blur, but is a more natural parameter. The higher the value of the degradation parameter the higher the edge degradation. When decreasing, it tends to the perfect edge. Fig.4 displays also another type of blurred edge as *stepped sigmoid functions*, showing interesting behaviour of their first and second derivatives (Fig.5).

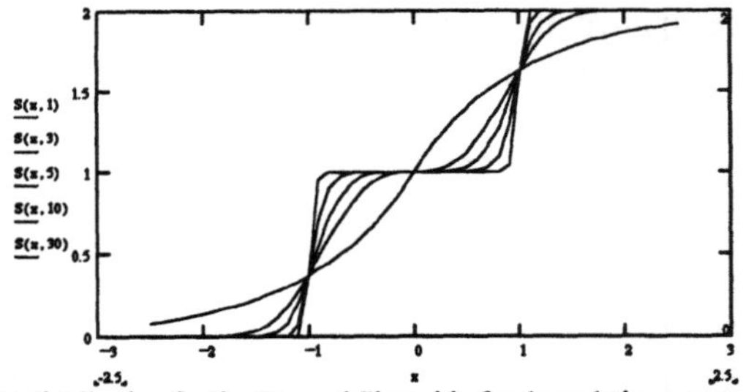

Fig. 4: Object intensity distribution for the Stepped Sigmoid, for degradation parameters 0, 1, 3, 5, 10, 30.

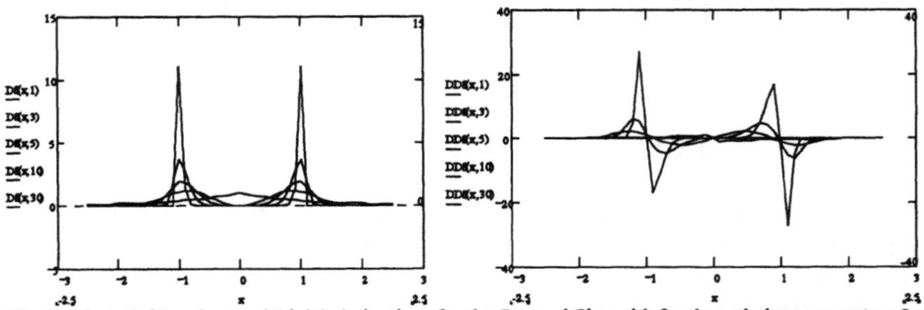

Fig. 5: First (left) and second (right) derivatives for the Stepped Sigmoid, for degradation parameters 0, 1, 3, 5, 10, 30.

Conclusions.

- We have given an alternate representation for saturated edges that appears to be convenient for generating a larger class of edges. As a main characteristic, all have in common a unique generator.
- Current proposal under development: applying Logan's theorem [8] in order to recognize the object edge distribution from which the image edge distribution comes. *Let $h_1(x)$ and $h_2(x)$ be two arbitrary analytical functions. Then, if h_1 and h_2 have no free zeros. i.e. no zero in common with their Hilbert transforms, we can conclude that: $h_1(x) = A\, h_2(x)$, where A is a constant.* In our present analysis the proposed functions seem more suitable since their Fourier spectra are given in terms of the Hilbert transform.
- Analysis of defining resolution criteria: Under current results, difficulties appear in establishing criteria for resolution of two highly saturated edges. We are designing simple experiments to compare with analytical results.

Acknowledgements.

The financial support of the Spanish Ministry of Health, the Institute of Health "Carlos III" and the Health Research Foundation, under project 95/1518 is acknowledged. A UMSL research grant is also acknowledged.

References.

1. Marr D, Hildreth E. Theory of edge detection. Proc R Soc Lon B 1980;207:187-217.
2. Marshall JA, Burbeck CA, Ariely D, Rolland JP, Martin K. Occlusion edge blur: a cue to relative visual depth. J Opt Soc Am A 1996;13:681-688.
3. Pentland AP. A new sense for depth of field. IEEE Trans Patt Anal Mach Intell 1987;PAMI-9:523-531.
4. Steel WH. Calcul de la répartition de la lumière dans l'image d'une ligne. Revue d'Optique 1952;31:334-340.
5. Barakat R, Houston A. Line Spread Function and Cumulative Line Spread Function for systems with rotational symmetry. J Opt Soc Am 1964;54:768-773.
6. Gaskill J. Linear systems, Fourier transforms and Optics. John Wiley and Sons, 1978. And: Hufnagel R. Simple approximation to Diffraction-limited MTF. App Opt 1971;10:2547-2548.
7. Shanmugam KS, Dickey FM, Green JA. An optimal frecuency domain filter for edge detection in digital pictures. IEEE Trans Patt Anal Mach Int 1979;PAMI-1:37-49.
8. Logan BF. Information in the zero-crossing of bandpass signals. Bell System Techn J 1977;B211:151-180.

CLINICAL IMPLICATIONS OF CHANGES IN LENS AND OCULAR IMAGING PROPERTIES

MELANIE C. W. CAMPBELL, ADRIAN GLASSER and AUSTIN ROORDA.
School of Optometry, University of Waterloo, Waterloo, CANADA.

Abstract

Our measurements of *in vitro* changes in the focal properties of the human crystalline lens as a function of accommodative state and age demonstrate that presbyopia is a lens based phenomenon and that there may be a lens mediated drift towards a more hyperopic refractive state with ageing. The blur of the image formed by the lens changes as a function of age and accommodative state. Ocular image quality varies with accommodative state and pupil size. Although changes in ocular image quality with accommodative state are analogous to lens changes, there are qualitative differences between lens and ocular image quality. Asymmetric ocular image quality, mediated in part by tilt and decentration of the optical elements, combines with symmetrical blur to influence all methods of retinal imaging. Confocal scanning laser ophthalmoscopy (CSLO) is degraded least by retinal blur followed by scanning laser ophthalmoscopy (SLO) and lastly by conventional fundus imaging. Optimisation of ocular image quality through the choice of pupil centration, has produced the first real-time video images of the human cones. These results also have clinical implications to the development of refractive error and to the design of refractive corrections.

Introduction

The optical properties of the crystalline lens and of the eye change as a function of age and of accommodative state. We will first describe some of the changes in image quality and then discuss clinical implications of these changes. We are particularly interested in the loss of accommodative ability with age (presbyopia), age changes in refractive state and image quality and implications to the development and correction of refractive error and to fundus imaging.

Optical Quality of the Crystalline Lens

With ageing beyond the teenage years, corneal shape changes to a small extent and eye length remains relatively fixed. The crystalline lens is the only component of the eye which grows continuously throughout life by the laying down of fibres on the lens surface. This leads to changes in anterior chamber depth, lens thickness [1] and lens curvatures [2] and possibly to changes in the refractive index distribution [3]. The lens is also the optical element that changes shape to increase the power of the eye and focus objects at near during accommodation. Thus, changes in power and image quality of the crystalline lens as a function of accommodation and age are most likely to affect the refractive state and image quality of the eye.

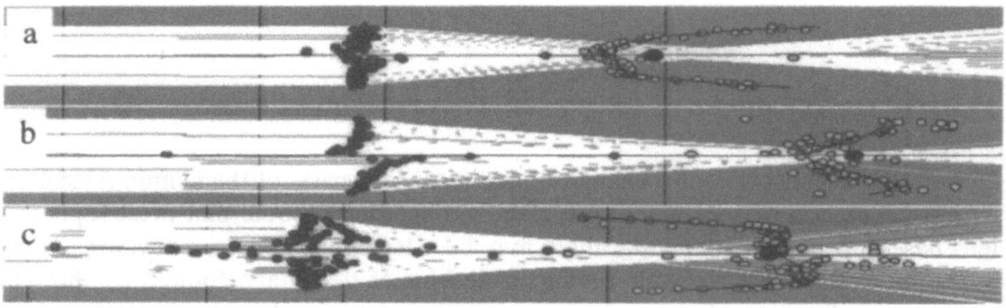

Figure 1. Laser scans of an unstretched 10 year old lens (a), the same lens when stretched (b), and an unstretched 66 year old lens (c). Small black symbols (left) represent the intersection of each parallel entrance beam with its corresponding refracted exit beam (the principle points of the lens). The small gray symbols (right) represent the intersection points of each exit beam with the optical axis and are well fitted with 4th order polynomials. The large black symbol (right) represents the mean focal length of the lens.

Human eyes were obtained from the Eye Bank of Canada. We studied the optical properties of 27 lenses as a function of age and accommodative state [4]. A scanning laser apparatus [5] was used to measure the focal lengths of the lenses and to assess the quality of the focus (Fig. 1). In an *in vitro* preparation, the zonular fibres are slack and the lens rounds up into the accommodated state. The ciliary body is glued to eight arms of a stretching apparatus such that an outwards force can be applied to the zonular fibres around the equator of the lens. Stretching the tissue flattens the lens surface curvatures to effectively unaccommodate the lens.

Younger lenses showed a larger change in power with zonular stretching than the older lenses (Fig. 2). The decrease in accommodative power change follows the same age dependence as Duane's [6] data on accommodative amplitude with age (Fig. 2). Beyond age 58, no matter how much the zonule is stretched, the lenses fail to change focal length. We have also measured a concurrent decrease in the deformability of human crystalline lenses as a function of age [7]. These results indicate that the loss of accommodative ability with age (presbyopia) is a lens based phenomenon. There may be concurrent ageing changes in the ciliary muscle but lens changes alone are enough to account for presbyopia.

The focal length of the unstretched lens increases continuously as a function of age (Fig. 3). If the other dioptric components are relatively fixed, this may represent the underlying mechanism of the observed drift in refractive state towards hyperopia in middle age [8]. Additional measurements on older lenses (> 80 years) are consistent with a shift in lens and ocular power towards myopia in the oldest lenses [7].

Image quality of both stretched and unstretched lenses changes as a function of age (Fig. 1). The spherical aberration in the younger lenses is negative or overcorrected, consistent with a spherical lens with a gradient of refractive index. Older lenses show positive or undercorrected spherical aberration of the type found for spherical lenses with a homogeneous refractive index. These changes in image quality are likely caused by simultaneous changes in the refractive index distribution within the lens and changes in the central spherical and peripheral aspheric curvatures of the lens surfaces. Some of the measured individual differences in lens shapes [9] may be age related differences. The image quality of the older lenses differs from the younger accommodated lenses. Thus, although these lenses appear similar in Scheimflug photography [10], older lenses are optically different from younger accommodated lenses. With accommodation there is a shift in spherical aberration towards overcorrected (negative) spherical aberration.

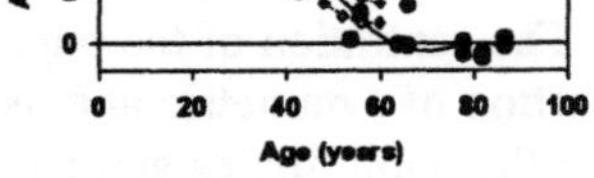

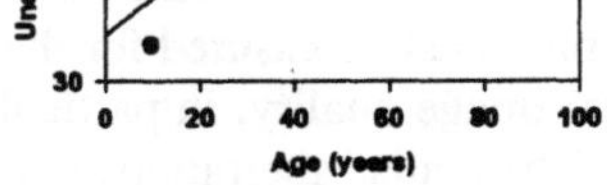

Figure 2. (Left) Change in lens power with stretching of 27 human lenses as a function of age (solid circles). This data plotted together with the maximum and minimum amplitudes of accommodation as a function of age as measured by Duane [6] (open diamonds).

Figure 3. (Right). The focal lenghts of unstretched human lenses as a function of age. Even beyond the age of presbyopia (58 years, from Fig. 2), at which time this represents the only state of the lens, the focal length of the lenses continues to increase.

Optical Quality of the Eye

The changes in image quality of the crystalline lens as a function of accommodative state and age would lead to an expectation of changes in ocular image quality as a function of age and accommodative state. Measurements to date of ocular image quality as a function of age have only considered and found a variation in spherical aberration [11] or scatter [12]. Our measurements [13] and others [14] of ocular image quality as a function of accommodative state have indicated a shift towards more overcorrected spherical aberration with accommodation. These results are consistent with the results found above for the lens alone.

The largest qualitative differences between the optical quality of the crystalline lens and the whole eye are the symmetry of the ocular aberrations, the presence of higher order aberrations and the variability among individuals. Whereas the crystalline lens is a symmetrical optical element, displaying only spherical aberrations, we and others [15,16,17] have found that the aberrations of the eye are highly asymmetric and often dominated by the comatic terms. This asymmetry in ocular blur has been apparent in subjective measurements for a number of years but objective, double pass point spread measurements of the eye had indicated a more symmetrical blur [18,19]. Roorda *et al.* [20] and Artal *et al.* [21] have independently shown that double pass point spread function measurements produce symmetric blur even when the single pass point spread is asymmetric. A fourth order polynomial provides a good fit to the longitudinal spherical aberration of the lens out beyond a diameter corresponding to an anatomical pupil size (Fig 1). This corresponds to a sixth order fit to wavefront aberration. Campbell *et al.* [15] found that sixth order was sufficient to fit ocular aberrations across a natural pupil. However for larger pupil sizes, Liang *et al.*[22] and Roorda [23] have found that higher order terms substantially improve the fit near the pupil edge.

The variability of ocular aberrations among individuals could in part be age related as many studies have measured young adults in whom the sign of spherical aberration of the lens is expected to reverse as a function of age. Additional factors may also cause variability among individuals while simultaneously producing asymmetric aberrations. Asymmetry and variability of the corneal surface curvature is one of these factors. There is some question of whether corneal topography can be measured accurately enough to allow derivation of the aberrations [24]. However, Howland [25] found that the low order aberrations of the cornea fell into the same range as the aberrations previously measured for the whole eye. The centration of the pupil will also affect optical image quality, in particular the proportion of symmetric and asymmetric aberrations. The ocular aberrations will also vary as the pupil dilates and its centration changes idiosyncratically [26,27]. The fact that the fovea is offset by angle alpha from the optical axis of the eye may introduce asymmetric aberrations into the system. Even if the aberrations of both the cornea and crystalline lens were symmetric, and angle alpha were zero, either decentration or tilt of one of the cornea or lens relative to the other will produce asymmetric aberrations. The fact that the Purkinje images do not in general align along an optical axis [28] indicates that the elements are misaligned. A tilt of 3 degrees or a pupil centre shift of 0.25 to 0.35 mm are sufficient to neutralize the asymmetric aberrations in a centred schematic eye model due to angle alpha [29].

Conditions for Optimal Image Quality in the Eye

Visual acuity at the fovea in an emmetropic eye with a diurnal pupil is well matched to the image sampling capabilities of the retinal elements [30]. However, in order to image these retinal elements in ophthalmoscopy, a higher optical quality is required. There are two means of achieving this higher optical quality; an active optical correction of the aberrations of the eye [31] or an optimisation of the imaging conditions to give the best ocular optical quality. In investigating the second approach, we explored the variation of optical image quality with accommodation. We did not find a single accommodative state which gave optimal image quality across individuals but we did find up to a factor of four improvement in the image quality measured across a single pupil meridian as a function of accommodative state between 0 and 4 dioptres [13].

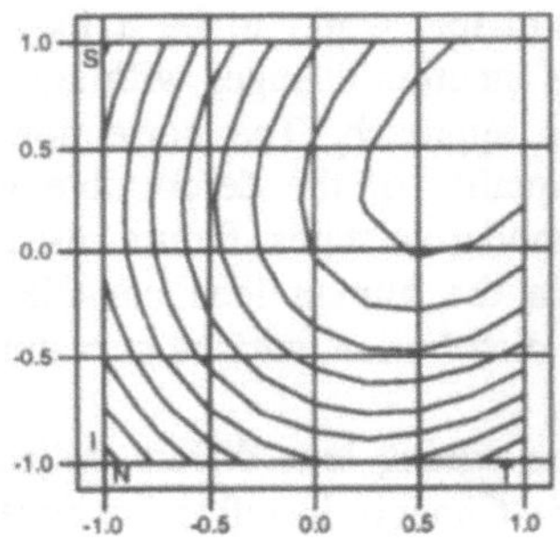

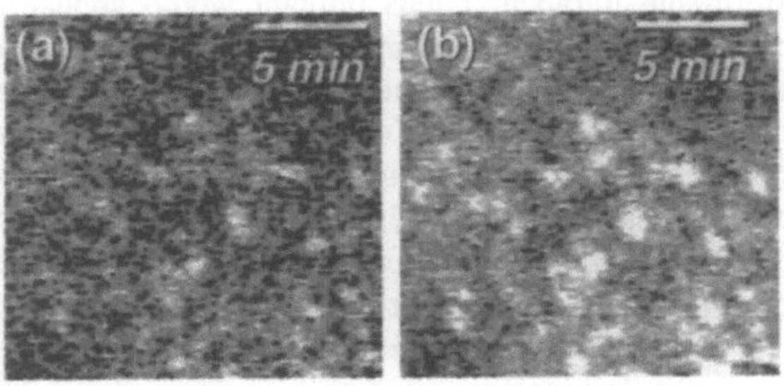

Figure 4. (Left) The contour plot shows how the RMS wavefront aberration changes as a function of the position of a 5mm artificial pupil (in mm). The origin of the plot is the location of the reference Purkinje image. Each contour line represents 0.05μm of RMS aberration.

Figure 5. (Right) Photoreceptor images at 1.85 degrees from the fovea. The single frame image (a) has a lot of noise due to speckle, electronic noise and small eye movements. An average of 4 frames (b) eliminated most of the noise and shows some resolved photoreceptors. The expected photoreceptor hexagonal array is not seen because of the coherent interaction between neighboring photoreceptors [33].

We investigated the sensitivity of the image quality of the eye to pupil centration in conjunction with an attempt to image individual photoreceptors using a CSLO. A two dimensional measurement of the aberration of the eye was performed using a method analogous to our previously developed one dimensional method [15]. Using the measured aberrations, the root mean square aberration (RMS aberration) was calculated as a function of position in the pupil (Fig. 4). For the eye shown, the RMS aberration drops by a factor of nearly two for a shift of the pupil centre by 0.5 mm temporally and by 0.25 mm upward from the reference Purkinje image. Roorda *et al.* [32] have shown that all fundus imaging techniques are affected by both asymmetric and symmetrical image blur. Conventional fundus imaging is affected by the single pass optical quality of the eye. In imaging with a SLO, improvement in image quality occurs if the detector is smaller than the extent of the blur due to scatter. A CSLO with a finite pinhole is still affected by the asymmetric blur, but less than an SLO. Images were taken with the

Waterloo CSLO through different, controlled areas of the pupil. The quality of the resulting images correlated with the RMS aberration at the corresponding pupil position. Individual photoreceptors were most visible for entrance pupil positions with the least aberration. These (Fig. 5) represent the first real-time video images of cones in the human eye.

Clinical Implications of Optical Changes in the Crystalline Lens

Optical changes in the crystalline lens produce changes in focal length and image quality with continued growth and ageing and with accommodation. From these measurements, we have established that presbyopia can be explained solely by changes in the crystalline lens. If ageing affects the ciliary muscle less than the lens, this finding could have profound implications for the search for methods to overcome presbyopia. A deformable intraocular lens implant would appear, from this work, to be a feasible approach. Further measurements on how ciliary muscle function changes with age are needed to establish the mechanical feasibility of this approach. The correction of presbyopia would still be optically complex. Image quality of the deformable lens implant needs to be maintained over a range of accommodative states. Future research will address the issue of how this is accomplished in the human lens considering concurrent changes in the lens gradient refractive index distribution, surface curvatures, object position and pupil size.

The lens measurements also established that the ageing lens differs optically from younger accommodated or unaccommodated lenses. Changes in refractive state in the middle aged and in the elderly may be mediated by age changes in lens power. In addition, we found that image quality of the lens changes as a function of age. The reversal in sign of spherical aberration that we have measured in the lenses as a function of age may maintain the overall image quality with ageing. These aberration changes occur in addition to a decrease in image quality in the older eye due to scatter [12]. However, indirect evidence has indicated that changing image quality is not responsible for contrast sensitivity losses in the elderly [34].

Optical blur is a signal to the reflex accommodative response [35] and contrast reduction has been implicated as a signal which maintains the eye in focus as it grows [36]. The chick eye grows towards emmetropia even when accommodation is prevented [37]. However, it is interesting that our lens results indicate that the power of the unaccommodated human lens shows a linear increase with age even after the loss of accommodative ability, which may produce a hyperopic shift in refractive state. Unfortunately, we had no refractive information of the individual eyes in the lens study.

Clinical Implications of Ocular Image Quality Changes

There is evidence of larger monochromatic aberrations in myopic versus emmetropic eyes [38]. It may be that these two effects are causally connected and produce a situation in which the age at which humans show an increasing spread in refractive errors [39] is also an age at which spherical aberration was previously seen to change character [11] (~age 6). It is possible that the blur due to aberrations disrupts the emmetropisation process, leading to refractive error or conversely that defocus error may lead to a breakdown in the maintenance of optical image quality and thus to higher aberrations. Alternatively, disruption of an additional feedback loop (e.g. accommodative oscillations) could disrupt both emmetropisation and image quality due to aberrations. Longitudinal measurement of ocular aberrations and refractive error as a function of age might help to define these relationships. Any involvement of the crystalline lens in such feedback loops remains speculative. Optical properties of the chick lens were identical for ametropic or emmetropic eyes [40], although in the fish eye, visual feedback appears to influence the optical quality of the lens without changing its focal length [41].

Ocular image quality is important to visual function. The falloff in visual acuity at large pupil diameters is attributed to the presence of monochromatic aberrations [42]. As discussed above, optical blur also provides a signal for accommodative responses and to eye growth. The demonstrated sensitivity of ocular image quality (particularly asymmetric aberrations) to the centration of the optical elements of the system has clinical implications to image quality during contact lens wear and as a result of refractive surgeries. Not only will changes to the shape of the refracting surfaces be important to image quality but the centration of the resulting refractive correction is also important. Some post PRK ocular complaints of ghosting are consistent with the presence of asymmetric, comatic blur.

Further understanding of the image quality of the eye and the factors that affect it will improve our understanding of the changes associated with ageing, with ametropia and with the correction of refractive errors. In addition, the quality of fundus imaging can be improved by optimising the conditions under which the images are taken.

Acknowledgements

We thank the Natural Sciences and Engineering Research Council of Canada for a grant to MCWC and International Fellowship to AG. Thanks to the Ontario Graduate Scholarship Program for a grant to AR. Thanks to Andy Lankin and Robina Clarke.

References

1. Cook CA, Koretz JF, Pfahnl A, Hyun J, Kaufman PL. Aging of the human crystalline lens and anterior segment. Vision Res 1994;34:2945-2954.
2. Brown N. The change in lens curvature with age. Exp Eye Res 1974;19:175-183.
3. Smith G, Atchison DA, Pierscionek BK. Modeling the power of the aging human eye. J Opt Soc Am 1992;9:2111-2117.
4. Glasser A, Campbell MCW. Changes in focal length and spherical aberration of the human lens with ageing. In: Vision Science and its Applications: Technical Digest. Washington, D.C.: Optical Society of America, 1996;1:246-249.
5. Kroeger RHH, Campbell MCW, Munger R, Fernald R. Refractive index distribution and spherical

aberration in the crystalline lens of the African cichlid fish, Haplochromis burtoni. Vision Res 1994;34:1815-1823.
6. Duane A. Normal values of the accommodation at all ages. J A M A 1912;59:1010-1013.
7. Glasser A, Campbell MCW. Physical and optical changes in the human crystalline lens with age and their relationship to presbyopia. Invest Ophthalmol Vis Sci 1996;37:S757.
8. Slataper FJ. Age norms of refraction and vision. Arch Ophthalmol (NY) 1950;43:468-481.
9. Howcroft MJ, Parker JA. Aspheric curvatures for the human lens. Vision Res 1977;17:1217-1223.
10. Brown N. The change in lens curvature with age. Exp Eye Res 1974;19:175-183.
11. Jenkins TCA. Aberrations of the eye and their effects on vision. Brit J Physiol Optics 1963;20: 59-91,161-201.
12. Westheimer G, Liang J. Influence of ocular light scatter on the eye's optical performance. J Opt Soc Am A 1995;12:1417-1424.
13. Lu C, Munger R, Campbell MCW. Monochromatic aberrations in accommodated eyes. In: Vision Science and its Applications: Technical Digest. Washington, D.C.: Optical Society of America, 1993;3:160-163.
14. Atchison DA, Collins MS, Wildsoet CF, Christensen J, Waterworth MD. Measurement of monochromatic ocular aberrations of human eyes as a function of accommodation by the Howland aberroscope technique.Vision Res 1995;35:313-323.
15. Campbell MCW, Harrison EM, Simonet P. Psychophysical measurement of the blur on the retina due to optical aberrations of the eye. Vision Res 1990;30:1587-1602.
16. Howland HC, Howland B. A subjective method for the measurement of the monochromatic aberrations of the eye. J Opt Soc Am 1977;67:1508-1518.
17. Walsh G, Charman WN, Howland, HC. Objective technique for the determination of monochromatic aberrations of the human eye. J Opt Soc Am A 1984;1:987-992.
18. Campbell FW, Gubisch RW. Optical quality of the human eye. J Physiol (Lond) 1966;186:558-578.
19. Santamaria J, Artal P, Bescos J. Determination of the point spread function of human eyes using a hybrid optical-digital method. J Opt Soc Am A 1987;4:1109-1114.
20. Roorda A, Campbell MCW. The relationship between double and single pass image quality of the eye. Invest Ophthalmol Vis Sci 1994;35:S1258.
21. Artal P, Marcos S, Navarro R, Williams DR. Odd aberrations and double pass measurements of retinal image quality. J Opt Soc Am A 1995;12:195-201.
22. Liang J, Williams DR. Effect of higher order aberrations on image quality in the human eye. In: Vision Science and its Applications: Technical Digest. Washington, D.C.: Optical Society of America, 1995;1:70-73.
23. Roorda A. Double pass reflections in the human eye [dissertation]. Waterloo: University of Waterloo, 1996.
24. Schwiegerling J, Greivenkamp JE, Miller JM. Representation of videokeratoscopic height data with Zernike polynomials. J Opt Soc Am A 1995;12:2105-2113.
25. Howland HC, Buettner J, Applegate RA. Computation of the shapes of normal corneas and their monochromatic aberrations from videokeratometric measurements. In: Vision Science and its Applications: Technical Digest. Washington, D.C.: Optical Society of America, 1994;2:54-57.
26. Wilson MA, Campbell MCW, Simonet P. Changes of pupil centration with change of pupil size. Optom and Vis Sci 1992;69:129-136.
27. Walsh G, Charman WN. The effect of pupil centration and diameter on ocular performance. Vision Res 1988;28:659-655.
28. Tscherning M. Physiologic Optics. (trans. Weiland G.). 4th ed. Philadelphia: Keystone Publishing Co.,1924.
29. Bing L, Campbell MCW. The change of monochromatic aberrations with lens tilt and pupil decentration in a four aspheric surface model eye. Invest Ophthalmol Vis Sci 1994;35:S1803.
30. Snyder AW, MillerWH. Photoreceptor diameter and spacing for highest resolving power. J Opt Soc Am 1977;67:696-698.
31. Liang J, Williams DR, Miller, D. Imaging photoreceptors in the living eye with adaptive optics. This volume

33. Roorda A, Campbell MCW. Comparison of the influence of ocular aberrations on three fundus imaging techniques. OSA Annual Meeting: Technical Digest. Washington D.C.: Optical Society of America, 1996; accepted
34. Atkinson MR, Roorda A, Campbell MCW. Imaging of individual photoreceptors: Optical possibilities beyond the incoherent resolution limit. Invest Ophthalmol Vis Sci 1995;36:188.
35. Elliott D, Whitaker D, MacVeigh D. Neural contribution to spatiotemporal contrast sensitivity decline in healthy ageing eyes. Vision Res 1990;30:541-547.
35. Cuiffreda K. Accommodation and its anomalies. In: Cronly-Dillon JR, editor. Vision and visual dysfunction. Vol 1: Visual Optics and Instrumentation. Charman WN, editor. London:The Macmillan Press, 1991:231-279.
36. Bartmann M, Schaeffel F. A simple mechanism for emmetropization without cues from accommodation or colour. Vision Res 1994;34:873-876.
37. Wildsoet CF, Howland HC, Falconer S, Dick K. Chromatic aberration and accommodation: Their role in emmetropization in the chick. Vision Res 1993;33:1593-1603.
38. Collins MJ, Wildsoet CF, Atchison DA. Monochromatic aberrations and myopia. Vision Res 1995;35:1157-1163.
39. Gwiazda J, Thorn F, Bauer J, Held R. Emmetropization and the progression of manifest refraction in children followed from infancy to puberty. Clin Vis Sci 1993;8:337-344.
40. Sivak JG, Ryall LA, Weerheim J, Campbell MCW. Optical constancy of the chick lens during pre- and post-hatching ocular development. Invest Ophthalmol Vis Sci 1989;30:967-974.
41. Kroeger RHH, Fernald RD, Campbell MCW. The refractive index distribution and optical quality of the crystalline lens of the African cichlid fish, Haplochromis burtoni, as a function of lens size and lighting condition during development. Vision Res submitted.
42. Bennett AG and Rabbetts RB. Clinical visual optics, 2nd ed. Toronto: Butterworths, 1989.

COLOR AND LUMINANCE: A 24 BIT ANALYSIS OF ECCENTRIC PHOTOREFRACTION COMBINED WITH THE BRÜCKNER RED REFLEX (VVDA)

GERHARD CIBIS, MELANIE CRANDALL, VALERIY PRUZHANOVSKIY, JUDITH LYND, TIMOTHY HUG,
Children's Mercy Hospital Departments of Surgery and Pediatrics, Section of Ophthalmology, School of Medicine, University of Missouri, Kansas City, MO.

Abstract

Brückner reflex, eccentric photorefraction contour plotting of separate red, green and blue channels gives a 24 bit analysis revealing minimal to no dead space. Patterns remain regardless of pupil size. Algorithms defining chromatic relationships for various refractive powers and pupil sizes are being developed.

Interpretation of eccentric photorefraction images depends on how "crescents" and non "crescent" reflexes are formed. It is well accepted that theoretical crescent sizes fail to conform to practical experience in the living eye [1]. The reasons for this may be multiple. The type of analysis used, namely "geometrical" versus a "physical" or "wave optics" theory, may provide some explanations [2]. Each method makes assumptions and simplifications that may or may not be justified in real life conditions. Another "real life" factor that causes variations in images is chromatic refaction. Theoretical calculations usually assume a single wavelength. The eye refracts different wavelengths differently however. Chromatic aberrations within the ocular structures themselves also play a role. Most specifically the absorption, reflectance and lateral spread of red, blue and green wavelengths differ in different ocular tissues, most specifically the retina, pigment epithelium and choroid [3].

We have developed a white light source eccentric video photorefractive system that combines the Brückner red reflex with dynamic examination of photorefractive crescents [4]. We call this system Video Vision Development Assessment (VVDA) [5]. Our choice of light source and system development was to most closely match the clinical experience with the direct ophthalmoscope. Fixation is determined from dynamic video observation of when Hirschberg reflexes, pupil size and fundus reflectance all indicate foveation. Those video frames are then analyzed for overall reflectance and crescent size comparing the two eyes using an 8 bit, 250 gray scale system. We did not analyze color but realized from observing images that color differs with different pupil sizes and refractive errors. Specifically, blue appears first inferiorly (myopia) and red superiorly (hyperopia) [4]. At low refractive powers overall reflex is a deeper red; at higher powers more yellow, at very high powers gray-white. Using commercially available software (Spyglass Transform) we have developed the ability to look at our VVDA images in 24 bit (64K) colors. Adobe Photoshop is used to break down the video image into its red, green and blue channels, each at 8 bit. Each channel is then graphed separately in Spyglass Transform providing 24 bit analysis (Figures 1&2).

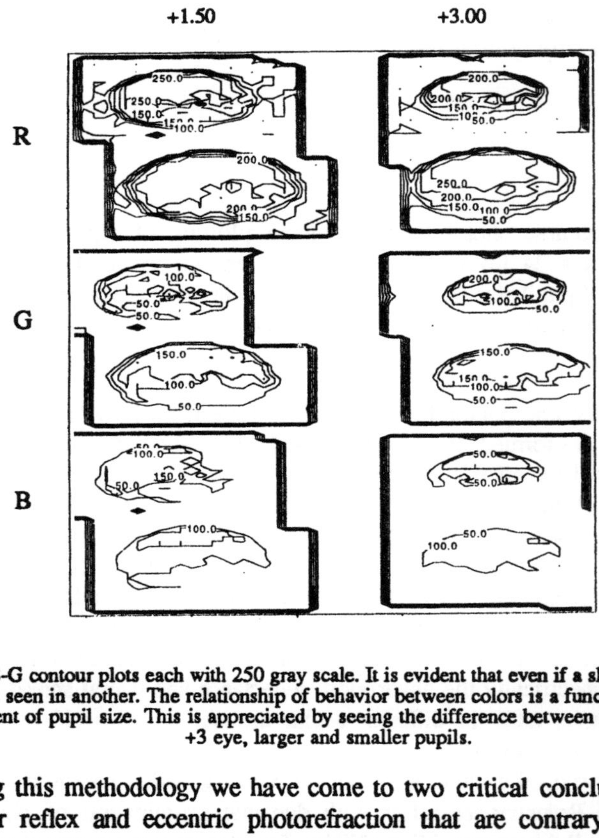

Figure 1. R-B-G contour plots each with 250 gray scale. It is evident that even if a slope is not present in one color, it is seen in another. The relationship of behavior between colors is a function of the refractive error independent of pupil size. This is appreciated by seeing the difference between the right +1.5 and left +3 eye, larger and smaller pupils.

Using this methodology we have come to two critical conclusions concerning the Brückner reflex and eccentric photorefraction that are contrary to conventional wisdom. First, pupil size does not matter within reason (>2mm). We find that refractive information concerning myopia or hyperopia is always present as the slope of the image, either superiorly for hyperopia or inferiorly for myopia (inferiorly decentered light source, the reverse for superiorly decentered), regardless of pupil size (Figure 1). If the pupil is very small, there is an inadequate number of pixels to provide the slope mathematics. The relationships of R-B-G slopes to each other is a function of refractive power. Second, there is no dead space with minimal light source eccentricity (Figure 2). There is always a slope for some wavelength of light even at very low refractive powers. True plano has no slope.

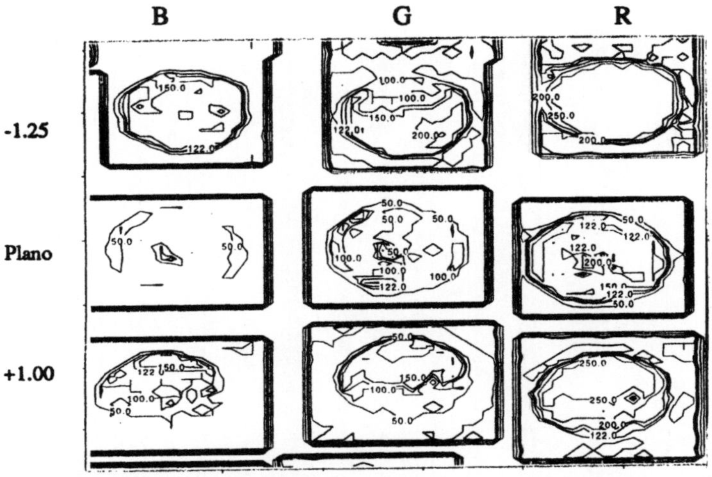

Figure 2. R-G-B contour plots each with 250 gray scale (8 bit). There is no dead space. A slope is always present in at least one color to determine sign. The relationships of colors to each other is a function of refractive error.

We are currently working on the development of algorithms to relate the behavior of red, blue and green light in VVDA to determine refraction independent of "crescent" measurements. We recognize that the traditional photorefractive "crescent" is actually the most luminous (red) wavelength and is a function of film speed and film color characteristics. The same analysis will reveal how the VVDA reflex changes with eccentric fixation to help in defining fixation.

References

1. Roorda A, Campbell MCW. Geometric theory to predict eccentric photorefraction intensity profiles in the human eye. J Opt Soc Am A 1995;12:1647-1656.
2. Kusel R. Models describing eccentric photorefraction crescents. In: Vision science and its applications. Technical Digest Series. Santa Fe: Optical Society of America, 1995;I:117-120.
3. Campbell MCW, Bobier WR, Roorda A. Effect of monochromatic aberrations on photorefractive patterns. J Opt Soc Am A 1995;12:1637-1646.
4. Cibis GW. Video vision development assessment (VVDA): Combining the Brückner test with eccentric photorefraction for dynamic identification of amblyogenic factors in infants and children. Tr Am Ophth Soc. 1994;XCII:644-685.
5. Cibis GW, Luke TP. Video vision development assessment. In: Cibis GW, Tongue AC, Stass-Isern. Decision making in pediatric ophthalmology. St Louis: C.V. Mosby Co, 1993: 202-203.

POTENTIAL ACUITY ON A SHOESTRING

THE USE OF ENTOPTIC IMAGERY

THEODORE E. COHN and JAY M. ENOCH
School of Optometry, University of California, Berkeley, CA 94720.

Abstract

The pre-operative determination of retinal function, "potential acuity", is assuming an increasingly important role in ophthalmic care under the joint pressures of maximizing visual function while minimizing health care costs. Quantitative potential acuity is obviously the most desirable approach but it can also be the most expensive. This communication introduces an inexpensive qualitative technique for measuring subjective potential acuity, and describes its use. Required are: optometrist's penlight, some tin foil, a pin, a paper hole punch, and good communication with the patient.

Introduction

Potential acuity is defined as the visual acuity that could be achieved, postoperatively, upon removal or correction of optical malfunction. Cataract, corneal opacity and a variety of other conditions can lower measured visual acuity despite an intact retina and visual pathway. It is often a challenge to the doctor to assess the acuity that might be achieved, if only the offensive optical element were repaired or removed. The purpose of this assessment is multifaceted. One wants to have patient's and surgeon's expectations at an appropriately realistic level.

Goldmann and Lotmar [1] made one of the first breakthroughs in this arena with the application of interferometric methods. Interference fringes imaged on the retina largely bypass media faults, but require a window through the opacity to function. Very high contrast fringes thus developed can be adjusted in size (or frequency) to give an indication of the best resolvable detail behind the optical fault. Such acuity was shown to be highly correlated with the postoperative acuity following cataract removal. Enoch has been working separately on the problem of assessmentof vision through dense media opacities (no window required) for some years [2,3], and has devised both a quantitative and a qualitative test of potential visual acuity applicable to such patients (as well as individuals where there is a window through the cataract or other media disorder).

The Potential Acuity Meter (PAM) is a commercially available instrument designed for this purpose. This device concentrates the stimulus beam into a narrow cone imaged in the plane of the pupil. There it must be positioned to occupy a tiny clear area, should one exist, and thus supply good imagery upon the retina. The endpoint is a letter acuity measurement. The PAM manufactured by Mentor Instruments requires some training for appropriate use. A less expensive alternative would be desirable, although in the present case, what must be sacrificed is quantitation.

A clue to the present approach can be found in Green's report [4] on interference based potential acuity measurement. He was concerned how the laser light from the two beams that were intended to undergo interference could gain access to the media behind the cataract. To this end he dilated the pupil with a mydriatic and searched about with his apparatus to find a point in the pupil where the two beams could be imaged so as to yield maximum fringe contrast. Many times, it was not clear whether "holes" were available in the cataract for this search to be successful. Nonetheless, fringes were always seen, indicating that "microscopic" paths for unimpeded light travel must exist. Perhaps of more significance, patients reported seeing "dark irregular shapes" upon which the fringes were superimposed. The existence of these shapes, probably shadows of the catarcatous mass, is what gave rise to the present startegy. After Goldmann [5], who described imaging the Purkinje tree on the retina, we sought to image the cataract itself on the retina and to use the ability of the patient to perceive its shape as a measure, albeit subjective, of the patient's retinal integrity.

Methods

The often cited observation that point sources of light allow one to visualize the lens sutures is a phenomenon similar to that Green reported which lies at the heart of our method. This was first described by Listing according to Helmoholtz [6]. The idea is to use this kind of entoptic imagery to allow the patient to visualize the detail of his/her own cataract or opacity, whatever its cause. Then if the detail can be described and appreciated by the patient, the doctor can be confident that subjectively, potential acuity is good.

The construction of the potential acuity stimulator is easy and fast enough that it can be done from scratch while attending the patient. A penlight flashlight is balanced upon its switch end and a white paper disc from a paper punch is placed over the lens. (This step deletes a confounding image of the bulb filament which will otherwise distract the patient). Then, a small (5cmx5cm) square of tin foil, pierced in its center by a single pin prick (or by two such holes side by side), is centered over the paper disc and shaped over the lightable end of the penlight.

The patient should remove his/her spectacles and be in a darkened room. Following a brief (several minute) adaptation period (during which the aforementioned construction can be undertaken) the patient is given the lit penlight and asked to position it within 1 cm (at less distance than the anterior focal point) of his/her cornea taking care of course not to touch the eye. As the doctor can verify with his/her own eye, this stimulus leads, in the normal eye with clear media, to the sensation of a disc of light whose size is in inverse proportion to the distance of the light from the cornea. Careful observation will reveal to the doctor the lens sutures, the pupillary border (iris shadow), and possibly the detail of interposed floaters or other extraneous debris within the media. The image of all such detail is quite sharp and distinct in the normal eye.

Under these conditions the patient is then asked to describe, or even to draw, his/her impression of the pattern of illumination formed. If a cataractous lens is present, the picture should show just what the slit lamp does: areas of opacity and areas of clarity, with the obvious difference that to the patient the image will be inverted. The patient should be asked whether the detail thus seen, compares in its clarity and sharpness to detail remembered in pre-cataract days. If the answer is yes, then the notation in the record can be that subjectively potential acuity is high. If the answer is no, and if the cataractous opacity is itself devoid of detail upon slit lamp examination, then the notation in the record must be equivocal, and no information was thus gained.

A second order observation to ask of the patient concerns fringes in the detail of the perceived shapes due to diffraction. Such fringes would be expected to be visible centrally if the foveal circuitry were intact. Thus the report of fringes lends credence to the view that potential acuity is high.

It is possible to elaborate the procedure for the purpose of obtaining a numerical (though still subjective) determination of potential acuity. With two points of light (from two adjacent holes in the foil) the patient will visualize two pupils slightly overlapped. The overall impression is one of a figure "8". The outline of the opacity thus appears twice, unless the opacity presents at or near the retina, for in that case, it will be imaged singly (Listing termed this *relative entoptical parallax*). By this strategy the doctor can assist his/her patient to distinguish opacity at the level of the lens or before, from opacity at the level of the retina. The indicator of acuity is then the angle of rotation of the tin foil cover upon the penlight (both of which can be marked with a pen) in order to yield the impression of a change of orientation of the "figure eight". This acuity, ordinarilly quite high in the normal eye, is, if in the normal range, a necessary, though not a sufficient, indicator of high potential acuity. It is not sufficient because the retinal processing required to conduct such a judgment remains intact in the face of 10 diopters of blur under normal viewing. That is an indicator that the acuity thus assessed may not reflect only detail vision, even if the acuity endpoint is in minutes of arc.

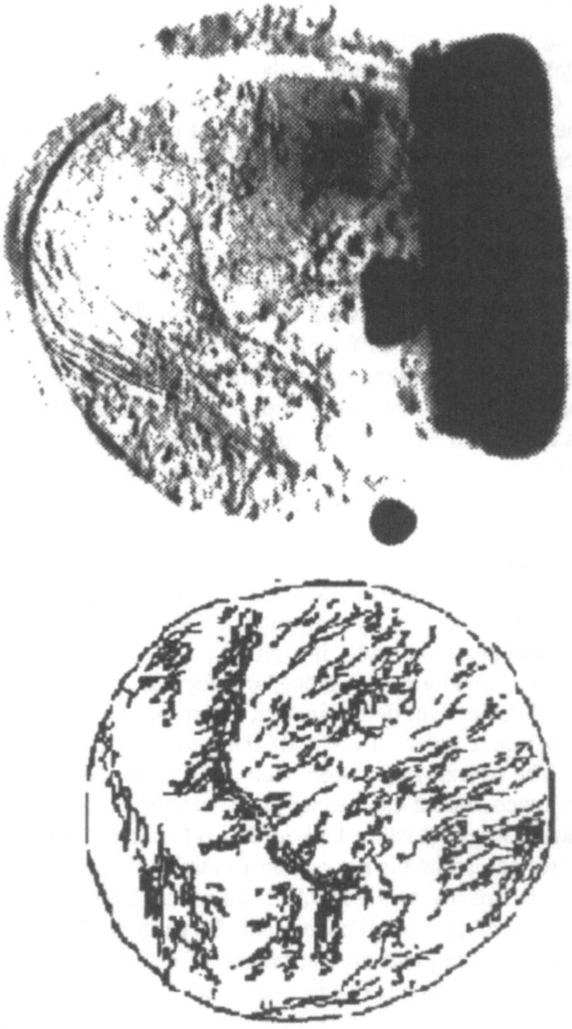

Figure 1. Slit-lamp photograph (top) of posterior capsule and sketch based on entoptic viewing (bottom). The photograph slide was scanned and digitized. The image was converted to a black and white with gray scale and this was contrast reversed and then processed to enhance detail. The pen and ink sketch was scanned and digitized. Two features are worthy of comment: the similarities between image and drawing are found in the low frequency information, which does not by itself establish a healthy retina. The level of detail conveyed in the drawing, its correlation with the patient's comments, and its comparison to that seen by slit lamp are what establishes the quality of the retina behind the optical defect.

Results

Case Study: One of us (JME) a then 63 year old male had a unilateral (RE) cataract procedure performed in 1994 to remove a posterior subcapsular and nuclear cataract. The lens was replaced with a foldable silicon lens implant which later proved to be disposed normally within the capsular bag. Nonetheless, by spring 1995, acuity, which had been 20/20 immediately postoperatively, had worsenned to 20/70 owing to the development in the posterior lens capsule of an array of irregular lens fibres and pearls from residual cells left by the operation. Elschnig pearls are clearly visible upon slit lamp examination in Fig. 1 (Top) Laser treatment of this opacity was scheduled for Fall 1995. Just prior to the procedure, subjective potential acuity was assessed by the means described above. The patient drew a picture to represent his opacity, as it appeared upon entoptic imagery (Fig. 1 Bottom). It is apparent that the basic features of what was seen and what was actually present are quite concordant. The patient, asked as to the clarity of detail in this entoptic image reported clarity comparable to that available to him through this eye prior to the formation of the opacity. Thus this potential acuity was subjectively assessed to be normal. Indeed, following the laser treatment his monocular VA improved from 20/70 to 20/20-.

Discussion

Subjective procedures carry disadvantages that are familiar to any eye doctor, but the compensating utility has often proven to be sufficient to overcome these. In the present case we have demonstrated and described a means of subjectively assessing potential acuity. The procedure is not dependent upon ones ability to locate and image a source in holes in the cataract or opacity as is the case with some potential acuity instruments. It is the fineness and clarity of the detail drawn which predicts potential central retinal acuity. In a single patient, this procedure supplied a useful indicator of the acuity that later proved to be accurate.

The materials and assumptions required to make use of this technique are straightforward, and, with one exception, quite easy to find in any office or clinic. The crucial ingredient in this technique, however, may not be in long supply. It is a ready and facile communication between doctor and patient. With that present, we conclude that inexpensive subjective potential acuity determination is a practical tool for the doctor to embrace.

Acknowledgments

This work was supported in part by EY 07606 to TEC. We thank Dr.'s Karen Walker, Mike Glazeski, Carl Jacobsen and Richard Knowles for assistance with Fig.1

References

1. Goldmann H, Lotmar W. Beitrag zum problem der bestimmung der retinalen sehscharfe bei katarackt. Klin Monnatsbl Augenheilkd 1969;154:324-329.
2. Enoch JM, Giraldez-Fernandez MJ, Knowles R, Huang D, Hunter A, LaBree L, Azen SP. Hyperacuity test to evaluate vision through dense cataracts: Research preliminary to a clinical study: I. Studies conducted at the University of California at Berkeley prior to travel to India. Optom Vis Sci 1995;72: 619-629.
3. Enoch JM, Knowles R. Hyperacuity test to evaluate vision through dense cataracts: Research preliminary to a clinical study: II. Initial trials of the India instrument and HASP protocol at Aravind Eye Hospital, Madurai, India. Optom Vis Sci 1995;72: 630-642.
4. Green DG. Testing the vision of cataract patients by means of laser-generated interference fringes. Science 1970;168:1240-1242.
5. Goldmann H. Examination of the fundus of the cataractous eye. Am J Ophthalmol 1972;73:309-320.
6. Helmholtz H v. Helmholtz's treatise on Physiological Optics. J. P. C. Southall, ed.. Washington DC: Optical Society of America, Third English Edition, 1924.

THE AXIAL LENGTH/CORNEAL RADIUS RATIO IN EMMETROPIA AND AMETROPIA: A REVIEW

THEODORE GROSVENOR & DAVID A. GOSS
School of Optometry, Indiana University, Bloomington, IN.

Abstract

The ratio of axial length to corneal radius (AL/CR ratio) has a value of approximately 3.0 in emmetropia eyes, <3.0 in hyperopic eyes, and >3.0 in myopic eyes. There is evidence that in emmetropic children an AL/CR ratio greater than 3.0 indicates a risk for the development of myopia. In adult eyes, variance in the AL/CR ratio has been shown to account for as much as 93% of the variance in the eye's refractive state. The results of 3 cross-sectional studies show that the AL/CR ratio, in emmetropic or near-emmetropic eyes, is remarkably stable with age.

Background

Stenstrom [1] was apparently the first investigator to report axial length/corneal radius ratios. In his landmark study of the refractive components of the right eyes of 1000 subjects between the ages of 20 and 35 years. Stenstrom reported a mean AL/CR ratio slightly greater than 3.0 for emmetropic eyes. For highly myopic eyes AL/CR ratios were from 3.6 to 3.8, and for highly hyperopic eyes AL/CR ratios were from 2.6 to 2.8. The correlation coefficient for refractive error with axial length was -0.76; and the correlation coefficient for refractive error with AL/CR ratio was -0.84.

The Axial Length/Corneal Radius Ratio as a Risk Factor for Youth Onset Myopia

When tabulating refractive component data for 625 emmetropic Melanesian children examined in the island nation of Vanuatu [2], Grosvenor [3] found that these children had flatter corneas and shorter eyes than one would expect for eyes of emmetropic Caucasian children. The AL/CR ratios for these children were considerably lower than 3.0, which would normally indicate a moderate amount of hyperopia. Mean AL/CR ratios for the 625 emmetropic Melanesian children were compared to those of 643 emmetropic British children whose data had been reported by Sorsby and his colleagues [4, 5], with the result that mean AL/CR ratios were found to be significantly greater for the British children (3.05 for boys and 3.04 for girls) than for the Melanesian children (2.88 for boys and 2.86 for girls).

Because the prevalence of myopia is much higher among British children than among Melanesian children, these results were interpreted as indicating that the eyes of the emmetropic British children had already begun to elongate, and that this elongation was compensated by a decrease in lens power. In such a case, further axial elongation or corneal steepening, if not compensated by a decrease in lens power, would be expected to bring about the onset of myopia. As a result of these findings it was suggested that a high AL/CR ratio is risk factor for the development of myopia [3].

In a 3-year prospective longitudinal study of 87 initally emmetropic children examined at Northeastern State University in Tahlequah, Oklahoma, Goss and Jackson [6] found that 88% of eyes that became myopic during the 3-year period had horizontal meridian AL/CR ratios of 3.00 or greater; and that 93% of the eyes having horizontal meridian AL/CR ratios less than 3.00 did not become myopic. Noting that the AL/CR ratio was the variable having the highest sensitivity and specificity for predicting the onset of myopia, Goss and Jackson [6] suggested that a greater corneal power may limit the capability of the crystalline lens to decrease in power to offset an increase in vitreous chamber depth. They concluded that greater corneal powers and greater AL/CR ratios are risk factors for youth onset myopia.

The Role of the AL/CR Ratio in Determining the Refractive State in Adult Eyes

In a report of a study of the refractive components of 125 medical students between the ages of 19 and 21 in Japan, Okamoto [7] published a graph showing that the AL/CR ratio gradually increased from approximately 3.0 for eyes having 1 D of hyperopia to 3.6 for eyes having 9 D of myopia.

White [8] reported on a study involving 61 optometry students and staff members at the Auckland University School of Optometry. Ages of subjects ranged from 32 to 68 years, and spherical equivalent refraction ranged from +4.00 D to -10.00 D. AL/CR ratios varied from approximately 2.80 for the highest hyperopes to 3.45 for the highest myopes. Regression analysis resulted in correlation coefficients of -0.84 for refractive error with axial length, and -0.95 for refractive error with AL/CR ratio. White [8] concluded that these results supported Okamoto's [7] contention that refractive error depends on the shape of the eye.

The role of the AL/CR ratio in determining the refractive state in young adults was investigated by Grosvenor and Scott [9]. Using refractive component data for 194 subjects between the ages of 18 and 30 years whose spherical equivalent refraction ranged from +7.91 to -13.32 D, they found that AL/CR ratios varied from 2.60 for the most highly hyperopic eye to 4.10 for the most highly myopic eye. Correlation coefficients were -0.76 for spherical equivalent refraction with axial length, and -0.92 for spherical equivalent refraction with the AL/CR ratio. The coefficient of determination of linear regression for the AL/CR ratio as a function of refractive error was $(-0.92)^2$, or 0.84, suggesting that 84% of the variance in refractive error for these subjects could be accounted for by variance in the AL/CR ratio.

Grosvenor and Scott [9] also calculated AL/CR ratios for 90 subjects examined by Sorsby et al. [10] between the ages of 18 and 30 years, with vertical meridian refraction from +7.50 to -20.00 D. The correlation coefficient for refractive error vs AL/CR ratio was -0.96, indicating that $(-0.96)^2$, or 92% of the variance in refractive error for the Sorsby et al. subjects could be accounted for by variance in the AL/CR ratio.

Using data from 176 young adult subjects [11] we calculated the AL/CR ratio in the vertical meridian for each subject. The correlation coefficient of AL/CR ratio with refractive error, expressed as the vertical meridian cycloplegic retinoscopy finding, was higher than that of any one ocular optical component or of any simple ocular metric. The correlations with refractive error were: AL/CR ratio, -0.86; axial length, -0.73; vitreous depth, -0.71; corneal radius, +0.28; anterior lens radius, -0.002; posterior lens radius, +0.13; axial length/anterior lens radius ratio, -0.24;. axial length/posterior lens radius ratio, +0.21.

The mean vertical meridian AL/CR ratio for 53 emmetropic eyes was 3.06 (SD = 0.09); and the mean vertical meridian AL/CR ratio for 115 myopic eyes was 3.23 (SD = 0.13). The level of agreeement between the results of the various studies is indicated in Table 1.

Table 1. Comparison of correlation coefficient data from 5 studies.

	Refractive Error with Axial Length	Refractive Error with AL/CR Ratio	Refr. Error Variance Due to Variance in the AL/CR ratio
Stenstrom [1]	-0.76	-0.84	71 %
White [8]	-0.84	-0.95	90 %
Grosvenor & Scott [9]	-0.76	-0.92	84 %
Sorsby [10]	-------	-0.96	93 %
Goss et al. [11]	-0.73	-0.86	74%

The Apparent Stability of the AL/CR Ratio with Age

Several investigators have published cross-sectional refraction and component data for populations of subjects of various ages. These data provide an opportunity to investigate the effects of age on the AL/CR ratio.

Leighton and Tomlinson [12] compared refractive component data for one eye of each of 36 pairs of subjects. Each pair consisted of one younger adult (mean age, 25.17 years) and one older adult (mean age, 61.83 years). Mean refractive errors were +0.37 D (range, +2.25 to -3.50 D) for the younger adults and +0.49 D (range, +3.00 to -3.00 D) for the older adults. Although the differences in mean axial length and mean corneal radius were statistically significant for the two groups of adults, the difference in mean AL/CR ratios was trivial. Mean axial lengths and spherical equivalent corneal radii for the younger adults were 23.42 mm and 7.86 mm, as compared to 22.15 mm and 7.67 mm for the older adults. Mean AL/CR ratios were 3.00 for the younger adults and 3.01 for the older adults.

Making use of refractive component data published by Sorsby et al. [10, 13], Grosvenor [14] tabulated data, in 10-year age groups, for right eyes of subjects having vertical meridian refractive errors between plano and +2.00 D. Mean vertical meridian corneal radius and mean axial length for 48 subjects 10-19 years old were 7.89 mm and 24.1 mm; as compared to 7.78 mm and 23.6 mm for 65 subjects 40-49 years old: these differences were statistically significant ($p<0.01$). Mean AL/CR ratios were 3.05 for the younger subjects and 3.03 for the older subjects.

In a third study designed to compare components of refraction on the basis of age, Ooi and Grosvenor [15] reported component data for 48 young adults (ages 19 to 31 years) and 48 mature adults (ages 49 to 61 years), with spherical equivalent refraction ranging from +2.50 D to -2.50 D. Mean corneal radius and mean axial length for the young adults were 7.78 mm and 23.52 mm; compared to 7.77 mm and 23.42 mm for the mature adults. Mean AL/CR ratios were 3.02 for the young adults and 3.01 for the mature adults.

It is worthy of emphasis that even though the Leighton and Tomlinson [12] data and the Sorsby et al. [10,13] data showed significant differences in mean corneal radius and mean axial length for younger subjects as compared to older subjects--while the Ooi and Grosvenor [15] data did not--for all 3 data sets the mean AL/CR ratios differed for the two age groups by no more than 2 units in the second decimal place: a difference of no more than 0.07%.

Conclusions

The AL/CR ratio is a simple numerical value derived from ocular optics. We conclude that the AL/CR ratio: (a) may indicate a risk for the onset of myopia in emmetropic children, if higher than about 3.0; (b) is more highly correlated with refractive error than any one ocular optical component; and (c) as shown by cross-sectional data, appears to change little with age for emmetropic or near-emmetropic eyes.

References

1 Stenstrom S. Investigation of the variation and covariation of the optical elements of human eyes. Transl by D Woolf. Am J Optom Arch Am Acad Optom 1948; 25: 218-32, 286-99, 340-50, 388-97, 438-49, 496-50.

2. Grosvenor T. Myopia in Melanesian school children in Vanuatu. In: Fledelius HC, Goldschmidt E, editors. Myopia Workshop. Copenhagen: Scriptor, 1988: 24-28.

3. Grosvenor T. High axial length/corneal radius ratio as a risk factor in the development of myopia. Am J Optom Physiol Opt 1988; 65: 689-696.

4. Sorsby A, Benjamin D, Sheridan J. Refraction and its Components during the Growth of the Eye from the Age of 3. London: Her Majesty's Stationery Office, 1961.

5. Sorsby A, Leary GA. A Longitudinal Study of Refraction and its Components during Growth.. London: Her Majesty's Stationery Office, 1970.

6. Goss DA, Jackson TW. Clinical findings before the onset of myopia in youth. I. Ocular optical components. Opt Vis Sci 1995; 72: 870-878.

7. Okamoto H. An idea for the measurement of the axial length of the eye with a laser as visual target. The correlation between the refractive error and the shape of the eye. In: Thijssen AM, Verbeek JM, editors. Ultrasonography in Ophthalmology, Proceedings of the 8th SIDUO Congress. Doc Ophthalmologica Proceedings Series 29, 1981: 205-210.

8. White M. The shape of the eye as the primary determinant of refractive error. University of Auckland, Auckland, NZ: unpublished manuscript, 1988.

9. Grosvenor T, Scott R. Role of the axial length/corneal radius ratio in determining the refractive state of the eye. Optom Vis Sci 1994; 71: 575-579.

10. Sorsby A, Benjamin D, Sheridan J. Davey M, Tanner J. Emmetropia and its Aberrations. London: Her Majesty's Stationery Office, 1957.

11. Goss DA, Van Veen HG, Rainey BB, Feng B. Ocular optical components measured by keratometry, phakometry, and ultrasonography in emmetropic and myopic optometry students. In preparation.

12. Leighton DA, Tomlinson A. Changes in axial length and other dimensions of the eyeball wih increasing age. Acta Ophthalmol 1972: 50: 815-826.

13. Sorsby A, Sheridan J, Leary GA. Refraction, Its Components in Twins. London: Her Majesty's Stationery Office, 1962.

14. Grosvenor T. Reduction in axial length with age: an emmetropizing mechanism for the adult eye? Am J Optom Physiol Opt 1987; 64: 657-63.

15. Ooi CA, Grosvenor T. Mechanisms of emmetropization in the aging eye. Optom Vis Sci 1995; 72: 60-66.

NEW PROGRESSIVE ADDITION LENSES WITH ASPHERICAL PRESCRIPTION SURFACES

GÜNTHER GUILINO
Optische Werke G. Rodenstock, Isartalstrasse 43, D-80469 Munich, GERMANY.

Abstract

The new Progressive life lens series - launched in the German market in '94 - more or less marked the end of the process of overall optimization of all-round progressive addition lenses (PALs) based on the present state of the art. This means that if we discount for the present the new versions based on different materials, there is relatively little room for the further development of conventional PALs for universal wear. However, new aspects are immediately opened up if it becomes possible to manufacture aspherical or atoric back surfaces under economically justifiable conditions.

Technical Realization of Multigressive

A brief look back at the beginnings of PALs will reveal a number of parallels to the current situation with regard to the prescription (Rx) surfaces: Lenses with a continuously increasing surface curvature on one side were known from patents for the correction of presbyopia before the 1950's. But only when the manufacturers designed their own surfacing machinery for this new kind of surface did it become technically possible to produce those PAL concepts which then became successful on the market. Today, numerically controlled lens working machines represent the state of the art. As a result, it is no problem from the grinding side to reproduce with sufficient precision a surface of a glass or plastic lens whose design parameters can be selected more or less freely. But just like before, we do have problems with the polishing of these non-rotationally symmetrical, aspherical surfaces.

But what does all this have to do with the aspherical/atoric back surfaces mentioned above? Quite simply: Particularly in the critical polishing process there are considerable differences in the working of the front and back sides. As the polishing process must always be linked to a motion of the polish carrier over the whole surface, with aspherical lenses the amount of polish applied can vary in size from point to point. The limited number of front surfaces, characterized by base curve and addition, means that once such systematic deviations from the surface design have been determined, correction values can be calculated and programmed.

With the almost unlimited number of possible prescriptions - sphere, cylinder, axis position, prism, base - it is, however, practically no longer possible to determine the same corrections values for specific surfaces for aspherically designed back surfaces. This means that different polishing processes are needed which can always immediately achieve the required surface faithfulness for a lot size of 1, i.e. single lens production. Intensive research activities have now put Rodenstock in a position where they can use in-house developments in production machinery and processes to manufacture the prescription surface economically in an aspheric and/or atoric version, too. The practical realization is found in the new lens series Multigressiv.

The Dual Concept Progressive life/Multigressive

A modern and highly demanding lens series is expected to combine the best possible cosmetic appearance with high optical performance. It is well-known that these contradictory demands can only be met by using additional design parameters. A good appearance really means a low arching of the lens vertex beyond the plane of the frame. This requires the lowest possible curvature. In contrast, high imaging quality requires a comparatively high curvature. For single vision (SV) lenses, for example, an aspheric design of the non-Rx surface solves this problem in a satisfactory manner, as demonstrated by the Cosmolit lens series introduced to the market as early as 1986. The aspherical design of the front surface compensates for the peripheral imaging defects caused by the flattening of the curvature.

This concept, which is so successful for SV lenses, can only be transferred in an analog process to PALs if the Rx surface can be used to compensate for those optically disadvantageous consequences which arise from the flat design. As can be seen from Table 1, this means that for a spherical prescription the back surface must have a rotationally symmetrical aspherical design. For an astigmatic prescription, the Rx design must logically be atoric.

Table 1. Front- and back surface design for the lens series Progressive life and Multigressive.

Front surface	Back surface	Lens series
Progressive	Spherical, torical	**Progressiv life**
Progressive »flat«	Aspherical, atorical	**Multigressiv**

A practical realization of these concept can be found in the Multigressiv lens series first introduced in May 1995. The front surface of Multigressiv has the same design as Progressiv life, but with a curvature which is 1 to 1.5 D flatter for the same power. The asphericity of each back surface, whether for a spherical or astigmatic prescription, is optimized together with the corresponding progressive power surface and stored for the control of the tool machines. This individual surface optimization means that losses in optical quality in the periphery such as otherwise have to be accepted by the wearer if his or her prescription values are at the end of the power range of a base curve, no longer occur.

Typical Properties

The effect of a better cosmetic appearance cannot only be described by means of diopter values of the flattening. It can also and better be described by the vertex or design height of the lens because this value also includes the rim thickness. The reduction in the design height still amounts to around 2 mm over the conventional design. If we look at the relationships between Multigressiv and Progressiv life in dependence on the cylinder power, then in accordance with Table 2 we find a design height reduction of up to 20 per cent for Multigressiv lenses in dependence on sphere and cylinder. The flattening effect is particularly pronounced in the spherical case, but also occurs, as can be seen, with increasing cylinder power. This difference in vertex is maintained even after glazing as the best-shape edging for the frame has the same effect on both products compared.

Table 2. **Design height relationship Multigressiv/Progressiv life for different combined powers, add 2.0.**

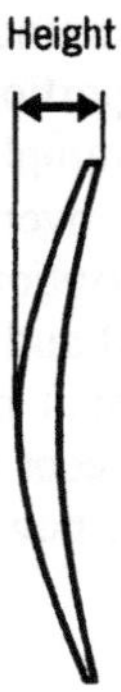

Different cyls for equal combined powers, add 2.0, dia 66/72 mm				
sphere	cyl 0.0	cyl -1.0	cyl -2.0	cyl -3.0
4.0	0.8	0.8	0.8	0.8
3.5	0.8	0.8	0.8	1.0
3.0	0.8	0.8	1.0	1.0
2.5	0.8	1.0	1.0	1.0
2.0	0.8	1.0	1.0	1.0

The astigmatic correction is not so easy to deal with as the unavoidable peripheral surface astigmatism of the progressive front surface has a great effect on the correction results. In any case, it is expected that an atoric surface will provide better correction for the astigmatic eye with fairly large eye movements than a conventional toric design. This assumption can be proven to be correct for the example of sph +4.0 cyl 1.0 A 0° in the Figure: The graphs show the available VA at the relevant points of vision in relation to the maximum VA. A comparison of the two graphs immediately reveals that with the selected cylinder value the optically available vision field without restriction ($VA_{rel} \geq 0.8$) is larger in the distance portion of the atoric Multigressiv version and even more so in the reading portion. With higher cylinder powers the optical benefit of Multigressiv becomes even greater .

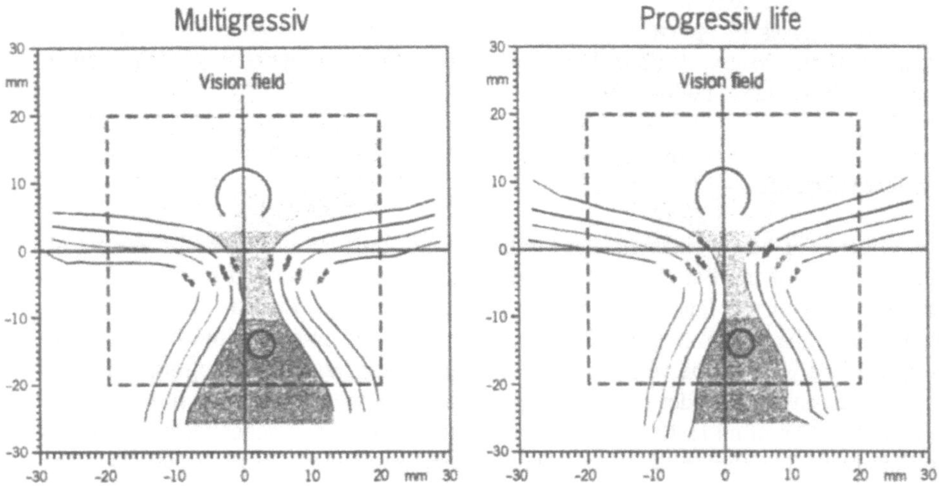

Figure 1. **Iso-line representation of the available relative VA for Multigressiv and Progressiv life with the acuity grades 0.8, 0.63, 0.5 and 0.4. The spatial coordinates of the lenses have their origin at the prism reference point. Distance portion, progressive corridor and reading portion are shown in different shades.**

To characterize quantitatively that benefit, the ratio of visual field extension calculated from the areas enclosed by the VA line 0.8 (20/25) for each design and the boundaries given dashed in the figure will be considered: These ratios are around 1.1 for the distance portion and progressive corridor and 1.3 for the reading portion. If we take the mean value over the three visual areas, we obtain for this example an extension of the total Multigressiv vision field of 1.17 or 17 per cent over the Progressiv life version.The following comparison for four cylindrical prescriptions e. g. with a combined power of 2 or 4 D respectively (sph -1.0 and 0.0; cyl 2.0 and 3.0) and cylinder axes varying in steps of 30° shows the increases in the visual areas typical for Multigressiv: The values fluctuate between around 5 and 55 per cent with the greatest gain found at an axis position of 0°; here the (positive) cylinder power is approximately flush with the direction of the principal meridian of the PAL's.

Summary

The concept for two PAL series is dealt with which allows the technical possibility of manufacturing optimized Rx surfaces for individual cases. The one series Progresšiv life works with conventional Rx surfaces. The other Multigressiv is equipped unconventionally with aspherical or atoric back surfaces whose surfacing data are calculated "just-in-time". This so to speak dual aspherical design produces a real benefit for the wearer in both cosmetic and optical regard.

CALCULATION OF ABERRATION COEFFICIENTS: A MATRIX METHOD

V. LAKSHMINARAYANAN[1,2] and S. VARADHARAJAN[2]
[1]School of Optometry, [2]Department of Physics and Astronomy, University of Missouri - St. Louis, St. Louis, MO 63121.

Abstract

We describe a matrix method to calculate the nonlinear terms in the refraction of a ray. An example involving a single elliptical refracting surface is provided.

Introduction

Matrix optics is traditionally restricted to Gaussian or paraxial optics ($\sin\theta=\theta$) [1]. To deal with higher order, i.e., nonlinear terms in the expansion of Snell's law, some type of linearization has to be done in order to utilize a matrix approach [2]. We describe the method below and show how this can be used to describe aberrations (both 3rd and 5th order) produced by an elliptical refracting surface.

An Algorithm

We give below a step by step procedure for calculating the aberration coefficients. In principle this technique can be applied to any order.

(a) A ray of light can be expressed as a vector with its position and direction as the components. An optical element transforms a vector into another vector. In fact we can define a ray vector field [3].Therefore the emergent ray is a (non-linear) function of the incident vector. When the system is a cascade of optical elements then the final emergent ray is function of the incident ray. If such functions are to be represented as operators that transform a vector into another vector then they must map the zero vector into a zero vector. Since any ray on the optic axis remains unaltered the lenses and mirrors can be represented by such operators.

(b) A ray can be represented by the vector $\mathbf{x}=(x,y,u,v)$ where (x,y) is the position of the incidence of ray on a plane perpendicular to the optic axis at the vertex of the surface and (u,v) is its slope ($u=dx/dz$, $v=dy/dz$, where z is coordinate along the optic axis.) The effect of an optical element can be written as $\mathbf{x_1}=f(\mathbf{x_0})$ where f is a non-linear function where $\mathbf{x_0}$ is the incident vector and $\mathbf{x_1}$ the emergent.

(c) The effect of any two lenses have the same functional form (though the parameters - like refractive index, radius of curvature - may differ). Therefore, when dealing with cascaded systems, it is sufficient to calculate upto the order of expansion that we are interested in, at each intermediate step. For example, suppose we have two lenses and we are interested in the third order expansion. Let's denote the effect of the first lens by the equation $x_1=f_1(x_0)$ where x_0 is the vector representing the ray incident on the first lens and x_1 the ray emerging from it and f_1 repersents the effect of the first lens. Similarly, let's denote the translation in the space between the first and second lens as $x_2=f_2(x_1)$ and the effect of the second lens by $x_3=f_3(x_2)$. We calculate x_1 up to third order in x_0, calculate x_1^2 and x_1^3, use these to find x_2 up to third order in x_1, calculate x_2^2 and x_2^3 and calculate x_3 up to third order in x_2.

(d) From (1) and (3) we can construct vectors X with components $x^i y^j u^k v^l$ with the maximum value of i+j+k+l=n, the order expansion we are interested in, and minimum equal to 1. Then f_1, f_2 and f_1 can be represented as an NxN matrix where $N={}^{(n+4)}C_n -1$. ${}^{(n+4)}C_n$ represents the total number of combinations of i,j,k,l possible with the constraint that the maximum value of i+j+k+l=n. The -1 appears to eliminate the possibility of i+j+k+l=0. For example $N={}^7C_3-1=34$ for third order and $N={}^9C_5 -1=125$ for 5th order.

(e) Many optical systems have some symmetry in them. These drastically reduce the number of allowed values of i, j, k and l and hence the dimension of N is reduced. For example, for a spherically symmetric system, N=8 for 3rd order and N=20 for 5th order.

(f) The matrix multiplication corresponding to step (c) results in the component x of the final emergent vector x as a polynomial of degree n (n= 3 in the example in (c)) of the object position x_0. The non-linear terms represent the aberrations.

Application to an Elliptical Surface

With this recipe we can do non-linear optics using the well known tools of matrix algebra. We apply this method to study the aberrations due to an aspheric surface which is ellipsoidal. To keep the calculation simple we assume the surface to be axisymmetric. A general ellipse is given by 'a' and 'b', the semi major and semi minor axis lengths. Figure 1 shows the refraction of a ray by the elliptical surface. To calculate the slope of the refracted ray, we first bring the incident ray to the vertex keeping the angle between the ray the normal to the curve the same, apply Snell's law at the vertex point A and then bring it back to the point of incidence P. Each of these step is a transformation as described in step (c) above. Let X_0 be the vector representing the incident ray. Let T_0 represent the rotation of the point of incidence to the vertex (a transformation matrix), (the result of this transformation is represented by the dashed line - - - - - - in the figure), T_1 a transformation matrix representing Snell's Law (dashed line -------), T_2 the rotation matrix back to the point of incidence (the thick line ▬▬▬▬). Let X represent the refracted ray. Then we have $X=T_2T_1T_0X_0$ (Figure 1 shows the results of all these various transformations). Doing the algebra and restricting the calculations to the 5th order, we get

$$U = k_1(\mu - 1)X_0 + \mu U_0 + A_1 X_0^2 \overline{X}_0 + A_2 X_0^2 \overline{U}_0 + A_3 X_0 \overline{X}_0 U_0 + A_4 X_0 U_0 \overline{U}_0 + A_5 \overline{X}_0 U_0^2 + A_6 U_0^2 \overline{U}_0$$
$$+ B_1 X_0^3 \overline{X}_0^2 + B_2 X_0^3 \overline{U}_0^2 + B_3 X_0^3 \overline{X}_0 \overline{U}_0 + B_4 X_0^2 \overline{X}_0^2 \overline{U}_0 + B_5 X_0^2 U_0 \overline{U}_0^2 + B_6 X_0^2 \overline{X}_0 U_0 \overline{U}_0$$
$$+ B_7 X_0 \overline{X}_0 U^2 \overline{U} + B_8 U_0^3 \overline{U}_0^2 + B_9 \overline{X}_0^2 U_0^3 + B_{10} \overline{X}_0 U_0^3 \overline{U}_0 + B_{11} X_0 \overline{X}_0^2 \overline{U}_0^2 + B_{12} X_0 U_0^2 \overline{U}_0^2$$

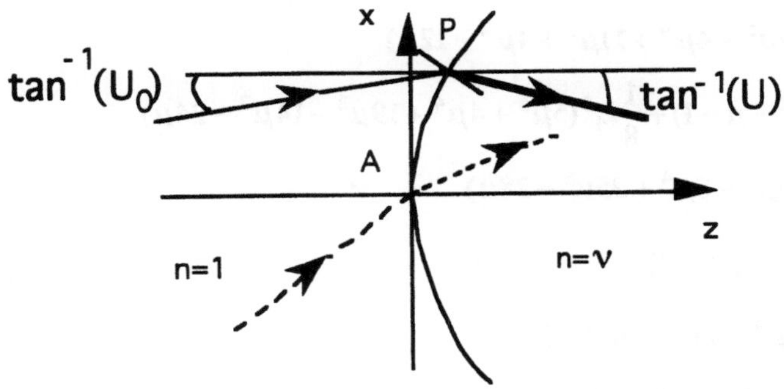

Figure 1: Refraction of a ray by an elliptical surface. See text for details.

where the bars over the letters denote complex conjugates, $X_0 = x_0 + iy_0$, $\mu = 1/\nu$ where ν is the refractive index of the medium to the right of the surface (to the left we assume the medium to be air, hence refractive index is 1), $U_0 = u_0 + iv_0$ is the complex slope of the incident ray, (similarly $U = u + iv$, the complex slope of the refracted ray), $k_1 = a/b^2$, and A_i-s and B_i-s are the various third and fifth order aberration co-efficients respectively which are polynomials in k_1 and μ. (We have used complex numbers for simplifying the mathematics). We list below these coefficients.

$$A_1 = (\mu - 1)(k_3 + \frac{k_1^3}{2}) + (\mu^2 - 4\mu + 2)\mu \frac{k_1^3}{4}$$

$$A_2 = (\mu - 2)\mu^2 \frac{k_1^2}{4}$$

$$A_3 = (\mu^2 - 3\mu + 1)\mu \frac{k_1^2}{4}$$

$$A_4 = A_5 = (\mu - 2)\mu^2 \frac{k_1}{4}$$

$$A_6 = (\mu^2 - 2)\frac{\mu}{4}$$

where $k_3 = (b^2 - a^2)\frac{a}{2b^6}$ and with $k_5 = (b^4 - 2a^2b^2 + a^4)\frac{3a}{8b^{10}}$

$$B_1 = k_5(\mu - 1) - \frac{3}{2}k_3 k_1^2(2\mu^2 - 3\mu + 1) + \frac{1}{8}k_1^5(5\mu^5 - 4\mu^4 + 8\mu^3 - 12\mu^2 + 14\mu - 3)$$
$$+ \frac{3}{4}k_3 k_1 \mu(\mu^2 - 2) + \frac{3}{8}k_1^4 \mu(\mu^2 - 2)$$

$$B_2 = \frac{1}{16}k_1^3\mu(10\mu^4 - 4\mu^3 + 5\mu^2)$$
$$B_3 = \frac{1}{2}k_3k_1(\mu^3 - 2\mu^2 - 2\mu + 2) + \frac{1}{16}k_1^4(10\mu^5 - 8\mu^4 + 21\mu^3 - 16\mu^2 - 4\mu)$$
$$B_4 = \frac{1}{2}k_3k_1\mu(2\mu^2 - 5\mu + 2) + \frac{1}{16}k_1^4\mu(10\mu^4 - 8\mu^3 + 30\mu^2 - 46\mu + 5)$$
$$B_5 = \frac{1}{16}k_1^2(10\mu^5 - 4\mu^4 + 11\mu^3 + 4\mu^2 - 12\mu)$$
$$B_6 = \frac{1}{2}k_3\mu(\mu^2 - \mu - 1) + \frac{1}{8}k_1^3(5\mu^5 + 4\mu^4 + 19\mu^3 - 14\mu^2 - 24\mu)$$
$$B_7 = \frac{1}{16}k_1^2(10\mu^5 - 8\mu^4 + 25\mu^3 - 28\mu)$$
$$B_8 = \frac{1}{8}\mu(5\mu^4 - 2\mu^2 + 3)$$
$$B_9 = \frac{1}{8}k_1^2\mu(5\mu^4 - 2\mu^3 + 5\mu^2 - 5)$$
$$B_{10} = \frac{1}{8}k_1^2\mu(5\mu^4 - 2\mu^3 + \mu^2 + 4\mu - 3)$$
$$B_{11} = \frac{1}{4}k_3\mu^2(\mu - 2) + \frac{1}{16}k_1^3\mu(10\mu^4 - 8\mu^3 + 13\mu^2 - 20\mu + 12) + \frac{1}{4}k_1\mu(\mu^2 - 2)$$
$$B_{12} = \frac{1}{8}k_1\mu(5\mu^4 - 2\mu^3 + \mu^2 + 4\mu - 3)$$

Discussion

We have outlined in this paper a matrix algebra to perform nonlinear calculations. We wish to stress that this approach is valid only to those physical systems the states of which can be represented as vectors in some suitable vector space. As an example we have applied the technique to the calculation of aberration co-efficients of an elliptical surface. Since the cornea can be modeled as an ellipse [4], this formalism is suitable for studying corneal aberration and can be extended to study aberrations due to, for example, corneas which have undergone RK procedures [5].

References

1. Gerrard A, Burch JM,.Introduction to matrix methods in Optics. Mineola, NY: Dover Publications, 1994.
2. Kondo M, Takeuchi Y. Matrix method for nonlinear transformation and its application to an optical lens system. J Opt Soc Am A 1996; 13(1): 71-89.
3. Lakshminarayanan V, Varadharajan S. Ray vector fields and representation of spherocylindrical lenses. Optom Vis Sci 1995; 72:396-402.
4. Lotmar W. Theoretical eye models with aspherics. J Opt Soc Am 1971; 61(11):1522-29.
5. Applegate RA, Howland HC, Buettner J, Cottinghan Jr AJ,Sharp RP,Yee KW. Corneal aberrations before and after Radial Keratotomy (RK) calculated from videokeratometric measurements. Vision Science and its Application, Technical Digest Series, Vol 2. Washington DC: Optical Society of America, 1994:62-66.

RESIDUAL STRESS IN PRK OPERATED CORNEA AND EVALUATION OF THE RETINAL IMAGE

H. OHZU[1], M.H. KHIN[1], M. MORI[1] and T. HATADA[2]
[1]*Dept of Applied Physics, Waseda University, 3-4-1 Ookubo, Shinjikuku, Tokyo 169, JAPAN*
[2]*Dept of Photo-optical Engineering, Tokyo Institute of Polytechnics, 1583 Iiyama, Atsugi, Kanagawa 243-02, JAPAN.*

Abstract

During and after PRK procedures on a cornea, both the deformation of the surface and the stress changes in the cornea should be carefully observed. This paper will report some clinical examples showing qualitatively the stress distribution changes in PRK operated cornea and the calculated retinal images due to the deformation of the corneal surfaces.

Introduction

Corneal area ablations in photorefractive keratectomy (PRK) procedures using the 193 nm excimer laser has been studied with cow [1] and human [2-4] eyes. The results have shown that excimer laser treatment of the cornea could be both safe and effective. However, during and after the PRK procedure, there are only limited data on stress changes in the cornea.

Since optical birefringence of the cornea is well known [5], by using a modified fundus camera, we measured the polarization patterns of several living eyes. We found that the stress conditions of the right and left eyes are, in general, not identical [6,7]. This measurement technique is very sensitive for detecting the stress distribution in a cornea due to deformation.

We report herein the results of not only the deformation of the surface but also the stress changes in the cornea, during and after the PRK procedure. The effect of the deformation of the corneal surface on the retinal image is also reported.

Methods and Subjects

A modified fundus camera was developed for the measurement of polarization characteristics of the overall ocular area. A set of polarizer and analyzer was inserted in the optical system so that it varies the state of polarization in the illumination and observation [6,7]. The output images were transferred to an Apple Power Macintosh computer on which the image processing and analysis were performed using the IP Lab Spectrum Program (Signal Analytic Corp., USA).

The 193 nm excimer laser apparatus (EC-5000, NIDEK Co., Ltd., Japan) was fully computerized and the scanning beam on the cornea created a smooth ablation surface. Laser delivery parameters were automatically calculated by entering the basic data. During the ablation procedure, the computer continuously monitored all the parameters of the operating system. Ablated areas were 6.0 mm in diameter for patients.

The PRK operated corneas from 12 eyes were studied with this method. This paper reports clinical examples from two subjects (OK; ablation thickness: 145.4mm, operated time: 83sec, and YJ; ablation thickness: 152.5mm, operated time: 87sec respectively). Qualitative changes of stress distribution in the cornea after PRK operation, and retinal images estimated due to the deformation of the corneal surface are shown.

Results and Discussion

1. Refractive data and Astigmatism: Table 1 shows refraction and astigmatism data for each subject pre- and post-operatively at 1 week and 4 weeks. One month after surgery, refractive data indicated significant flattening. However, astigmatism was not substantially affected by PRK, based on measurements of refractive and keratometric cylinders (Table 1). Observation of corneal polarization effect in both subjects, 4 weeks postoperatively showed that a significant residual stress remained.

Table 1. Changes in refractive data and astigmatism from preoperative to postoperative visits

Subjects	Preoperative	Attempted Correction	Postoperative (D)	
Name/Sex/Age	Refraction/Astigmatsim	Refraction/Astigmatsim	Refraction/Astigmatsim	
(yrs)	(D)	(D)	1wk	4wk
OK/F/36	-13.00/-2.25	+10.00/+2.00	+2.25/-2.00	+0.25/-5.75
YJ/M/32	-9.50/-4.75	+8.00/+4.50	+3.00/-3.75	+0.00/-1.75

2. Changes in stress distribution: Figure 1(a) shows the changes in corneal polarization patterns before and after PRK for subject OK, and 1(b) demonstrates the polarization patterns pre- and post-operatively at different thicknesses, respectively. Arrows in the figure show the change of ring pattern in the corneal thickness following PRK. The postoperative cornea in the peripheral area shows a clearly different polarization pattern from that pre-operatively because of changes in stress distribution after PRK procedure (Figure 2). In other words, when the central cornea had been deeply excised, normal polarization patterns [6,7] are lost, and a significant residual stress due to PRK operation remains. These results demonstrate that excision of the central cornea affects stress over the entire corneal surface which suggests not only the eye refraction but also the image quality on the retina (for example, the MTF) may change significantly. The changes may also show a different degree of astigmatism [8].

In conclusion, as the PRK may cause pressure (stress) over the entire cornea, careful decisions should be made before PRK surgery on a patient.

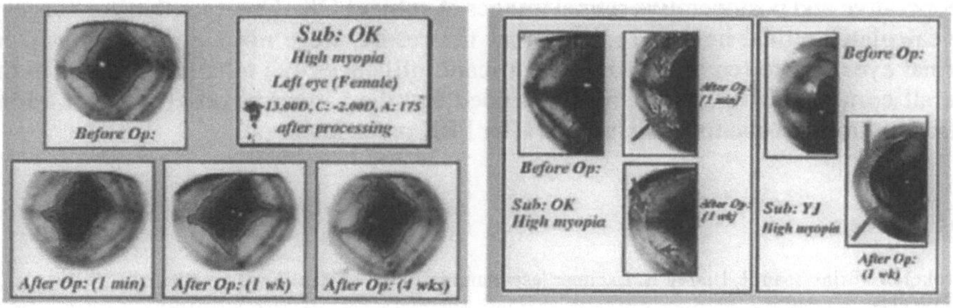

(a) (b)

Figure 1. (a) Changes in corneal polarization patterns before and after PRK (subject OK) (b) Polarization patterns pre- and post surgically at different thicknesses.

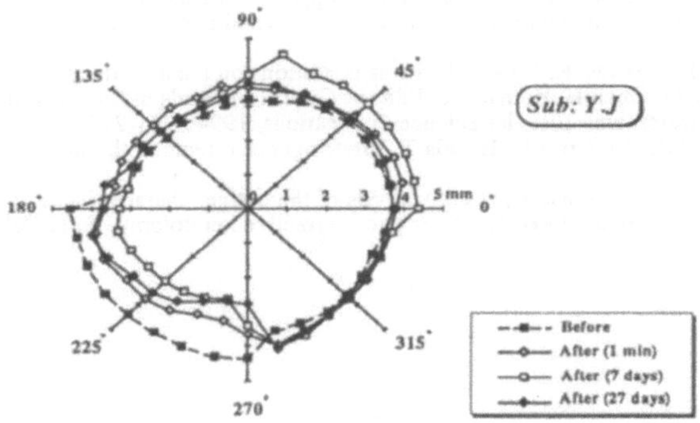

Figure 2. The changes in peripheral corneal polarization patterns before and after PRK.

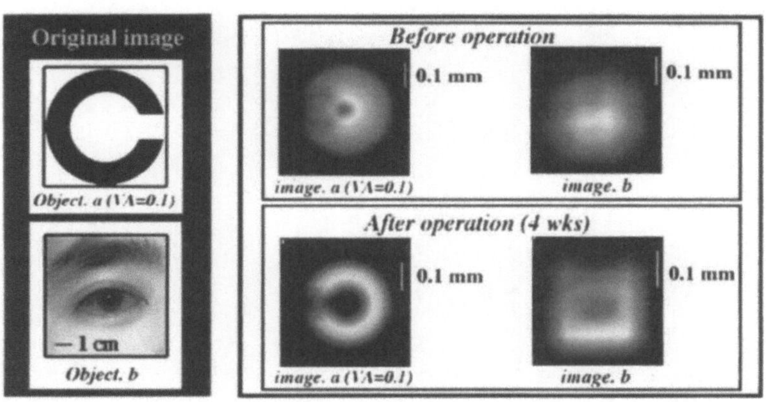

Figure 3. The calculated retinal images pre- and post-operatively (subject OK).

3. Calculated retinal images: The calculated retinal images were generated by ray-trace analysis of some PRK operated human eye optical data. Figure 3 shows the calculated preoperative and postoperative retinal images of subject OK. One month after surgery, the calculated retinal images indicate that the results were not similar to that from normal eyes. There remained some significant influences due to strain changes in the overall cornea. It is, therefore, recommended that the patient be observed over a long period of time and continuously treated after PRK procedures.

References

1.Trokel SL, Srinivasan R, Braren B. Excimer laser surgery of the cornea. Am J Ophthalmol 1983; 96:710-715.
2.McDonald MB, Frantz JM, Klyce SD, et al. Central photorefractive keratotomy for myopia: The blind eye study. Arch Ophthalmol 1990; 108: 799-808.
3.Sher NA, Barak M, Daya S, et al. Excimer laser photorefractive keratotomy in high myopia. Arch Ophthalmol 1992; 110: 935-943.
4.Wilson SE, Klyce SD, McDonald MB, Liu JC, Kaufman HE. Changes in corneal topography after excimer laser photorefractive keratotomy for myopia. Ophthalmology 1991; 98: 1339-1347.
5.Stanworth A, Naylor EJ. The polarization optics of the isolated cornea. Br J Ophthalmol 1950; 34: 201-211.
6.Khin MH, Ohzu H, Ishikawa K, Hatada T. Stress conditions on the human eye measured by corneal polarization effects. In: Ohzu H, Komatsu S, Editors. Optical Methods in Biomedical and Environmental Sciences. Vol III. Amsterdam: Elsevier Science Publications, 1994: 211-215.
7.Ichihashi Y, Khin MH, Ishikawa K, Hatada T. Birefringence effects of the in vivo cornea. Opt Engg 1995; 34: 693-700.
8.Khin MH, Yoshida Y, Nakayasu K, et al. Analysis of the optical characteristics of the cornea after surgery: Effect on the cornea of excimer laser photorefractive keratotomy. Folia Ophthalmol Jpn 1996; 47: 57-64.

THE ROTATING DANDELION: A NEW ENTOPTIC PHENOMENON?

LOTHAR SPILLMANN,
Institute of Biophysics and Radiation Biology,
University of Freiburg,
Hansastrasse 9, 79104 Freiburg, GERMANY.

Abstract

The star-like pattern perceived around a bright point source and its rotation with head tilt are attributed to diffraction within the vitreous body.

The phenomenon:

When looking at a bright point source such as a clear electric bulb, one perceives a corona of crisp, densely spaced, rays emanating from the filament. My 9 year old daughter likened it to a *Pusteblume* or puffball, hence the dandelion effect. The phenomenon is reminiscent of the ancient artists' rendition of stars, in which the radiating lines were thought to be of stellar origin. Of course, we now know that these arise in the eye, easily demonstrated by placing an occluder between the "rays" and the observer. The scattered rays are visible on the occluder.

The dandelion effect was possibly described as early as 1801 by Thomas Young (see Figure 29, Plate VI of reference 1; personal communication by Nick Wade). It is easily observed in department stores and art galleries where bright, small iodine lamps are frequently used, but also in distant street lights and car headlights. Minnaert [2] writes: "When the glaring lights of a motorcar a long way off shine towards us, we can see the entire field of view around the intense point of light covered by a haze of light, which is speckled, and sometimes striped radially." Although a dark uniform background is favorable, the effect is also observed during daylight. It is most spectacular when the sun is reflected from the curved window of a car. Long brilliant rays will be seen "streaming out to a distance of several degrees from the centre" [3].

The rays number anywhere between 150 and 300, and they are about equally bright. Their length varies in proportion to the observation distance. Simpson [3] using aperture sizes from 2-4 mm in diameter found that the largest angular size for which the rays were still perceived was about 20 min arc in each case. Although luminance is an important parameter, a systematic study on the visibility and length of the rays has not been conducted to the best of my knowledge. The dependence on wavelength has also not been investigated. It should be noted, however, that with a monochromatic light (Sodium,589 nm) source, instead of rays, a pattern of spots is seen [3].

Curiously, with a brisk head tilt the entire corona will appear to rotate slowly in the same direction (by as much as 150 deg), come to a stop and then counterrotate (but not all the way). There is a brief delay before the rotation sets in followed by a longer delay preceding the counterrotation. What may be the origin of this phenomenon? Let us examine the possible sources of the radial rays and their perceived rotation one by one.

Torsional eye movements: Counter-rolling of the eyes can be ruled out as a potential explanation because it would occur in the opposite direction and would traverse a much smaller angular extent.

Cornea: The cornea is known to be the origin of several entoptic phenomena which are circular, due to the roughly circular shape of the corneal epithelial cells. There is the well known theorem in diffraction called Babinet's principle which says that the diffraction effects of many small apertures superimpose into a single pattern [4]. However, what I describe here is a starlike appearance of the pattern, not a concentric halo. The tearfilm may be similarly ruled out as it is unclear how it would cause rotation of the phenomenon under consideration.

Pupil: Let us assume the phenomenon originates by diffraction from the serrated edge of the iris. One can eliminate the iris shape by using a very smooth round artificial pupil. If this is done, the ray structure should disappear. Indeed, when the pupil is dilated to 8 mm in diameter and a 2 mm artificial pupil is then placed in front of the eye, the strength of the radial rays is much weaker than in the nondilated eye. This may suggest that the effect arises from the less than perfect edge of the iris. The idea that the dandelion phenomenon has a pupillary origin dates back to von Helmholtz [5] (quoted after Emsley and Fincham, [6]) who called it "ciliary corona" (see also reference 3). Helmholtz [5] mentions a corona consisting of numerous, very fine and colored radial lines which he called corona of hair lines, "*ein aus unzähligen, äusserst feinen und bunt gefärbten Linien bestehender Strahlenkranz.*" However, as in the case of the tearfilm, there is a problem with this kind of explanation: how can a pupillary diffraction pattern be set into motion by a head tilt?

Lens: The histological structure of the crystalline lens can cause radial diffraction lines and so is a plausible origin for the dandelion phenomenon. Being presbyopic I can see the rays with glasses as well as without glasses. However, the starlike pattern is clearly diminished and approaches a large round halo when I render myself myopic by looking through an additional lens of +3 diopters. Rotation under this condition is only slight. Studies by van den Berg [7] suggest that a high contrast light source scatters over more than a few degrees (see also Vos [8]). It follows that pseudophakes should lack this phenomenon. However, the rays were also reported by two elderly patients with an intraocular lens implant. More patients with IOLs should be studied. Even if the star pattern were of lenticular origin, why would it rotate when the head is tilted toward one's shoulder?

Vitreous: There remains the vitreous. Simpson [3] discusses why he thinks the "bright, fibre-like rays of light" may be due to diffraction caused by small particles (less than 10 μ) in the eye. He concludes that "The nature of these particles and their exact location in the eye are as yet undetermined."

It seems I can now suggest a location. By looking slightly off the light source, I was able to observe that the perceived rotation of the dandelion was coincident with the rotation of nearby floaters (mouches volantes) in my eye. It thus appears that the histological structure of the vitreous body or any particles dispersed therein are the source of the dandelion phenomenon. If so, the phenomenon might be expected to become stronger with age due to the deterioration of the vitreous body. This I did not find. In 50 optometrists ranging in age from 20 to 65 years, there was little difference in the number and clarity of the rays. However, the counterrotation was reported more often by the older observers. It might be interesting to look at patients who have undergone a vitrectomy.

Minnaert [2] reports parallel line diffraction patterns originating from tube-like sodium street lamps and showing fine hatching. I have not yet attempted to induce rotation of those gratings.

Acknowledgment

I thank Drs. Arthur Bradley, Gerald Westheimer, Tom van den Berg. Larry Thibos and Walter Ehrenstein for their helpful comments and V. Lakshminarayanan for his encouragement.

References

1. Young TH. On the mechanism of the eye. Phil Trans Royal Soc 1801;91:23-88.
2. Minnaert, M. The Nature of Light and Color in the Open Air. Translated by Kremer-Priest HM, revised by Brian Jay KE. New York: Dover, 1954.
3. Simpson GC. Ocular halos and coronas. Br J Ophthalmol 1953;27: 450-486.
4. Klein MV, Furtak TE. Optics. Second ed. New York: John Wiley & Sons,1986:345.
5. von Helmholtz H. Handbuch der Physiologischen Optik. First Ed. Leipzig: Leopold Voss, 1867:138.
6. Emsley HH and Fincham EF. Diffraction halos in normal and glaucomatous eye. Trans Opt Soc 1922;23: 225-240.
7. van den Berg TJTP. Analysis of intraocular straylight, especially in relation to age. Optom Vis Sci 1995;72:52-59.
8. Vos JJ. Disability glare - a state of the art report.. Commission International de l'Eclairage Journal 1984;3/2:39-53.

SAMPLING THEORY OF VISUAL RESOLUTION AND ITS CLINICAL APPLICATIONS

LARRY N. THIBOS,
Indiana University, Bloomington, IN

Abstract

Visual resolution appears to be limited by neural sampling everywhere in the visual field except the very center, where optical limitations dominate. Consequently, visual acuity represents a non-invasive estimate of the spatial density of the mosaic of photoreceptors (in parafoveal retina) or ganglion cells (in peripheral retina) of the living human eye. Recent experiments have paved the way for clinical applications of this approach to the problem of monitoring the spatial densities of neurons in a variety of retinal diseases.

Introduction

Helmholtz laid the foundation for the sampling theory of visual resolution over a century ago when he argued that resolution requires at least one relatively unstimulated neuron between two relatively stimulated neurons [1]. Although Helmholtz formulated his rule in the context of resolving two points of light, it applies equally well to the case of resolving the bars of a sinusoidal grating, illustrated in Fig. 1. Figure 1A depicts a sinusoidal grating being sampled by three rows of visual neurons. The spatial pattern of neural responses constitutes a "neural image" that represents the stimulus within the visual system. The neurons in the top row are packed tightly enough to exceed the requirements of Helmholtz's rule, the minimum sampling density required is shown in the middle row, but the bottom row of neurons are too widely spaced to satisfy Helmholtz's rule and consequently the pattern is undersampled. In one respect the neural image and the optical image it represents are fundamentally different: the optical image formed on the retina is continuous whereas the neural image is discrete. Therefore, to appreciate the spatial content of the neural images depicted in Fig. 1A, it is helpful for the reader to mentally interpolate between sample points to form an envelope of modulation. Clearly this envelope accurately represents the spatial frequency of the stimulus for the upper and middle neural images illustrated. In fact, given the proper method of interpolation [2], the envelope will exactly reconstruct the original signal provided that the sampling process is error-free and that the sampling density satisfies Helmholtz's Rule. On the other hand, if Helmholtz's Rule is violated then the envelope of modulation in the neural image will yield a false representation of the stimulus waveform, as occurs in the bottom neural image of Fig. 1A. This unavoidable misrepresentation of the stimulus due to undersampling is called aliasing.

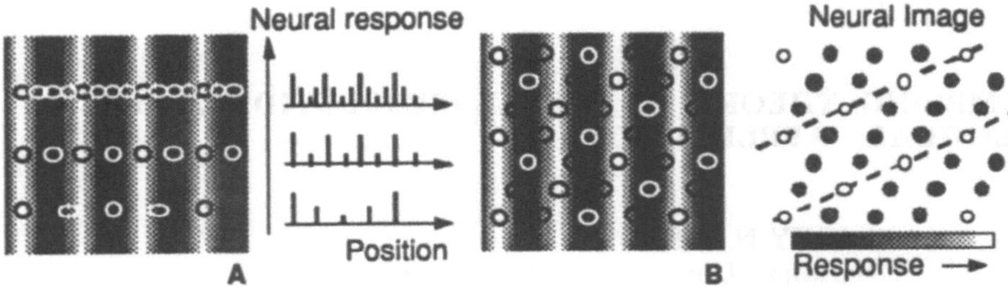

Figure 1. (A) Three sampling regimes. Top row, oversampled; middle row, critically sampled; bottom row, undersampled (B) Neural undersampling of a two-dimensional grating misrepresents orientation (dashed lines) and spatial frequency.

In short, according to the sampling theory of visual resolution, the highest spatial frequency which a neural array can faithfully represent (the Nyquist frequency) is one-half the neural sampling frequency. Stimuli beyond the Nyquist frequency may still modulate the neural image, but the resulting pattern of neural activity will misrepresent the physical stimulus as a lower-frequency alias. Thus, *the sampling limit to visual resolution is characterized by the onset of aliasing*. In the case of undersampling by two-dimensional sampling arrays, the neural image may also misrepresent the orientation of the stimulus pattern, as shown in Fig. 1B (where the strength of neural response is coded by the luminance of the circles at each sample point). For the example illustrated, the neural image indicates the presence of an obliquely oriented pattern with a lower spatial frequency than is actually present on the retina.

Evidence that visual resolution is sampling-limited

Although Helmholtz's Rule is well known to every student of visual science, until relatively recently there was little evidence that the rule actually applies to human vision. That is, there was scant evidence that the tell-tale signs of aliasing accompanied the end of visual resolution as we know it. In the absence of compelling evidence

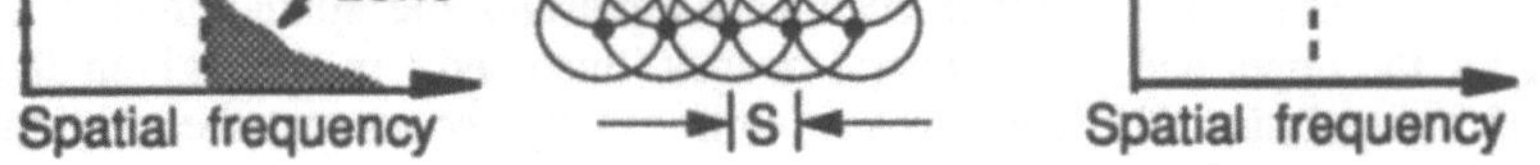

Figure 2. Filtering model of the limit to visual resolution. The spatial frequency spectrum of the object (left) is sampled by an array of overlapping receptive fields (middle) resulting in the attenuation of contrast sensitivity of the observer (right) for frequencies beyond the Nyquist limit f_N of the sampling array. Dashed curve at right excludes the effect of filtering, solid curve includes filtering.

of neural undersampling, numerous competing theories rose to prominence which implied that the sampling limit is never attained in vision because spatial filtering attenuates high frequencies, thus preventing aliasing. According to this filtering model of the limit to visual resolution, contrast sensitivity is less than the absolute threshold of unity for spatial frequencies above the Nyquist limit. One physiological arrangement consistent with the filtering model is illustrated in Fig. 2. Individual receptive fields of sampling units in this model are relatively large when plotted in object space, perhaps due to large anatomical dendritic fields or to blurring by the eye's optical system. Consequently, receptive fields overlap extensively to provide redundant coverage of the visual field. Spatial summation over such receptive fields will reduce the cutoff spatial frequency of individual cells to zero before the Nyquist limit of the array is exceeded [3]. Although aliasing is avoided in a filtering-limited visual system, the penalty is a loss of contrast sensitivity at frequencies below the Nyquist limit [4] (right-hand panel of Fig. 2). Conversely, for neural undersampling to be the limiting factor for visual resolution, contrast sensitivity must be greater than unity over a range of spatial frequencies beyond the Nyquist limit. This would be achieved by an array of sampling elements with relatively small receptive fields with a low coverage factor, as illustrated in Fig. 3.

Qualitative evidence that peripheral resolution is sampling limited is provided by reports of both spatial and motion aliasing reported independently by several groups using a variety of test stimuli and viewing conditions (see [5] for refs.). Quantitative support for the sampling hypothesis includes evidence that detection acuity can exceed resolution acuity by an order of magnitude in peripheral vision and that contrast sensitivity is much greater than unity at the resolution limit [5]. Saturation of resolution acuity as contrast increases is additional evidence that peripheral resolution is limited by undersampling [5]. Finally, the close correlation between psychophysical and anatomical estimates of sampling density of the cone mosaic in the parafoveal retina [6] and the ganglion cell mosaic in the periphery [7] suggests that not only is visual resolution sampling-limited, the limiting array is in the retina itself.

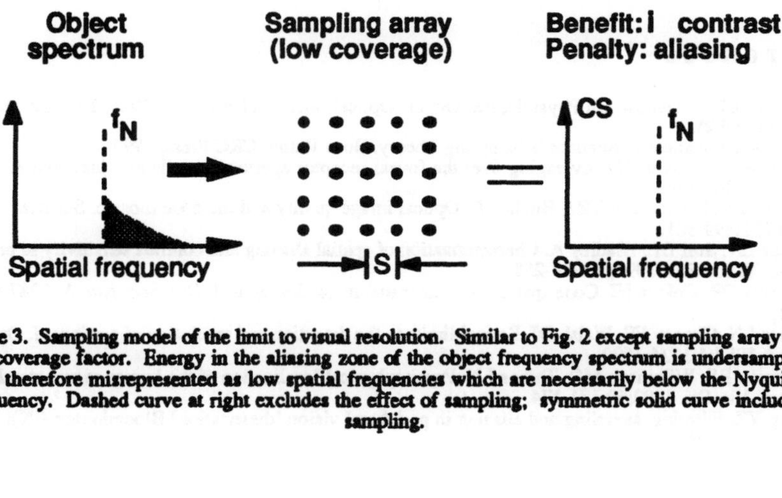

Figure 3. Sampling model of the limit to visual resolution. Similar to Fig. 2 except sampling array has low coverage factor. Energy in the aliasing zone of the object frequency spectrum is undersampled and therefore misrepresented as low spatial frequencies which are necessarily below the Nyquist frequency. Dashed curve at right excludes the effect of sampling; symmetric solid curve includes sampling.

Clinical applications

The rationale for clinical applications of the sampling theory of resolution is that acuity, when measured with a sampling-limited task, is an estimate of the density of retinal neurons. Clinical exploitation of this approach for the detection and monitoring of photoreceptor loss in central retina, or ganglion cell loss in peripheral retina, will require additional research to determine the sensitivity of the technique to various clinical conditions. Experience with normal observers gives us reason to be optimistic since even subtle features of retinal anatomy such as naso-temporal asymmetry and the visual streak, a region of slightly elevated density of retinal ganglion cells near the horizontal meridian, are revealed by peripheral acuity measurements [8]. Another concern is whether the measurement of resolution acuity using a sampling-limited technique is reliable enough for clinical use. For trained subjects, changes in acuity as small as 10% are measurable [5] but the reliability of measurements obtained from untrained patients remains to be discovered. Whether it is necessary to correct the sizable refractive errors of the peripheral field in order to achieve sampling-limited performance must also be determined. Recent experiments have shown that although detection acuity varies strongly with defocus, resolution acuity for high contrast targets is robust against refractive blur, being independent of defocus over a range of several diopters [9]. This suggests that careful correction of peripheral refractive error may not be necessary in practice, provided targets are of high contrast and approximately in focus. Fortunately there is a built in check to see if close enough is good enough: so long as detection acuity exceeds resolution acuity, aliasing is indicated and we infer that resolution remains sampling limited. Optimal target configuration and psychophysical methods for clinical work also need to be determined by future research.

In short, much work remains to be done to develop these emerging ideas from laboratory science into useful tools for patient care. There could be no more auspicious time to begin that work than now, at this celebration of the career of Jay Enoch.

References

1. Helmholtz HV. Treatise On Physiological Optics. Optical Society of America, 1924, 1911:32. (Southall JPC, ed. vol 2).
2. Zayed AI. Advances in Shannon's Sampling Theory. Boca Raton: CRC Press, 1993.
3. Miller WH, Bernard GD. Averaging over the foveal receptor aperture curtails aliasing. Vision Res. 1983;23:1365-1369.
4. Snyder AW, Bossomaier TRJ, Hughes A. Optical image quality and the cone mosaic. Science 1986;231:499-501.
5. Thibos LN, Still DL, Bradley A. Characterization of spatial aliasing and contrast sensitivity in peripheral vision. Vision Res. 1996;36:249-258.
6. Williams DR, Coletta NJ. Cone spacing and the visual resolution limit. J. Opt. Soc. Am. A. 1987;4:1514-1523.
7. Thibos LN, Cheney FE, Walsh DJ. Retinal limits to the detection and resolution of gratings. J. Opt. Soc. Am. A 1987;4:1524-1529.
8. Anderson RS, Wilkinson MO, Thibos LN. Psychophysical localization of the human visual streak. Optom. Vis. Sci. 1992;69:171-174.
9. Wang YZ. Filtering, sampling and aliasing in peripheral vision [dissertation] Bloomington (IN): Indiana University, 1996

A NEW METHOD FOR MEASUREMENT OF CYCLODEVIATION IN DIAGNOSTIC POSITIONS BY THE NEW CYCLO TESTS

SHINOBU AWAYA, MIHO SATO, TOSHITAKE KORA and MASASHI ARAI
Nagoya University, School of Medicine Department of Ophthalmology, 65 Tsurma-cho, Showa-Ku, Nagoya 466 JAPAN

Abstract

One of the authors (S.A.) developed the "New Cyclo Tests" in 1982 for quick quantitative measurement of cyclodeviation, in order to quantitatively measure the amount of cyclodeviation in various positions of gaze for diagnostic evaluation as well as for comparison of the deviation before and after treatment. We have found a new way of presenting a pair of halfmoons of this test in a position such that the rectilinear edges of the halfmoons are at a right angle to the visual direction without artifact.

Introduction

Among several tests or methods to evaluate ocular torsion or cyclodeviation, some methods measure ocular "torsion" which means monocular cycloduction, while others measure "cyclodeviation", which implys an addition of cyclodeviation in both eyes or a difference of cycloductions between the two eyes when one eye shows incycloduction and the other eye excycloduction with a head tilted to one side. Thus, we should clearly distinguish the words, "torsion" and "cyclodeviation", though these two words are often confused.

In dealing with cyclovertical or A-V pattern strabismus, it is important to measure cyclodeviation in 9 diagnostic positions of gaze not only for proper surgical planning, but also for correct evaluation of the surgical effects. For this purpose, one of the authors (S.A.) developed the New Cyclo Tests for easy quantitative measurement of cyclodeviation[1,2].

Methods and Materials

In this New Cyclo Tests, a pair of halfmoons, one red and the other one green are placed, facing each other at the rectilinear edges with an interval of 10 mm between them. When viewed through a pair of red-green glasses, the red halfmoon is visible to the eye with the green glass, while the green halfmoon is seen by the eye with the red glass. Figure No. 0 presents a pair of halfmoons placed exactly in parallel position at their rectilinear edges and

Figure No. 1 shows the right green halfmoon tilted clockwise by 1 degree and Figure No. 2 by 2 degrees likewise, and the green halfmoon is tilted by 1 degree in a stepwise fashion in each of the following figures. Thus, the number of the figures coincides with the degree of the clockwise tilting of the right green halfmoon (Fig. 1).

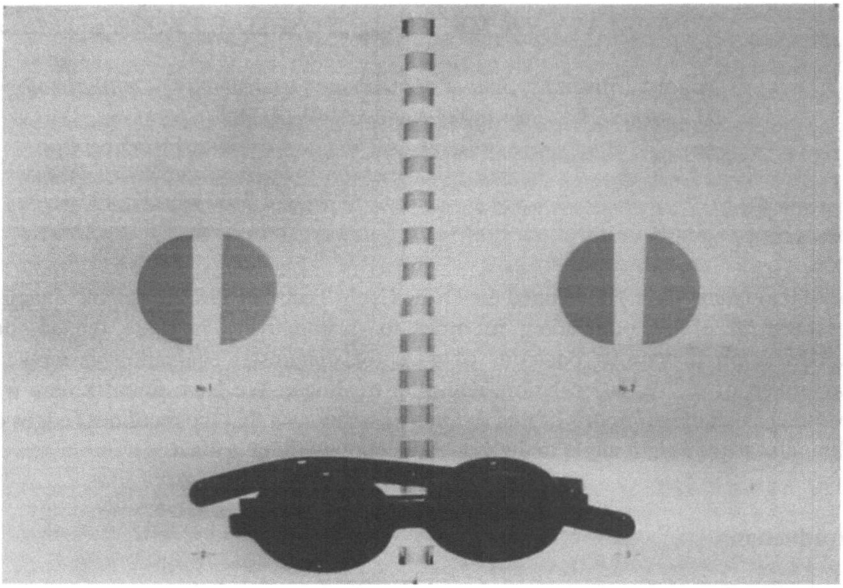

Figure 1. The New Cyclo Tests (Awaya), presenting a pair of halfmoons, one red and the other one green to be seen through a pair of red-green glasses.

When measurement is performed, it is very important to hold this test chart parallel to the frontal plane of the patient, for if the test chart is tilted forward or backward, the halfmoons printed in parallel will appear tilted aside, presenting false or erroneous evaluation. Therefore, when we measure cyclodeviation in 15 degrees upward gaze, if we hold the test chart at the 15 degrees upward position on the perpendicular wall, it causes 15 degrees backward tilting of the test chart, resulting in an artificial incyclodeviation. Likewise, if we hold the test chart at the 15 degrees downward position on the wall, the test chart will appear to the examinee in 15 degrees forward tilting, naturally causing an artificial excyclodeviation. However, we have reached the conclusion that we could measure the amount of cyclodeviation in 9 diagnostic positions of gaze without any artificial deviation, if we present a pair of halfmoons such that the rectilinear edges of the halfmoons are placed at a right angle to the visual direction (Fig. 2).

By this method we measured the cyclodeviation in 9 diagnostic positions of gaze in 12 normal subjects who had good visual acuity in both eyes, good sensory and motor fusion and no overaction or no underaction of oblique muscles.

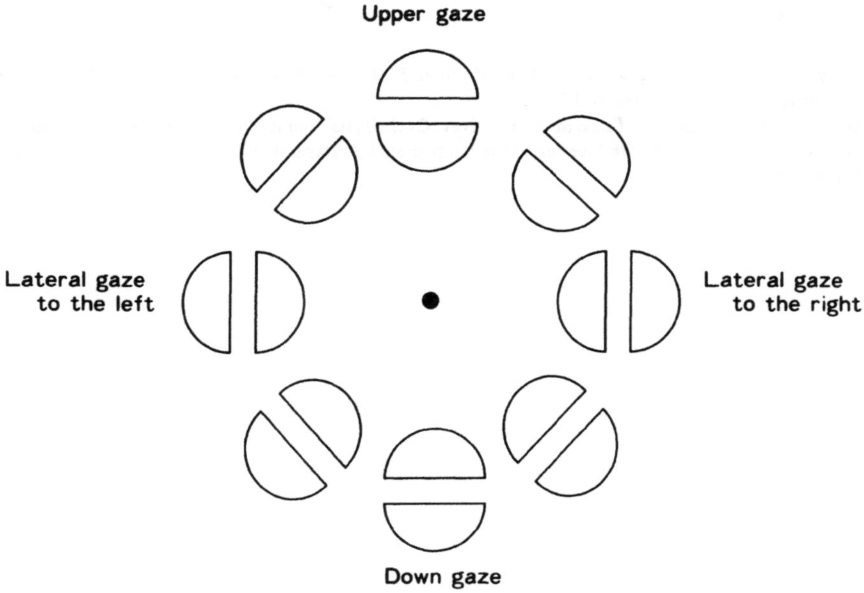

Figure 2. A method of presenting a pair of halfmoons so that the rectilinear edges of the halfmoons are placed at right angle to the visual direction.

Results and Discussion

We measured cyclo deviations in 9 diagnostic positions of gaze with upright headposition in 12 normal subjects. Cyclodeviation was essentially null in all subjects except in the three upward gazes where statistically a significant amount of excyclodeviation of approximately 1.5 degrees was observed. A slightly, less significant amount of incyclodeviation of around 0.5 degrees was observed in straight downward gaze.

When we measured cyclodeviation in 9 diagnostic positions of gaze with headtilt by 15 or 30 degrees to the right or left, in three upward gazes, a significant similar amount of excyclodeviation occurred, while a slight but essentially the same amount of incyclodeviation was encountered in downward gaze, as with upright head position.

We have concluded that this method of presenting a pair of halfmoons enables us to measure quantitative amount of cyclodeviation in any position of gaze without simulated artifact.

Summarizing these 5 sets of measurement of cyclodeviation in 9 diagnostic positions of gaze with upright head position or 15 or 30 degrees headtilt either to the right or to left, that is, 45 diagnostic positions of gaze, slight, but significant amount of excyclodeviation was observed in three upward gazes under any circumstance of head posture and a more slight and less significant amount of incyclodeviation, was observed in straight downward gaze in normal subjects.

References

1. Awaya S, Majima A, Sugawara M, Miura M, Hirai T. On the "New Cyclo Tests(Awaya)" J Jpn Assoc Strabismus and Amblyopia. 1984;10:83-86.
2. Awaya S, Iwata M, Miura M, Mizukami Y. The "New Cyclo Tests" and its clinical application. In: Campos E, editor. The Proceedings of the 5th Meeting of the International Strabismological Association. Modena: Athena Publishing Co., 1986: 225-231.

ACTIVITY OF THE HUMAN PRIMARY MOTOR CORTEX DURING MOTOR PERFORMANCE AND MOTOR IMAGERY : A FUNCTIONAL MAGNETIC RESONANCE INVESTIGATION

P. BARALDI[1], V. CETTOLO[2], M.P. FRANCESCATO[2],
M.E. DIAMOND[2], C.A. PORRO[2]
[1] *Dip. Scienze Biomediche, Universita'di Modena, Via Campi 287, 41100 Modena, ITALY.*
[2]*Dip. Scienze e Tecnologie Biomediche, Universita'di Udine, Via Gervasutta 48, 33100 Udine, ITALY.*

Abstract

Functional activity levels of the human primary motor cortex during motor performance and motor imagery were investigated by a functional magnetic resonance imaging technique, sensitive to local changes of blood oxygenation. Subjects repetitively performed three different tasks: sequential finger-to-thumb opposition movements of the right hand, mental imagery of the same motor sequence, and mental imagery of a visual scene (taken as a reference state). A significant increase in signal intensity relative to the control condition was found in the precentral gyrus during both motor performance and motor imagery tasks. Even if the intensity of activation was much less during motor imagery, these results suggest a functional involvement of the primary motor cortex during mental imagery of sequential motor acts, not previously detected by mapping techniques with coarser spatial resolution.

Introduction

Functional MRI (fMRI) is a quite new, noninvasive technique increasingly used by researchers and clinicians to study brain activity. fMRI techniques, sensitive to the local changes of blood flow, volume, and oxygenation which occur during neuronal activity [1,2], have the advantage over other brain mapping methods, such as PET, of combining a good temporal resolution, fine spatial resolution and the capability to acquire multiple scans of the same individual over varying time intervals and multiple conditions. The study of neural correlates of mental activity, such as the internal representation of sensory events or motor acts, is one of the most interesting application of fMRI.

It is currently debated to what extent brain networks activated during internal motor imagery, that is a mental rehearsal of motor acts without overt body movements, overlap those involved in the preparation and execution of real motor acts [3]. This issue has been addressed using a variety of brain mapping techniques, but even the more recent studies yielded conflicting results [4].

The aim of the present study was to assess by high-resolution fMRI the activity pattern of the perirolandic region during execution and imagery of a sequential motor task.

Methods

Twelve right-handed volunteers (4 males, 8 females, aged 20-39 years) with no history of neurological disease were studied. The experiments were performed using a 1.5 Tesla whole body MR system (Magnetom SP 4000, Siemens, Erlangen, Germany). The functional images were acquired from oblique planes including the putative hand representation area of the contralateral primary sensorimotor cortex, using a gradient-echo FLASH sequence (TR/TE=91/60 ms, FA=40°; FOV=220mm; 128x128 acquisition matrix, interpolated to 256x256; slice thickness=4mm; scan time 14 s). Two contiguous planes were investigated: the more superficial plane covered the convexity of the pre- and post-central gyri, and the deeper one the depth of the central sulcus.

Dynamic data sets were acquired in blocks of 4 images, each lasting 14x4=56 s, while subjects performed one of the three following tasks, sequentially: 1) Visual Imagery (VI) - that is mental representation of a stationary visual scene. 2) Motor Imagery (MI) - mental representation of a simple sequence of self-paced, sequential finger-to-thumb opposition movements of the right hand. 3) Motor Performance (MP) - actual execution of the same motor sequence. Subjects started the execution of the next task immediately after the end of each block. However, the functional sequence started 12 s later to avoid the transition phase of the hemodynamic response. A total of 36 images were acquired for each plane. To minimize motion artifacts, an adjustable padded head-holder was used and functional images were aligned by a software procedure based on a previously described algorithm [5]. To control for unintential muscle contraction during the motor imagery task, in a separate experimental session, performed outside the MR equipment, electromyographic activity was recorded by surface electrodes while subjects performed the three tasks in the same order as during the fMRI experiment.

Functional images were normalized by dividing the intensity value of each pixel by the mean intensity of the same pixel in the 12 images acquired during the control condition. Three regions of interest were manually outlined on anatomical images : the anterior portion of the precentral gyrus (PreCG-ant), the posterior portion of the precentral gyrus (PreCG-post) and the postcentral gyrus (PostCG).

Mean values of functional signal intensity of pixels lying within each of such regions were analyzed by repeated-measures analysis of variance (ANOVA). Activity maps were created, on a pixel by pixel basis, combining two different methods: a) correlating the signal time courses in each pixel with a square wave function [6], thus obtaining maps based on correlation coefficient *r* (possible range -1 to 1) and b) computing unpaired Student's t statistics. In both cases comparisons regarded motor imagery versus visual imagery and motor performance versus visual imagery.

Results

The mean normalized signal intensity in the three regions of interest was differently modulated during the three tasks (ANOVA: Task: $p < .001$; Task by Region: $p < .005$), and it was higher in PreCG than PostCG ($p < .005$). Figure 1 reports the mean signal time course in the PreCG-post over all the subjects. Significant higher values were found both during the motor performance task and the mental representation of the same motor sequence than during the control (visual imagery) condition (MP: $p < .001$; MI: $p < .05$). In the PostCG, a significant increase was found only during motor performance ($p < .01$).

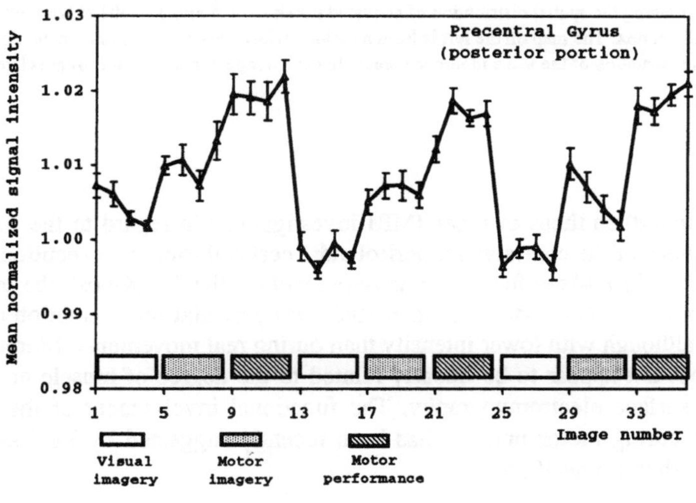

Figure 1. Time course of mean signal changes in the posterior portion of the precentral gyrus during the execution of the three tasks. Each point represents the mean ± S.E.M. (over the 12 subjects) of the normalized value of all pixels included in such region.

Representative statistical maps are shown in Fig. 2.. Activated foci were found during motor performance in the whole subject population, whereas 10/12 subjects displayed activated clusters during motor imagery. Mean extent of the activated area in PreCG-post was on average 15% as great during motor imagery as during motor performance.

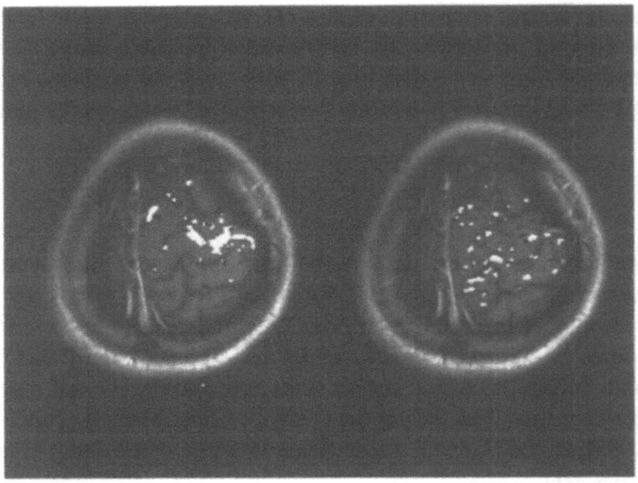

Figure 2. Statistical maps of one subject, overlaid on T1-weighted anatomical images of planes along the left central sulcus, showing the spatial distribution of activated pixels ($r > .6$ and $p < .001$ at Student's t test) in the perirolandic cortex. The map on the left is from a motor performance task, the one on the right from mental representation of the same motor sequence. In each image, top is anterior, right is lateral.

Discussion

Our results strengthen those of other fMRI investigations in regard to the functional activation pattern of the contralateral perirolandic cortex during the execution of hand movements (e.g.[7]). Mean functional activity levels in the PreCGpost, the presumed site of the primary motor cortex, are increased during mental representation of finger movements, although with lower intensity than during real movements. Moreover this activation does not appear to be linearly related to the degree of muscle activity, as recorded by surface electromyography. The functional involvement of the primary motor cortex during motor imagery has been recently suggested by PET and fMRI studies from other groups [8,9].

Acknowledgements

We thank R.Cox, Biophysics Research Institute, Medical College of Wisconsin, USA, for providing software for image registration and analyses. Supported by funds of CNR and MURST, Italy, and by a grant from Siemens Italia SpA to V.C.

References

1. Kwong KK. Functional magnetic resonance imaging with echo planar imaging. Magn Reson Quart 1995; 11:1-13.
2. Le Bihan D, Karni A. Applications of magnetic resonance imaging to the study of human brain function. Curr Opin in Neurobiol 1995; 5:231-237.
3. Jeannerod M. The representing brain: neural correlates of motor intention and imagery. Behav Brain Sci 1994; 17:187-245.
4. Decety J. Do imagined and executed actions share the same neural substrates?. Cogn Brain Res 1996; 3:87-93.
5. Irani M, Peleg S. Improving resolution by image registration. Comput Vision Graphics Image Process 1991; 53:231-239.
6. Bandettini PA, Jesmanowicz A, Wong EC, Hyde JS. Processing strategies for time-course data sets in functional MRI of the human brain. Magn Reson Med 1993; 30:161-173.
7. Kim S, Ashe J, Georgopoulos AP, et al. Functional imaging of human motor cortex at high magnetic field. J Neurophysiol 1993; 69:297-302.
8. Leonardo.M, Fieldman J, Sadato N, et al. A functional magnetic resonance imaging study of cortical regions associated with motor task execution and motor ideation in humans. Human Brain Mapping 1995; 3:83-92.
9. Stephan KM, Passingham RE, Silbersweig D, et al. Functional anatomy of the mental representation of upper estremity movements in healthy subjects. J Neurophysiol 1995; 73:373-386.

BINOCULAR CHROMATIC RIVALRY AND CHROMATIC GRID STIMULI

MICHAEL C. BARRIS
College of Optometry, Nova Southeastern University,
North Miami Beach, FL.

Abstract

Amblyopic humans have reported spatial distortions of Amsler grids while viewing them monocularly with their affected eyes. I asked 170 orthophoric observers and 20 observers with visual disabilities to view two heterochromatic but isoluminant displays through OD-red, OS-green anaglyphic goggles. Both displays were produced by equal proportions of red and green phosphors which appeared yellow through color addition. One display was a spatially-unstructured rectangle while the other was a grid with dots in each grid element. I hypothesized that spatial distortion in one eye must prevent binocular chromatic fusion of these grids when viewed through anaglyphic goggles. Forty-four percent of 116 orthophoric observers (the FUSERS) reported chromatic fusion of the spatially-unstructured display more than 50% of the time. I define chromatic fusion as a yellow percept. Fifty-six percent (the RIVALERS) reported binocular chromatic rivalry, defined as alternating red, green, and yellow percepts. Upon viewing the grid, the FUSERS decreased fusion dwell time while the RIVALERS increased fusion dwell time. None of the 8 observers with histories of strabismus reported spatial distortion of the grids viewed monocularly with the affected eye. Seven reported rivalry, one reported fusion, while three reported simultaneous perception of both red and green elements as well as rivalry. This may indicate interstimulus rather than interocular competition.

Introduction

Sireteanu et al. [1] have reported monocular spatial distortion in the visual perception of amblyopic humans viewing stimuli with their affected eyes. These stimuli resemble Amsler grids [2,3].

I have asked both ortho- and heterophoric individuals to report their perceptions of binocularly-viewed heterochromatic but isoluminant grids in order to evaluate these stimuli as screening devices for spatial distortions. We reasoned that spatial distortions in one eye must prevent binocular fusion of these grids. I have elicited no reports of monocular spatial distortion of grids from heterophoric observers. However, I did elicit reports of simultaneous perception of both red and green elements in binocular chromatic grids viewed with red-green anaglyphic goggles. This may indicate panoramic perception and the absence of rivalry and suppression in heterophoric observers [4,5].

Method

I presented heterochromatic spatially-unstructured fields and heterochromatic grids by using OD-red, OS-green anaglyphic goggles (Model BC1180, Bernell Corporation, South Bend, IN 46634, U.S.A.) to view a 345 mm diagonal color display on a video display terminal (Model CSJ4927A, Samsung SynMaster 3[a], Suwon, Korea). This display is created by the activation of red, green, and blue phosphors to produce a gamut of hues through color addition. Both stimuli were produced by a DisplayMate Video Display Utilities software program (Sonera Technologies, Rumson, NJ 07760, U.S.A.) operating on a Vextrec Model BB4DGLD Personal Computer, an IBM-clone. The spatially-unstructured display was the "bright yellow" panel of the "Mode Colors" screen of this program. When viewed at 60 cm, the full screen subtended 29.9 deg diagonally. Each of the 16 panels of different hues (ordered in a 4 x 4 square) subtended 5.4 x 3.6 deg on a white background. Blocks of red hues appeared dark when viewed through the green filter of the anaglyphic goggles while blocks of green hues appeared dark when viewed through the red filter. The GRID stimulus was the "Cross-Hatch Convergence Test" screen of the DisplayMate program with the apparent hue and luminance matched to the "bright yellow" panel of the "Mode Colors" screen on the dark background of the screen. Each of 30 vertical lines subtended 0.05 deg while each of 22 horizontal lines subtended 0.1 deg with the entire grid extending 23.5 deg horizontally by 17.5 deg vertically. In the center of each grid element was a filled circle subtending 0.05 deg.

One hundred eighty-six optometry students ranging in age from 22 to 40 years of age viewed the stimuli and reported their perceptions. Four additional observers ranging in age from 7 to 30 years of age were recruited from the college binocular vision clinic.

Each observer first centrally viewed the BLOCK for 5 minutes (This procedure essentially replicates the work reported by Breese in 1899 [6].) and then the yellow GRID for 5 minutes.

Results

When viewing the BLOCK stimulus with OD-red, OS-green anaglyphic goggles, 116 orthophoric observers reported that the chromatic percepts rivaled among yellow, green, and red hues [7, Fig. 1]. The left half of Fig. 1 illustrates the proportion of dwell time in each hue percept. Fifty-one orthophoric observers were categorized as FUSERS as they reported a yellow percept more than half of the viewing time. The remaining 65 orthophoric observers were classified as either SUPPRESSORS or RIVALERS. Of these, 6 were classified as SUPPRESSORS because they alternated between the dominant eye percept (red if OD dominant and green if OS dominant) and a yellow percept.

Thirty-seven OD-DOMINANT RIVALERS perceived yellow less than half of the time and red most of the rest of the time. Twenty-two OS-DOMINANT RIVALERS perceived yellow less than half of the time and green most of the rest of the time. Twenty observers had compromised visual systems; 8 had strabismus histories, 1 had an eye trauma history, 1 had convergence insufficiency, 1 had optic nerve atrophy, 8 had color vision anomalies, and 1 had amblyopia without a history of strabismus. Fifty-four observers reported data that could not be analyzed due to clerical errors.

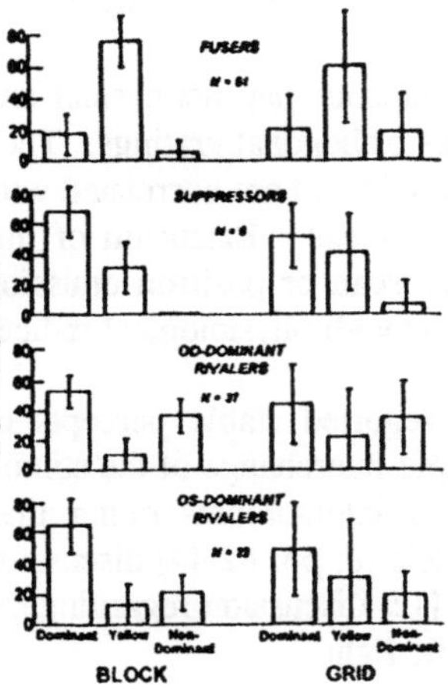

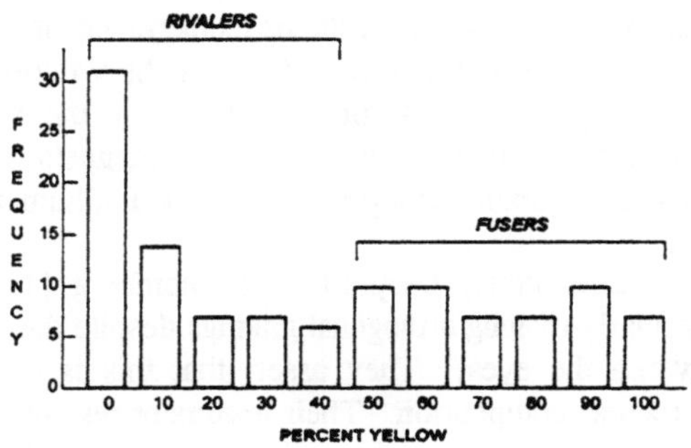

Figure 1. (Left) Mean (±1 sd) temporal dwell propotion for 116 viewers of BLOCK and GRID stimuli.

Figure 2. (Right) Frequency of observers reporting a yellow percept by temporal dwell proportion.

The dwell time proportions of red, green, and yellow for the GRID stimuli are presented on the right side of Fig. 1. FUSERS decreased the proportion of time during which they perceived yellow hues relative to their percepts with the BLOCK stimuli, and SUPPRESSORS and RIVALERS increased the proportion of time they perceived yellow hues.

Fig. 2 represents the frequency of orthophoric observers binned by the proportion of time they reported yellow percepts. The bimodal distribution suggests two populations of orthophoric observers, here classified as RIVALERS and FUSERS.

Discussion

When viewing chromatic BLOCKS with red-green anaglyphic goggles, 44 percent of orthophoric observers (the FUSERS) chromatically fuse the hues presented to each eye more than half of their viewing times while 56 percent (the RIVALERS) rival among red, green, and yellow hue percepts at approximately 40 times/minute [8]. When viewing chromatic grids under the same conditions, the FUSERS decrease their proportion of fusion while RIVALERS increase their fusion time.

Observers with a history of heterophoria report a variety of complex percepts under these conditions. These percepts include: 1) left and right hemifields chromatically rivaling at a slow (approximately 1/minute) rate; 2) field centers and field surrounds chromatically rivaling at a slow (approximately 1/minute) rate; and 3) simultaneous perception of both red and green hues without rivalry or suppression. Cooper et al. [4,5] have described this phenomenon in patients with intermittent exotropia and labeled it panoramic vision, a reference to a hypothesized ontogenetically earlier stage where the eyes were placed not parallel but opposite.

Leopold and Logothetis [9] have compared simultaneous psychophysical and electrophysiological data in rhesus monkeys viewing rivalrous orthogonal gratings. They report that a higher proportion of cells in the V4 cortical area of brain are correlated with psychophysical reports of rivalry than in the V1 and V2 areas. Extension of this paradigm to a noninvasive functional magnetic resonance scan or positron emission tomogram of brain might permit correlation of human percepts with physiological indices [10].

Logothetis, Leopold, and Sheinberg [11] have reported stable percepts of binocularly-rivaling orthogonal gratings despite the more rapid interchange of the stimuli between the eyes. They assert that this is evidence for interstimulus rather than interocular competition. Their argument resembles Breese's [6, pp. 42-44] discussion of monocular rivalry and Enoch, Goldmann, and Sunga's [12] discussion regarding the ability to distinguish which eye was stimulated by a specific light.

Acknowledgements

I gratefully acknowledge the intellectual assistance of Susanna Tamkins, O.D., Rachel Coulter, O.D., and the Classes of 1997 and 1998 of the Nova Southeastern University College of Optometry as well as the financial assistance of the Health Professions Division of Nova Southeastern University.

References

1. Sireteanu R, Lagreze W-D, Constantinescu DH. Distortions in two-dimensional visual space perception in strabismic observes. Vision Res 1993; 33: 677-690.

2. Amsler M. L'examen qualitatif de la function maculaire. Ophthalmologica 1947; 1142: 248-261. Cited in [3, p. 110].

3. Wall M, Sadun AA, editors. New methods of sensory visual training. New York: Springer-Verlag, 1990.

4. Cooper J, Feldman J. Panoramic viewing, visual acuity of the deviating eye, and anomalous retinal correspondence in the intermittent exotrope of the divergence excess type. Am J Optom Physiol Opt 1979; 56: 422-429.

5. Cooper J, Medow N. Intermittent exotropia: Basic and divergence excess type. Binocular vision and

eye muscle surgery quarterly 1993; 8: 185-216.
6. Breese BB. On inhibition. Psychol Rev 1899; 3: 1-65.
7. Wolfe JM. Resolving perceptual ambiguity. Nature 1996; 380: 587-588.
8. Fox R, Herrmann J. Stochastic properties of binocular rivalry alternations. Perception and Psychophysics 1967; 2: 432-436.
9. Leopold DA, Logothetis NK. Activity changes in early visual cortex reflect monkeys' percepts during binocular rivalry. Nature 1996; 379: 549-553.
10. Crick F. Visual perception: Rivalry and consciousness. Nature 1996; 379: 485-486.
11. Logothetis NK, Leopold DA, Sheinberg DL. What is rivaling during binocular rivalry? Nature 1996; 380: 621-624.
12. Enoch J, Goldmann H, Sunga R. The ability to distinguish which eye was stimulated by light. Invest Ophthalmol 1969; 8: 317-331.

MODELING MAGNO- AND PARVO-LIKE CONTRIBUTIONS FROM CONTRAST-RESPONSE FUNCTIONS USING NEUROMAGNETIC MEASURES

HAI-WEN CHEN, CHERYL AINE, EDWARD FLYNN and C.C. WOOD
Biophysics Group, D454, Los Alamos National Laboratory, Los Alamos, NM 87545.

Abstract

In our recent study [1], we have measured the spatial frequency (SF) tuning functions as well as the contrast-response (CR) functions at different contrast levels (from near threshold to suprathreshold) and different eccentricities of the visual field in humans using noninvasive magnetoencephalography (MEG) techniques. In the current study, the estimated CR functions and SF tuning curves were further fitted by a two-stream (M & P) model for all 4 subjects at 3 different eccentricities. The 5 parameters in equation (2) for each of the M- and P-like systems were also estimated.

Introduction

M and P pathways: Parallel pathways in cat and monkey visual systems have been studied extensively. Two major parallel pathways have been identified: (a) The magnocellular (M) pathway appears to project to much of the parietal lobe of cortex, and has been associated with analysis of movement (motion) and visual location of objects; and (b) The parvocellular (P) pathway appears to project to much of the temporal lobe, and has been associated with identification or recognition of different objects (color/form). The neurons in the M and P pathways respond very differently to various stimulus parameters. For instance, the M cells have high contrast sensitivity, prefer low spatial frequency and high temporal frequency, but are relatively color blind. On the other hand, the P cells have low contrast sensitivity, and are sensitive to chromatic contrast, high spatial frequency and low temporal frequency. Therefore, by manipulating stimulus parameters such as the stimulus contrast, spatial and temporal frequencies, we may be able to differentiate between P and M contributions in certain areas of visual cortex. Theses regions may be preferentially activated, depending upon the nature of the stimuli on the retina.

Contrast-response functions: In cat and monkey studies, the contrast-response (CR) functions at different contrast levels have been measured for M and P cells in the retina and LGN as well as cortical neurons in V1 and MT. A Michaelis-Menten-like equation can be used to describe the contrast-response function well

$$R(c) = R_{max}\, c^n/(c^n + c^n_{50}) + M \qquad (1)$$

where R is the amplitude of the response, c is contrast, R_{max} the maximum response, c_{50} the contrast at which the response reaches half of its maximum value, n the steepness (gain) of the curve, and M the dc level (spontaneous discharge). Equation (1) provides a quantitative way to describe the contrast-response relationship. For example, the parameter c_{50} can be used as an index for contrast sensitivity. The lower the c_{50} value, the higher the contrast sensitivity of the CR function will be. Although equation (1) can generally fit the measured data well, the fitting errors will be large if the CR functions are super-saturated (i.e., the response decreases when contrast increases, which may be caused by inhibition between mechanisms at high contrast levels). In order to reduce the fitting errors and to obtain a quantitative measure of the inhibition at high contrast, we introduce a fifth exponential parameter, in addition to the 4 parameters in (1)

$$R(c) = e^{-ac}\, R_{max}\, c^n/(c^n + c^n_{50}) + M \qquad (2)$$

where, a is the exponential parameter. Equation (2) reduces to equation (1) when $a=0$, and the larger the a value, the stronger the super-saturation.

Ratio of M to P cells in Retina and LGN at Different Eccentricities: It is still a controversial issue whether the ratio of M to P cells in the retina and LGN of macaque varies with eccentricities of the visual field. Some reports claim that a ratio of 1:8 does not change from the central to peripheral visual field [2-4]. However, there are conflicting reports stating that this ratio changes 10-20 times as a function of eccentricity of the visual field at both the retina [5] and LGN [6]. A recent report on the study of human retina *in vitro* [7] suggests that the M/P cell ratio ranges from about 1:3 in the retinal periphery to about 1:30 at 3° eccentricity. Their results also show evidence that the ratio of human M/P cell receptive field size increases from about 3:1 in the retinal periphery to about 10:1 at 3° eccentricity, and that the receptive field of M cells in humans are larger than those in macaques. These results suggest that the human M cells should have a higher contrast sensitivity and a lower spatial resolution than those in macaques. It is of interest to investigate this problem in the human visual system using noninvasive MEG techniques (neuromegnetic measures).

Methods

Experiments: Evoked magnetic fields were recorded with a BTi 7-channel SQUID-coupled gradiometer system in a magnetically-shielded chamber. Four subjects with normal vision participated in this study. Transient target stimuli (circular sinusoid, 266 ms duration and ~1 Hz rate of presentation) were presented one at a time in a sequential fashion to 3 different eccentricities (1.6°, 3°, and 6°) and three SFs (1.5, 4.5

and 8.5 c/d). For each specific SF and eccentricity, there were 5 different contrast levels (10%, 25%, 50%, 75%, and 99%). Please see [1] for a more detailed description of the experiments.

Data analysis: The SF tuning curves and the c_{50} values were obtained from the averaged power of the whole waveform (0-500 ms) or from a fraction of the waveform (90 ms duration around the 1st negative peak (with latency ~180 ms)). The averaged power was calculated by first taking the Fourier transform of the waveform, and then averaging the spectral power of different temporal frequencies.

For each eccentricity, there were 5 SF tuning curves at 5 different contrast levels, and each curve had 3 data points at 3 different SFs (i.e., 3x5=15 data points). To more quantitatively describe potential contributions of the M and P systems to the responses, we propose a two-stream model whose parameters were estimated by fitting the model to the data using a least-square-error program (Matlab, Signal processing toolbox). The model is expressed as:

$$R(sf, c) = M(sf)CR_m(c) + P(sf)CR_p(c) \qquad (3)$$

where $R(sf,c)$ is the response at 3 different SFs (sf) and 5 different contrast levels (c); $M(sf)$ and $P(sf)$ are SF tuning functions for the M- and P-like systems, respectively; and $CR_m(c)$ and $CR_p(c)$ are the contrast-response (weighting) functions for the M- and P-like systems, respectively. There are 3 unknown parameters (at 3 SFs) for each $M(sf)$ and $P(sf)$, and 4 unknown parameters (at 4 contrast levels) for each $CR_m(c)$ and $Cr_p(c)$. The values at contrast level 0.1 can be normalized as a unit for $CR_m(c)$ and $CR_p(c)$ (i.e., $CR_m(0.1) = Cr_p(0.1) = 1.0$). The total unknowns in equation (3) is 14, and the independent data values in the data set is 15. Therefore, we can uniquely estimate the 14 unknowns using a least-square-error fitting program. Equation (2), then, was used to estimate the 5 parameters (R_{max}, c_{50}, n, M, and a) from the obtained $CR_m(c)$ and $Cr_p(c)$ for the M- and P-like systems.

Results

The estimated SF tuning curves were fitted by a two-stream (M & P) model (equation (3)) for all the 4 subjects. The results at 3° eccentricity are shown in Fig. 1. The 1st-row in Fig. 1 shows the fitting accuracy: the minimum-square-error (MSE) is 9.3% for HWC (Fig. 1a), 5.6% for CA (Fig. 1b), 11.7% for WEN (Fig. 1c), and 6.9% for JE (Fig. 1d). The estimated SF tuning functions for the M- and P-like systems ($M(sf)$ and $P(sf)$) are shown in the 2nd-row of Fig. 1. The estimated $CR_m(c)$ and $CR_p(c)$ (the contrast-response (weighting) functions for the M and P systems) are shown in the 3rd-row of Fig. 1 as the 'o' and '+' symbols, respectively. Equation (2) was then used to fit the obtained $CR_m(c)$ and $Cr_p(c)$. The fitting curves are shown in the 3rd-row of Fig. 1 as the dashed curves. The estimated parameters in equation (2) are listed in Tables 1 and 2 [The parameter $V_{max}(m)$ (or $V_{max}(p)$) is not expressed in equation (2). It represents the maximum value of the estimated $CR_m(c)$ or $CR_p(c)$]. The fitting curves for the two other eccentricities (1.6° and 6°) are shown in the 1st- and 2nd-row of Fig. 2, respectively. The fitting results in Figs. 1 and 2 show similar features for all the 4

subjects. The ratio of the maximum values $R_{m/p}$ (= $V_{max}(m) / V_{max}(p)$) may serve as an index for the relative contributions of the M- and P-like systems. These ratios at 3 different eccentricities are listed in Table 3.

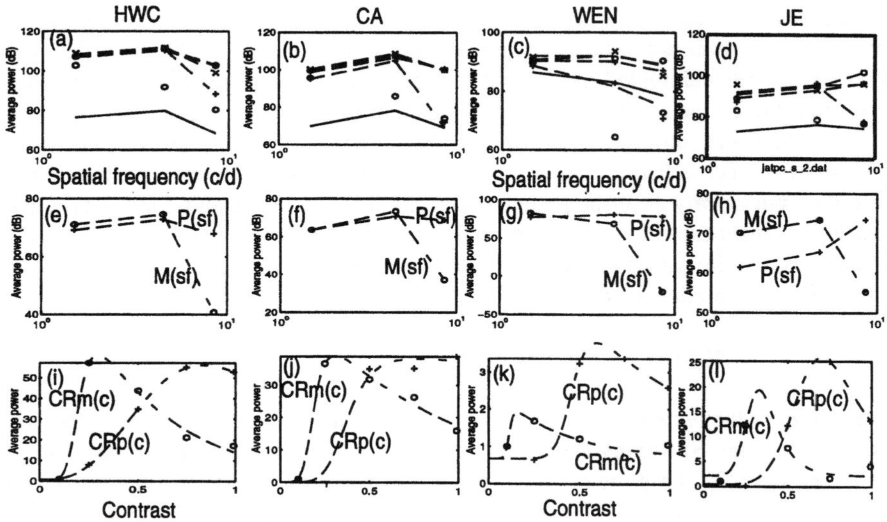

Figure 1. 3.0° eccentricity. Data from averaged power analysis (waveform duration: 90 ms; latency ~ 180ms) and fitted by a two-stream (M&P) model (equation (3)). 1st column: Subject HWC; 2nd column: CA; 3rd column: WEN; 4th column: JE. 1st row: Data were plotted as symbols; the curves were predictions from the model (equation (3)). 2nd row: Estimated M(sf) and P(sf) for the 4 subjects. 3rd row: Estimated $CR_m(c)$, $CR_p(c)$, and fitted curves (by equation (2)) for the 4 subjects.

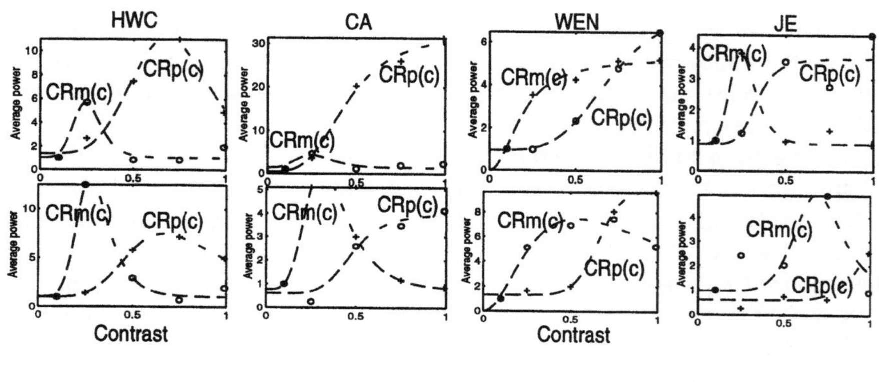

Figure 2. Estimated $CR_m(c)$, $CR_p(c)$, and fitted curves (by equation (2)) at different eccentricities. 1st row: 1.6° eccentricity; 2nd row: 6.0° eccentriciy.

Table 1. Parameters estimated from $CR_m(c)$; 3° eccentricity.

Subjects	$V_{max}(m)$	R_{max}	c_{50}	n	M	a	MSE
HWC	60	135	0.21	6.0	0.0	2.29	3.6%
CA	37	63	0.19	5.5	0.0	1.29	3.7%
WEN	1.7	2	0.11	10.0	1.0	2.74	8.6%
JE	12.5	983	0.33	7.0	2.0	10.24	9.1%

Table 2. Parameters estimated from $CR_p(c)$; 3° eccentricity.

Subjects	$V_{max}(p)$	R_{max}	c_{50}	n	M	a	MSE
HWC	57	480	0.81	3.2	1.0	1.81	0.4%
CA	39	44	0.39	5.5	0.0	0.15	6.1%
WEN	3.3	8	0.47	10.0	1.0	1.48	4.4%
JE	26	664	0.66	7.0	0.0	3.93	1.5%

Table 3. $R_{m/p}$ (=$V_{max}(m)/V_{max}(p)$) at 3 different eccentricities.

Subjects	$R_{m/p}$ at 1.6°	$R_{m/p}$ at 3.0°	$R_{m/p}$ at 6.0°
HWC	0.55	1.05	1.67
CA	0.15	0.95	1.22
WEN	0.81	0.52	0.77
JE	0.88	0.48	2.0

Discussion and Conclusions

As predicted by the two-stream model (the 2nd-row of Fig. 1), the M system shows a narrow-band low-pass SF tuning property, whereas the P system shows a broad-band band-pass SF tuning property, which is consistent for all the 4 subjects. As shown in Tables 1 and 2 (also in Fig. 2 and the 3rd-row of Fig. 1), the c_{50} value of $CR_m(c)$ (the M system) is lower (i.e., higher contrast sensitivity) than that of $CR_p(c)$ (the P system). These results are consistent with magno-parvocellular distinctions derived from single-unit monkey studies.

The results in Table 3 indicate that the techniques developed in this study may provide useful information about the relative strengths of the M- and P-like systems at different eccentricities of the visual field in humans. For three subjects (HWC, CA, and JE), the index $R_{m/p}$ is higher at more peripheral locations of the visual field (6° eccentricity). These results suggest that the M/P ratio is higher at more peripheral locations than at more foveal locations of the human retina, which supports some previous results from human [7] and animal [5,6] studies. Further analyses are needed for more quantitative studies of the M/P ratio changes at different eccentricities of the visual field.

It is worth noting that both M- and P-like systems show super-saturation at high contrast levels as evidenced by the exponential *a* values in the Tables 1 and 2, which may be caused by inhibition between mechanisms at high contrast levels. The super-saturation is generally stronger (higher *a* values) for the M-like system (the higher *a* values relate to the stronger response decreases as contrast increases in Figs. 1 and 2).

Single-unit studies in nonhuman primates indicate that different cortical areas may be differentially innervated by M or P streams. Based on our previous retinotopy studies using source localization strategies and our current results (i.e., SF tuning curves and CR functions), noninvasive MEG techniques may be able to shed more light on functions of neural groups in different cortical areas related to the two stream (M vs. P) theory.

ACKNOWLEDGMENT

This work was supported in part by a grant from NEI (EY08610) and by the United States Department of Energy (DOE) Contract W-7405-ENG-36.

References

1. Chen H-W, Aine CJ, Flynn E, and Wood CC. Spatial frequency tuning functions and contrast sensitivity at different eccentricities in the visual field. Biomag96:Advances in Biomagnetism Research. Springer-Verlag, 1996 (In press).
2. Perry VH, Oehler R., and Cowey A. Retinal ganglion cells that project to the dorsal lateral geniculate nucleus in the macaque monkey. Neuroscience 1984;12:1101-1123.
3. Silveira LCL and Perry VH. Topography of magnocellular projecting ganglion cells (M-ganglion cells) in the primate retina. Neuroscience 1991;40:217-237.
4. Livingstone MS and Hubel DH. Do the relative mapping densities of the magno- and parvocellular systems vary with eccentricity? J Neurosci 1988;8:4334-4339.
5. Schein SJ and de Monasterio FM. Mapping of retinal and geniculate neurons onto striate cortex of macaque. J Neurosci 1987;7:996-1009.
6. Connolly M and Van Essen DC. The representation of the visual field in parvocellular and magnocellular laminae of the lateral nucleus in the macaque monkey. J Comp Neurol 1984;226:544-564.
7. Dacey DM and Petersen MR. Dendritic field size and morphology of midget and parasol ganglion cells of the human retina. Proc Natl Acad Sci 1992;89:9666-9670.

EQUIVALENCE OF TEMPORAL FREQUENCY AND MODULATION DEPTH FOR FLICKER RESPONSE SUPPRESSION: PRELIMINARY RESULTS

ALVIN EISNER
R. S. Dow Neurological Sciences Institute and Devers Eye Institute, Portland, OR.

Abstract

For a wide range of temporal frequencies and modulation depths, stimulus conditions can be chosen so that flicker threshold decreases abruptly (i.e. flicker response becomes enhanced) with small increases of adaptation field illuminance [1]. At test illuminances sufficiently above this reduced flicker threshold, flicker again becomes subthreshold [1]. The adaptation field illuninances at which flicker response is enhanced or suppressed depend strongly on the temporal frequency and modulation depth of the test [1]. In the present report, data are presented to show that for both enhancement and suppression, reductions of modulation depth for 11 Hz stimuli can be operationally equivalent to increases of temporal frequency for fully modulated, higher frequency flicker.

Introduction

It is well-known that the temporal modulation depth required for flicker to be visible increases with temporal frequency across a wide range of sufficiently high temporal frequencies [2]. Thus, it might be assumed that an increase of frequency across this range generally may be regarded as equivalent to a decrease of the physiologic modulation depth of some appropriate flicker response. However, this assumption requires either a) that the suprathreshold flicker response remains linear as it ascends afferent visual pathways, or else b) that any nonnegligible time-dependent response nonlinearities be redressed or otherwise made irrelevant. Given the prevalence of time-dependent adaptation processes that can be inferred from a wide array of experiments conducted in the so-called "aperiodic tradition" [2], it would be highly unlikely for the linearity requirement to be satisfied generally. Thus, when an equivalence between temporal frequency and modulation depth does hold, particularly under conditions that exacerbate flicker response nonlinearities, that equivalence is likely to provide useful information regarding dynamic response or adaptation properties at restricted stages or sites in the visual pathway.

Although flicker response does appear to act linearly or quasi-linearly under many conditions [3], and has been exploited for this reason, the high degree of linearity appears to be achieved at a price. In particular, the useful flicker response range can become quite restricted at operationally dim ambient illuminances, with flicker response towards the end of its operating range becoming highly nonlinear, even nonmonotonic [4]. As suggested above, this constitutes a situation for which an investigation of the potential equivalence of temporal frequency and modulation depth may be especially fruitful.

Methods

Stimulus conditions and flicker-increment-threshold methodologies have been described in detail previously [1,4]. As before, the test stimulus was a 13' diameter, foveally centered disc presented for 750 msec every 2250 msec; the surrounding adaptation stimulus again was a 660 nm, 18' inner diameter, 60' outer diameter concentric annulus. For this study, the test stimulus was produced by a long wavelength LED (wavelength of peak emittance at 662 nm) combined with a 660 nm interference filter. Surround and test illuminances were incremented separately, each in 0.1 log unit steps. Full threshold vs. illuminance (tvi) curves were not obtained. Instead, to make data collection feasible for all the temporal frequencies and modulation depths that were tested, only enough tvi data were collected to determine the surround and test illuminances for which flicker threshold first decreased abruptly and flicker subsequently disappeared. Temporal frequencies and modulation depths were manipulated only between threshold excursions. Temporal frequencies for 99.5% modulation depth flicker were incremented in 1 Hz steps, starting at 14 Hz. Modulation depths for 11 Hz flicker were decremented in approximately 0.1 log unit steps, starting at 51%. Presentations for frequency and modulation depth were interspersed using an ABBA... sequence. One highly trained subject, subject TQN [1,4], has been tested.

Results

Figure 1 graphs the test and surround illuminances for which flicker threshold decreased abruptly and for which flicker then became subthreshold. Details regarding symbolism and other information are given in the Figure legend. The data may be regarded as portraying the test and surround illuminances that would define the corners of full flicker tvi curves [1] obtained for separate sequences of temporal frequencies and modulation depths. Thus, each data curve in Fig. 1 constitutes a 2-valued parametric function of temporal frequency or modulation depth. For brevity, the data in Fig. 1 will be referred to as "corner data".

Despite appreciable variation from session to session, there are important similarities among all four sets of corner data. Most notably, the data obtained as a parametric function of frequency are superimposable on the data obtained as a parametric function of modulation depth. Any differences are neither large nor systematic. The superimposition holds across all three distinct portions of the corner data curves. The superimposition holds a) at relatively dim surround illuminances where test illuminance is fairly constant, b) across a substantial range of intermediate surround illuminances where the ratio of test to surround illuminance is approximately constant, and c) at relatively high surround illuminances where test illuminance begins to level off again.

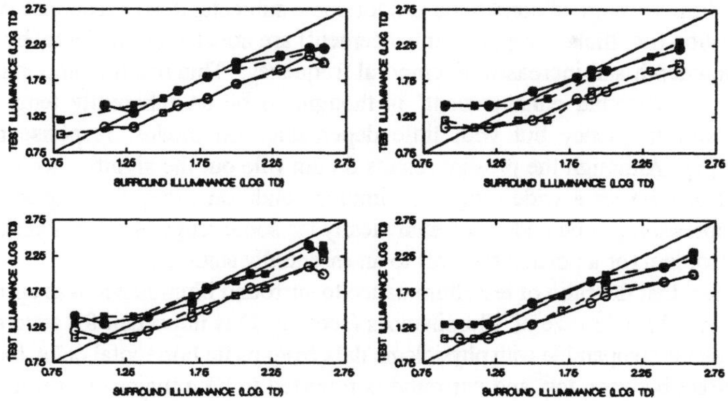

Fig. 1. Test illuminance dc component vs. surround illuminance for which flicker threshold abruptly decreased (open symbols) and for which flicker subsequently became subthreshold (filled symbols). The four panels constitute one subject's data from four separate sessions. Circles represent data for a fixed modulation depth of 99.5% at temporal frequencies of 14–20 (and sometimes 21) Hz, from lower to higher surround illuminances respectively. Squares represent comparable data for a fixed temporal frequency of 11 Hz at modulation depths of 51%, 40%, 32%, 25%, 20%, 16% and (sometimes) 13%. Axis scales differ by factor of 2.

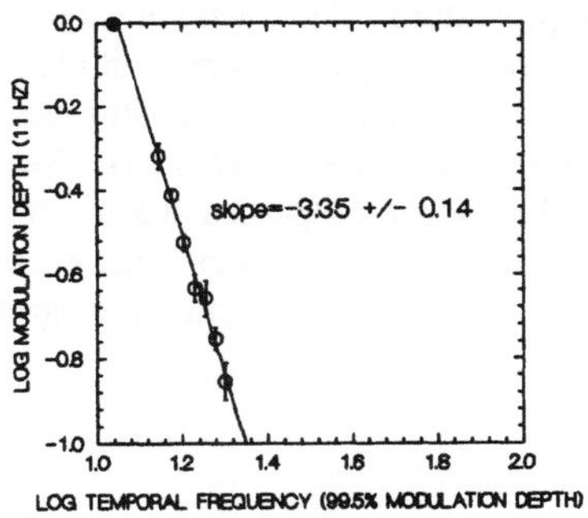

Fig. 2. Log modulation depth (at 11 Hz) vs. the log temporal frequency (at 99.5% modulation depth) to which the corner data of Fig. 1 correspond. Correspondence is based on linear interpolations of log modulation depths along the surround illuminance axes of Fig. 1. Straight line is a linear regression line derived from data for 14–20 Hz. Error bars are $\pm$ 1 standard deviation. Filled symbol represents 11 Hz, 99.5% modulation depth.

Although the curves for the two types of corner data superimpose, the frequency data and the modulation depth data might conceivably have progressed at non-corresponding rates with increasing surround illuminance. However, they did not; they are operationally equivalent. This is apparent in Fig. 2, which plots the log modulation depth (for 11 Hz flicker) vs. the log temporal frequency (for 99.5% modulation depth flicker) to which the corner data correspond. The resulting equivalencies are well-described by a linear regression line with a slope of -3.35. Note that this line nearly intersects the self-equivalent point on the upper axis that corresponds to 11 Hz, 99.5% modulation depth.

Discussion

For at least a limited range of conditions and for some subjects, flicker response suppression and its alleviation (i.e. flicker response enhancement) are affected equivalently by reductions of modulation depth and increases of temporal frequency. This result is important because "cone-mediated surround enhancement" is thought to be an inherently temporal effect, increasing with frequency but with little dependence on modest response modulation amplitudes [5]. Although the present results do not rule out the significance of inherently temporal effects across a wide range of stimulus conditions, they do suggest that flicker response suppression can be addressed analytically for some range of conditions by reducing a dynamic problem (or a portion thereof) to an essentially static one.

The fact that the ratio of test illuminance to surround illuminance was approximately constant over a broad range of illuminances (see Fig. 1) is important for several reasons. First, this result is comparable with physiologic data from turtle horizontal cells, for which the spatial contrast between test and surround is reported to be a major determinant of cone-mediated surround enhancement [5]. Since for the present study there was a gap between test and surround, it probably is more correct to say that some other illumination-dependent difference between test and surround has greater salience than actual contrast. Second, the identification of illuminance ratio as an important determinant of flicker response suppression helps to refine an earlier conclusion drawn from psychophysical data, that the dc component of the test stimulus helps cause flicker response suppression [1].

Interpretation of the linear relation between log temporal frequency and log modulation depth (see Fig. 2) now would be premature. The fractional slope does preclude the simple application of a cascade of first-order low-pass filters with identical time constants [2]. However, Cadenas *et al* [5] were able to fit small-test-stimulus data from horizontal cells by postulating post-receptoral changes to two first-order filters. The slope of -3.35 in Fig. 2 could have depended on temporal response properties entirely at post-receptoral site(s) of suppression (which presumably include(s) outer plexiform synapses [5]) only if flicker response changed steeply with test illuminance at the multiple psychophysical thresholds.

Acknowledgments

Supported by NIH grant EY05047 and a grant from Alcon Laboratories.

References

1. Eisner A. Suppression of flicker response with increasing test illuminance: roles of temporal waveform, modulation depth, and frequency. J Opt Soc Am A 1995; 12:214-224.
2. von Wiegand TE, Hood DC, Graham N. Testing a computational model of light adaptation dynamics. Vision Res 1995;35:3037-3051.
3. Lennie P, Pokorny J, Smith VC. Luminance. J Opt Soc Am A 1993;10:1283-1293.
4. Eisner A. Nonmomotonic effects of test illumiance on flicker detection: a study of foveal light adaptation with annular surrounds. J Opt Soc Am A 1994;11:33-47.
5. Cadenas ID, ReifsniderES, Tranchina D. Modulation of synaptic transfer between retinal cones and horizontal cells by spatial contrast. J Gen Physiol 1994;104:567-591.

HAEMOSTATIC EFFECTS OF THE CW-Nd:YAG LASER

FRANZ FANKHAUSER, SYLWIA KWASNIEWSKA
Lindenhofspital Bern
Bremgartenstrasse 117, CH-3012, Bern, SWITZERLAND

Abstract

Vessel occlusion may be effected as a consequence of the heating which ensues upon irradiating tissue with laser light. The conversion of radiated into thermal energy is realized within absorbing substances, the most important naturally occuring ones being melanin and haemoglobin. Both of these chromophores may play a role in photothermal thrombosis albeit by recruiting different mechanisms. In the current presentation, these two energy transfer pathways are elucidated by ultrastructural analysis of mesenteric (haemoglobin-based mechanism) and chroidal tissue (haemoglobin- and melanin-based mechanisms implicated) irradiated with cw-Nd:YAG laser.

Introduction

The Nd: YAG-, like its forerummer the argon, laser has now become an established energy source in ophthalmology. One of the principal assets of the Nd: YAG laser light lies in its great optical penetration depth, which renders possible its delivery across the sclera to such tissues as the ciliary body. In general, the effects elicited by laser light depend upon the nature of the absorbing chromophores. The most obvious contenders in the eye are melanin, contained with the neuroectodermal epithelia and uveal tract, and macular xanthophyl, but haemoglobin is also an important one. The extinction coefficients for melanin and maemoglobin are high at the principal argon wavelengths (488 & 514 nm) [1], but such is not the case with respect to Nd: YAG laser light (1064 nm), particularly not where haemoglobin and oxyhaemoglobin are concerned [1,2]. And it is for this reason that the Nd:YAG laser is sometimes considered unsuitable for photothermal haemostatis.

Methods

We have pursued this latter consideration using the following experimental set-up. In three pigmented rabbits, choroidal and mesenteric vessels of similar calibre were irradiated with a 10 W, cw-Nd:YAG laser, and the treated areas then processed for morphological analysis. Using pulse durations of 100-200 ms and a spot diameter in air of 200 mm, threshold effects (indicated by tissue blanching) were produced in choroidal vessels using pulse energies between 100 and 200 mJ; in order to elicit a similar response in mesenteric vessels, a five-fold higher input was necessary, namely one of between 500 and 1000 mJ.

Results

Choroidal vessels: Choroidal arteries (35-40 um) are characterized by a relatively narrow muscle cell layer, and adventitial melanocytes therefore lie within fairly close proximity to the lumen. The endothelium, (Figure 1) and melanocytes all evince signs of damage following irradiation. Adventitial collagen fibrils undergo a heat-induced increase in cross-sectional diameter with concomitant loss of periodicity, and such a manifestation indicates that the local temperature attained here was about 70 degree C. Within vessel lumina, partially degranulated platelets are seen to be amassed protruding many cytoplasmatic processes (Figure 2). The thrombocytes are free to move because the blood column is still in a fluid state. In regions where integrity of the endothelium is compromised, platelets build up a "psdudoendothelial" lining, delimiting the lumen from the surrounding tissue (Figure 1); in zones of contact with subendothelial collagen fibrils, their cytoplasm appears condensed. Blood flow stasis is thus realized by the formation of an occluding platelet plug, the morphological features of which closely resemble those characterizing the intravascular haemostatic plug produced at the onset of arterial thrombosis [3].

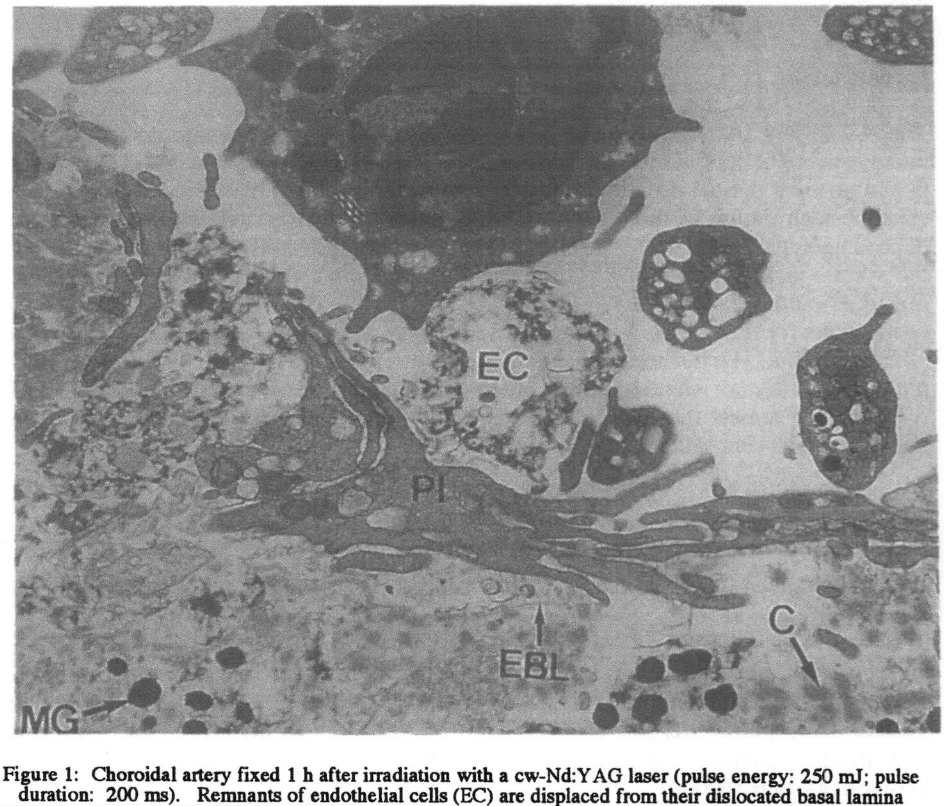

Figure 1: Choroidal artery fixed 1 h after irradiation with a cw-Nd:YAG laser (pulse energy: 250 mJ; pulse duration: 200 ms). Remnants of endothelial cells (EC) are displaced from their dislocated basal lamina (EBL) by platelets (Pl) which interdigitate with one another via long cytoplasmic processes, thereby building a "wall" against the subendothelial connective tissue. Within the surrounding connective tissue, melanin granules (MG) released from destroyed melanocytes are dispersed amongst collagen fibrils, most of which exhibit signs of destruction (C). (Electron micrograph; x 6,800).

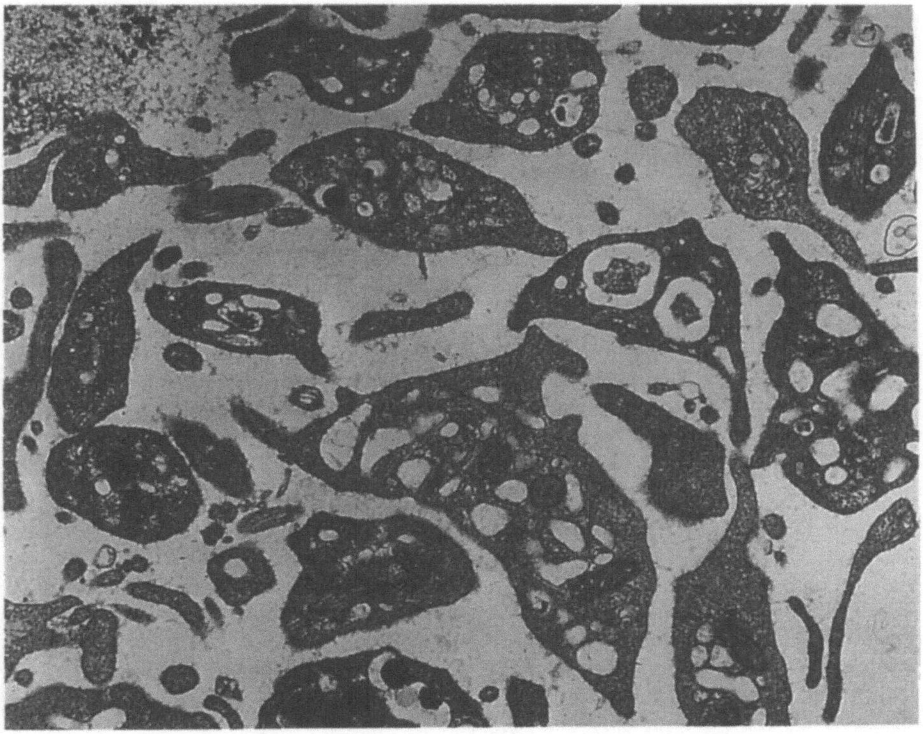

Figure 2: Lumen of larger vessels in vascular lamina of rabbit choroid 20 minutes after irradiation with Nd-YAG laser (pulse energy 100 mJ; pulse duration 100 ms). Aggregation of platelets show long pseudopods and are completely degranulated (Electron micrograph, x 9,000).

Mesenteric vessels: Blood flow statis must be effected by a different mechanism in vessels of the mesentery (Figure 3), since, owing to this tissue's containing no stromal melanocytes, haemoglobin becomes the principal absorbing chromophore. And, indeed, morphological analysis bears this expectation out. The thrombogenetic effect observed in choroidal vessels is absent. In mesenteric vessels, the lumen itself represents the absorption centre, and the temperature attained here is sufficiently high to induce precipitation of plasma proteins, which effectively form an occluding plug. Trapped within this mass, erythrocytes evincing signs of severe damage may be seen, and, in extreme cases, they are apparent only as membrane ghosts from which all haemoglobin has leaked out. Platelets are never observed within the centre of such plugs and they are presumably destroyed beyond recognition. They may, however, sometimes be seen peripherally, where they exhibit signs of degranulation (figure 3). Muscle cell filaments exhibit partial clumping. Subendothelial and adventitial collagen fibrils evince a heat-induced increase in cross-sectional diameter, but to a lesser degree than is observed in the choroid.

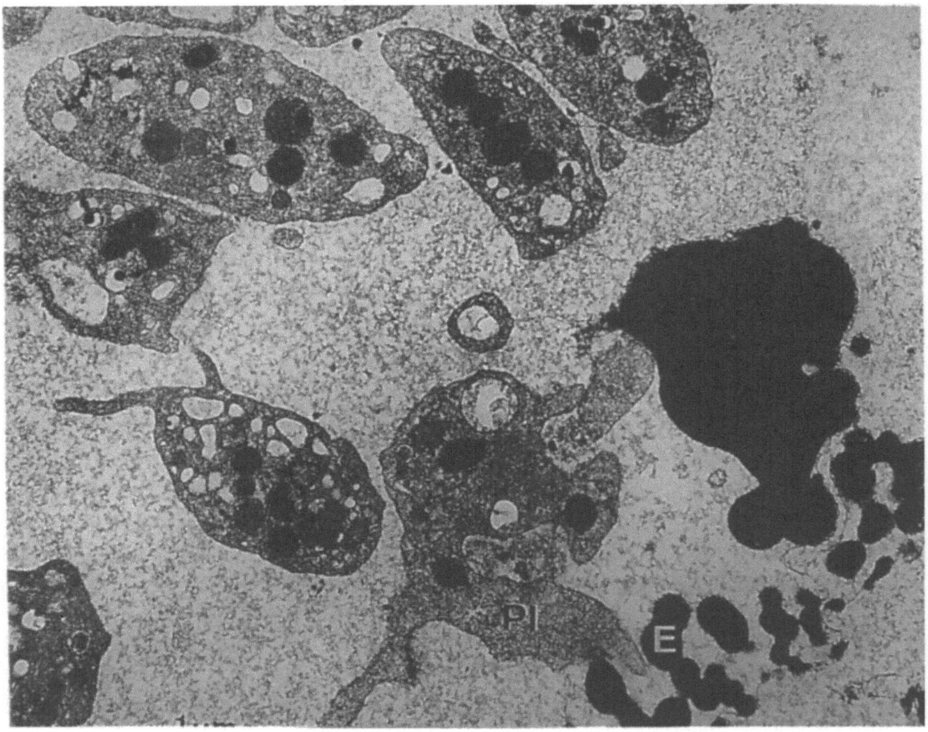

Figure 3: Lumen of mesenteric artery at periphery of impact zone, fixed 20 min after irradiation with a cw-Nd:YAG laser (pulse energy 1 J; pulse duration 100 ms). Platelets (P1) in a partially degranulated state are apparent in this region; they protract rudimentary pseudopodia which may be seen to contact damaged erythrocytes (E). (Electron micrograph; x 10,300).

Conclusions

The results presented here demonstrate that two basically different mechanisms subserve blood flow stasis induced by Nd: YAG laser light. The end result is achieved via a complexity of interrelated phenomena, which are summarized in simplified form in Figure 4.

In the first model (A, Figure 4), exemplified by choroidal vessels, blood flow stasis is induced by heat damage to the vessel wall, thermal energy being supplied by extravascular absorbers (melanin). As a consequence of this heat effect, a process involving blood platelets, and finally blood coagulation, is induced, which in every respect is comparable to the response induced by mechanical injury to the wall.

In the second model (B, Figure 4) represented by the mesenteric vessels, cellular and enzymatic processes are abruptly arrested when thermal energy is generated by absorption in the erythrocytes themselves, i.e., when haemoglobin is the major absorber. A firm vessel occusion may, nonetheless, still be achieved, provided pulse energy is increased approximately five-fold above that required to induce stasis according to the first model. In this second model, which involves an immediate inactivation of metabolic processes, the time constant is much shorter than that required to effect vascular occlusion via the classic haemostatic pathway.

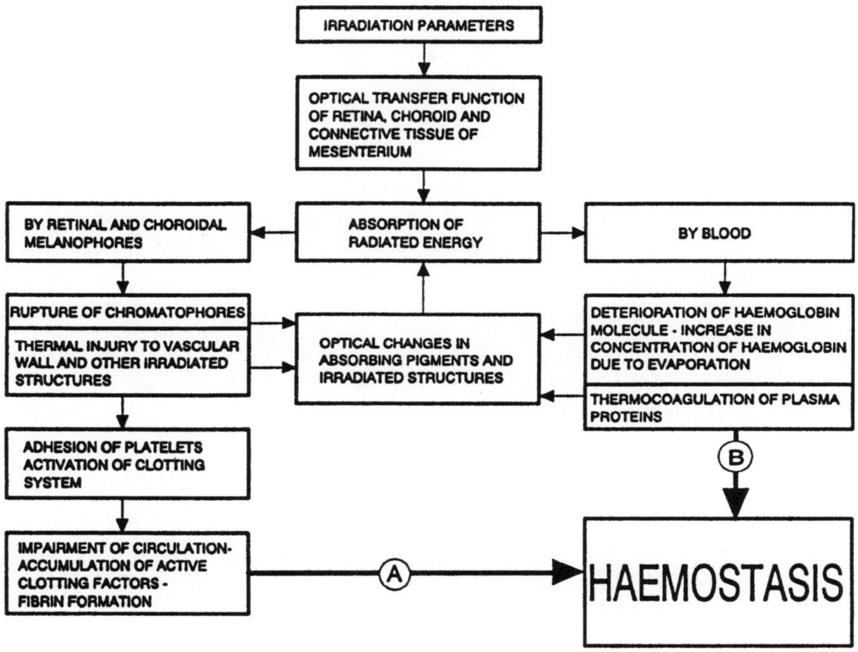

Figure 4: Scheme summarizing the various physical and biological effects operating to produce blood flow stasis in choroidal (A) and mesenteric (B) vessels irradiated with a cw-Nd:YAG laser.

References

1. Welsch H, Birngruber R, Boergen K-P, Gabel V-P, Hillenkamp F. The influence of scattering on the wavelength dependent absorption in blood. Symposium Laser Med Biol. Proceedings. GSF-Bericht BPT 5, 1977.
2. Hayes JR, Wolbarsht ML: Thermal model for retinal damage induced by pulsed lasers. Aerospace Med 1968; 39:474-480.
3. DeGroot PG, Sixma JJ. Role of von Willebrand factor in the vessel wall. Semin Thromb Hemost 1987; 13:416-424.

DEVELOPING MAGNOCELLULAR PATHWAYS IN CHILDREN SHOW REDUCED SENSITIVITY TO MOVEMENT DISCRIMINATION

Teri Lawton,
Nano Tech Services (NTS), 591 Katherine Ave, OakView, CA .

Abstract

A large number of children who have problems reading, even though they have 20/20 visual acuity, have a loss in their magnocellular or movement system, that can be measured with the CSF for brief or moving patterns. Therefore, to assess the integrity of each child's magnocellular pathways, direction discrimination thresholds were measured. The Contrast Sensitivity Functions (CSF) of a random sample of 56 students, ages 5 to 8 years old, all having 20/20 visual acuity, were measured to evaluate the sensitivity of their magnocellular pathways. CSFs for a 4 octave range of test and background spatial frequencies were measured using a temporal 2AFC task. All children had significantly lower CSFs for direction discrimination when compared with a practiced adult. Following practice, some good readers in grades 1-3 showed no difference in their direction discrimination CSFs, when compared to an adult's CSF at low test spatial frequencies. However, children classified as dyslexic had significantly decreased CSFs over all frequency combinations even after practice. Following practice, the CSFs of dyslexic readers were lowest for patterns where the test and background frequencies were equal in spatial frequency, whereas for good readers, CSFs were highest for these patterns. Arrested development of magnocellular and inhibitory pathways in dyslexic children are suggested by the frequency combinations that reveal the greatest CSF losses. In conclusion, movement discrimination develops over time, and is not present at full capacity when the child begins to read. Direction discrimination CSFs provide a definitive test for discriminating between borderline normal and borderline dyslexic children. Moreover, practice improves the CSFs of all children and adults tested, providing rapid remediation.

Introduction

This study extends Jay Enoch's approach using layer by layer perimetry in the retina to studying the magnocellular pathways in the dorsal cortical stream. We have two major goals in this research: 1) to examine the relationship between reading, that involves brief glimpses of letters between each saccade, and the magnocellular pathways, and 2) to provide vision screening at the elementary school level, enabling early detection and remediation of vision and reading problems. Recent studies [1,2] show that the mechanism used to detect brief patterns, required when reading, is one that develops over time, and is not present at full capacity when the child begins to read. These studies found that children who are learning to read: 1) have large CSF losses when detecting brief 150 msec patterns, their CSFs were 3 to 9 fold lower than an adult's CSF, and 2) have reading rates that were much faster when CSF losses were compensated for by presenting Normalized CSF (NCSF) based filtered text. Reading rates were 2 to 8 fold faster for all children tested when reading filtered text that compensates for CSF losses, than when reading unfiltered text. Moreover, mean reading rates were 3 to 4 fold faster for first grade readers and dyslexic children, instead of 2 fold faster as found for the average normal child in grades 2 and 3. Since all children have the lowest CSFs, relative to an adult's CSF when detecting briefly presented intermediate and high spatial frequencies, this suggests that all children have magnocellular and inhibitory pathways that are still maturing. In addition, dyslexic children have lower CSFs, at least 2 fold lower, than normal children to detect brief patterns. Previous research [1-3] suggests that dyslexic children have underdeveloped magnocellular and inhibitory pathways when detecting brief patterns. This study was conducted to determine whether dyslexic children also show underdeveloped magnocellular and inhibitory pathways when discriminating the direction of movement.

Methods

Vision testing was conducted on a Sun IPC SPARCstation. The screen was calibrated using a Spectra Pritchard 1980A photometer, under the same viewing conditions that were used for vision testing. A monochrome grayscale, using Pseudocolor from XWindows X11-R5, was used to display 150 msec patterns. A linear gamma function was used to increase contrast linearly. The mean luminance of the screen was maintained at 67 cd/m^2 during this study. Each child sat 57 cm from the screen, so that vertical sinewave test patterns subtended 4 deg visual angle surrounded by 20 deg circular vertical sinewave backgrounds. A total of 56 children, 5 to 8 years old: 8 in Kindergarten (K), 13 in grade 1 (7 Normal (N), 6 Dyslexic (D)), 14 in grade 2 (7N, 7D), 21 in grade 3 (10N, 11D), who were obtained from a random sample at a local elementary school, participated in this study. Only children with 20/20 visual acuity and normal intelligence, having no learning or attention deficits, participated in this study. The adult's CSF was the mean CSF of a 42 year old male and female, both adult's having 20/20 acuity and normal visual function. Initially, CSFs to detect whether 150 msec sinewave grating patterns, spanning a five octave range of spatial frequencies, from 0.25 to 8 cyc/deg, had stripes that were up-down or sideways were measured using a spatial 2AFC double staircase procedure [1,2]. These CSFs were used to assess each child's ability to detect spatial detail and to provide the image enhancement transfer function [1,2] for filtering text. Each child's reading level and reading problems were diagnosed using The Dyslexia Screener (TDS) [4] for children in grades 2 and 3, and the speed of reading rates was used to divide first graders into good and poor readers. Reading rates for unfiltered and NCSF-based filtered text [1,2] were also measured to evaluate each child's reading performance. Direction discrimination thresholds were measured to assess the integrity of each child's magnocellular pathways. Four test spatial frequencies, 0.25, 0.5, 1, and 2 cyc/deg were each presented on backgrounds consisting of a sinewave grating over a range of spatial frequencies spanning 4 octaves, each background frequency being 1 octave apart. The test sinewave grating was presented within a round fish shape, 160 pixels wide, to provide an interesting pattern. Sample patterns can be seen by connecting to http://www.west.net/~nanotech. Background patterns were always presented at 5 % contrast to maximally activate magnocellular pathways [5]. Test and background patterns were presented in two 150 msec intervals, since: 1) 150 msec prevents eye movements from affecting discrimination [6], 2) direction discrimination thresholds are equal for 150 and 750 msec [7], 3) brief durations are not detected as easily by dyslexic children [1-3], and 4) short durations speed up data collection. Test and backgrounds were presented abruptly using simultaneous metacontrast. The test spatial frequency was shifted 90 deg relative to the background spatial frequency, between the first and second pattern interval, since this is the optimum spatial phase shift for discriminating the direction of movement [7]. The child's task was to push one of two buttons to indicate whether the stripes in the test patterns moved to the left or to the right. Auditory feedback, 1 or 3 short beeps, was provided to train the child. A temporal 2AFC task was used to interactively measure each child's CSF. Following a short practice session, that set the initial contrast, the test run was initiated. A double staircase procedure [7] was used to measure the contrast required for 79% correct responses.

Results

All children had significantly lower direction discrimination CSFs, 2 to 10 fold lower, when compared with the CSF of an adult, see Figs. 1a-d. Normal children have CSFs that are 2 to 3 fold lower than the adult's CSF. Dyslexic children have CSFs that are 5 to 10 fold lower than the adult's CSF, and 2 to 4 fold lower than the normal child's CSF at the same grade level. These differences were all significant at $p<0.003$, when analyzed using Students t test for paired comparisons. For test frequencies higher than 0.25 cyc/deg, the CSFs of dyslexic children ressemble the CSFs of a 5 year old child in K, suggesting arrested development of magnocellular and inhibitory pathways.

By examining Figs. 1a-d, showing the CSFs of dyslexic (d) children, normal (n) children, and practiced (p) normal children, it can be seen that movement discrimination is a mechanism that develops over time. With one to two practice thresholds for each frequency combination, some good readers in first, second, and third grades showed no difference in their direction discrimination CSFs, when compared to an adult's CSF at low test spatial frequencies. When the background frequency was 2 octaves higher than the test frequency, all children had CSFs that were at least 2 to 3 fold lower than an adult's CSF. Lower direction discrimination CSFs for all children, compared to adults, reveal that magnocellular and inhibitory pathways are still maturing in all children in grades K-3. The CSFs of dyslexic readers were always lowest for patterns where the test and background frequencies were equal in spatial frequency, whereas for good readers, CSFs were highest for these patterns. The relative CSF when test and background frequencies are equal provides the definitive test for discriminating between borderline normal and borderline dyslexic children, since dyslexic children always have a lower CSF for these test and background frequencies. We know of no other test that can divide borderline dyslexic and borderline normal children into two disjoint groups with 100% accuracy.

Patterns having the largest difference between normal and dyslexic children, when test and background frequencies are equal, suggest magnocellular and inhibitory pathways are underdeveloped in dyslexic children. When dyslexic children practiced discriminating whether the fish stripes moved to the left or to the right, reading rates for filtered text doubled again [1,2]. Following practice discriminating the direction of movement, all children said that reading was much easier, the individual letters in a word were easier to identify, and spelling and pronunciation were also much easier. In addition, following practice, all children noticed that speed and depth discrimination had also improved. Since strengthening magnocellular pathways improves the reading performance of all children, in addition to improving speed and depth discrimination, this data provides further support that normal and dyslexic children have magnocellular and inhibitory pathways that are still maturing and can be improved by practice.

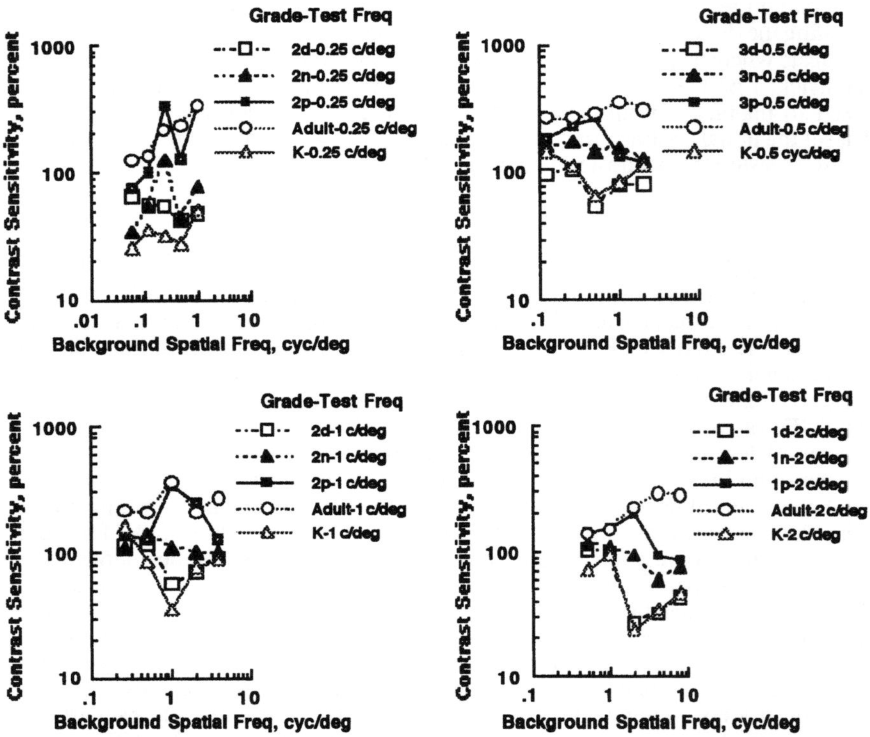

Figure 1: Mean direction discrimination CSFs for children in: grade 2 where test spatial frequency is 0.25 cyc/deg in Fig. 1a, grade 3 where test spatial frequency is 0.5 cyc/deg in Fig. 1b, grade 2 where test spatial frequency is 1 cyc/deg in Fig. 1c, and grade 1 where test spatial frequency is 2 cyc/deg in Fig 1d. The suffix d denotes the mean CSF for a dyslexic child, n denotes the mean CSF for a normal child, and p denotes the mean CSF for a practiced normal child. On each graph, the data from a single grade level is bracketed by the mean CSF of the normal adult and the normal child in K.

Discussion

It is likely that the CSFs measured in this study are determined predominantly by the output of magnocellular pathways, since the adult's CSF is determined by the output of magnocellular neurons [5] and the patterns used in this study maximally activated magnocellular neurons. The lowered CSFs of all children, when compared to an adult, that are measured when either detecting brief patterns or discriminating the direction of movement indicate that magnocellular pathways are still maturing in all children. Additional evidence that the magnocellular pathways are still developing comes from finding significantly lower flicker sensitivities, spanning temporal frequencies from 5 to 50 Hz, for 5 to 10 year olds [9]. Losses in the responsiveness of the magnocellular pathways early in development will affect all subsequent levels of processing that receive input from these magnocellular neurons [10]. For example, reduced magnocellular processing in dyslexic readers causes higher contrast thresholds not only to detect movement, but also depth [11,12]. These studies found that dyslexics have an impaired ability to see the visual direction of moving patterns, unstable binocular control, and unstable depth localization. It is likely that the dyslexic reader's poor vergence and binocular control, and impaired sense of visual direction, causing letters to appear to change position within the word, may be the result of a disordered development of the visuospatial processing function of the right posterior parietal cortex [11,12], the highest center of the dorsal magnocellular cortical stream. Compensating for CSF losses improves reading performance when children read NCSF-based filtered text [1,2]. Since strengthening the magnocellular pathways by having the child practice the direction discrimination task improves reading performance even more, this provides more evidence that reading relies on magnocellular pathways.

The increase in the CSF that is found as the child increases in age from 5 to 8 years may be a result of the corpus callosum becoming more functional, enabling the inhibitory interactions mediated by magnocellular pathways to develop a complex interactive network, that will be used for reading. Reading involves computations performed by both right and left cortical hemispheres, dependent on interactions mediated by the corpus callosum [13]. Not until the child is 5 years old does the corpus callosum become noticeably myelinated [14], the myelination continuing until the child reaches puberty. The gain of neurons that innervate the portion of the corpus callosum connecting visually related areas are controlled predominantly by large fibers in the corpus callosum having a phasic response [15], *i.e.* magnocellular neurons. Moreover, callosal projections exert predominantly inhibitory responses by synapsing with local inhibitory interneurons [16]. The portion of the corpus callosum where posterior parietal and superior temporal fibers cross over seems to be a nodal point in the widespread system of ipsilateral and contralateral connections that control attentional and other complex functions such as reading [17].

The inhibitory component of the Visual Evoked Potential (VEP) matures until puberty [18]. It is likely that the improvement in the child's CSF to detect brief patterns and discriminate the direction of movement as the child's reading ability improves is, in part a result of the maturation of inhibitory pathways, enabling the output response of individual cells to be more sharpley tuned. In addition, these developing inhibitory pathways appear to be arrested in their development in dyslexic children. When measuring the VEP to low contrast patterns, that maximally activate magnocellular neurons, the inhibitory component of the cortical VEP in dyslexic readers is delayed by 50 msec when compared to the latency of the VEP's inhibitory component for normal observers [10]. Anatomical studies [19] examining the cortex of dyslexic adults indicate that they have a lack of columnar structure, indicating underdeveloped inhibitory circuits. In addition to the lack of cortical structure, the magnocellular layers in the lgn of dyslexic readers were 27% smaller and more disorganized in dyslexics [10]. Since cortical inhibitory networks are developed as a result of activity dependent wiring [20], as are callosal projections [16], and dyslexic children have more cortical mass that is more diffusely organized, lacking a well defined columnar organization, on the left side (primary language hemisphere) where inhibitory circuits usually cause pruning [16,21], this supports the assertion that dyslexic children have underdeveloped inhibitory pathways. Direction discrimination was most difficult for dyslexic children when test and background frequencies were equal, requiring inhibitory interactions, whereas these patterns were easiest for practiced observers to detect. In conclusion, we found that movement discrimination develops over time, and is not present at full capacity when the child begins to read. Since the CSF to detect brief patterns, and the CSF to discriminate the direction of movement are at least 2 to 3 fold lower than an adult's CSF for the same patterns, this indicates that magnocellular and inhibitory pathways are still developing in children. Dyslexics show arrested development of magnocellular and inhibitory pathways, since the CSFs for dyslexic children in grades 1-3 approximate the sensitivity of the normal child in kindergarten at most test and background frequencies. We found that strengthening the magno pathways using the task in this study improves the reading performance of all children tested. The results from this study are consistent with inhibitory interactions mediated by magnocellular pathways being needed to develop the complex interactive network used for reading. In addition, this study found that when the direction discrimination masking function for different background frequencies is mapped out, then thresholds when the test and background frequency are equal provide the definitive test for discriminating between borderline normal and borderline dyslexic children. This project shows that it is possible to provide inexpensive and effective vision screening at the elementary school level, enabling early detection and remediation of vision and reading problems.

This project was supported by NTS and Jet Propulsion Laboratory, Caltech, Pasadena, CA.

References

1. Lawton T, Barker N. All children show contrast sensitivity losses at high spatial frequencies and a doubling in reading rates when reading filtered text. Suppl Investig Ophthal Vis Sci 1996; 36: 4907.
2. Lawton, T. Comparison of contrast sensitivity functions to detect brief patterns and reading ability in children with a specific reading disability and normal readers. Vision Res 1996; in review.
3. Lovegrove W, Bowling A, Badcock D, Blackwood M. Specific reading disability: differences in contrast sensitivity as a function of spatial frequency. Science 1980; 210: 439-440.
4. Griffin JR, Walton HN, Christenson GN. The Dyslexia Screener (TDS). Culver City, CA: Reading and Perception Therapy Center, 1988.
5. Shapley R. The importance of contrast for the activity of single neurons, the VEP, and perception. Vision Res 1986; 26: 45-62.
6. Westheimer G. Eye movement response to a horizontally moving visual stimulus. Arch Ophthal 1954; 52: 932-941.
7. Lawton TB. Outputs of paired Gabor filters summed across background frame of reference predicts direction of movement. IEEE Trans Biomed Eng, 1989; 36: 130-139.
8. Lawton TB. The effect of phase structures on spatial phase discrimination. Vision Res 1984; 24: 139-48.
9. Tyler CW. Two processes control variations in flicker sensitivity over the life span. J Opt Soc Am A 1989; 6: 481-490.
10. Livingstone M, Rosen G, Drislane F, Galaburda A. Physiological and anatomical evidence for a magnocellular defect in developmental dyslexia. Proc. Natl. Acad. Sci. USA 1991; 88: 7943-7947.
11. Stein JF, Riddell P, Fowler MS Disordered right hemisphere function in developmental dyslexia. In: von Euler C, Lund I, Lennerstrand G, editors. Brain and Reading. NY: Macmillan Press, 1989: 139-157.
12. Stein JF. Visuospatial sense, hemispheric asymmetry and dyslexia. Stein JF, editor, Vision and Visual Dyslexia. BocaRaton, Fl: CRC Press, 1991; 13: 181-188.
13. Rosen GD, Sherman GF, Galaburda AM. Interhemispheric connections differ between symmetric and asymmetric brain regions. Neurosci 1989; 33: 525-533.
14. Stein JF. Physiological differences between the hemispheres. In: Rose C, editor. Aphasia. London: Whurr Wyke, 1988: 131-169.
15. Aboitiz F, Scheibel AB, Fisher RS, Zaidel E. Fiber composition of the human corpus callosum. Brain Res 1992; 598: 143-153.
16. Innocenti GM. General organization of callosal connections in the cerebral cortex. In: Jones EG, Peters A, editors. Cerebral Cortex. N.Y: Plenum, 1986; 5: 291-353.
17. Pandya DN, Seltzer B. The topography of commissural fibers. In: Lepore F, Ptito M, Jasper H, editors. Two Hemispheres, One Brain, Functions of the Corpus Callosum. Liss, NY: Liss, 1986: 47-73.
18. Spekreijse H. Comparison of acuity tests and pattern evoked potential criteria: Two mechanisms underly acuity maturation in man. Behavior Brain Res. 1983; 10: 107-117.
19. Sherman GF, Rosen GD, Galaburda AM Neuroanatomical findings in developmental dyslexia", In: von Euler C, Lund I, Lennerstrand G, editors. Brain and Reading. NY: Macmillan Press, 1989: 3-15.
20. Shatz CJ. Emergence of order in visual system development. Proc Natl Acad Sci 1996; 93: 602-608.
21. Galaburda AM, Sherman GF, Rosen GD, Aboitiz F, Geschwind N. Developmental dyslexia: four consecutive patients with cortical anomalies. Ann Neurol 1985; 18: 222-233.

AN ANATOMICAL METHOD FOR MONITORING EXPERIENTIALLY-INDUCED CHANGES IN EYE-RELATED COLUMNS IN KITTEN VISUAL CORTEX

DONALD MITCHELL and CHRISTOPHER BEAVER
Psychology Department, Dalhousie University, Halifax NS B3H 4J1 CANADA

Abstract

A method is described for visualizing the 3-dimensional arrangement of eye-related columns in the extragranular layers of the kitten visual cortex during postnatal development.

Introduction

The development by Hubel and Wiesel of animal models for deprivation and strabismic amblyopia provided the first opportunity to explore the neural basis for the perceptual deficits associated with these two forms of amblyopia [1]. Nevertheless, despite nearly 30 years of electrophysiological and anatomical study [1,2], the neural basis of amblyopia is still only partly understood. One factor contributing to the slow progress in this endeavor has been the absence of anatomical or other methods that permit observation of changes induced by early selected visual deprivation across large populations of cells as compared to the extremely small samples that can be examined by electrophysiological methods. Although anatomical methods for study of normal and abnormal development within the geniculorecipient or granular cell layer (layer 4) of area 17 have existed for many years, these methods do not permit observation at a cellular level of the anatomical correlates of the more substantial functional changes that occur concurrently in the extragranular cortical layers as documented in electrophysiological investigations. Metabolic mapping methods that depend upon autoradiographic techniques or optical imaging can provide some of this information but are limited by respectively, low resolution or by the small size and depth of the sampling area. Recently, a number of groups [e.g. 3,4,10] have exploited the rapid sensory-evoked expression of certain immediate-early genes (IEGs) as a means for metabolic mapping of specific neuronal populations. Methods based on immuno-histochemical detection of the protein product of IEGs hold promise for allowing visualization, at cellular levels of resolution, of the three-dimensional layout of neural populations within the visual cortex that are activated by specific visual stimulation. In this paper we describe the use of immunodetection of Fos, the protein product of the IEG, *c-fos*, as a means for detection of cortical cells that are activated by visual stimulation of one eye, specifically the deprived eye of monocularly deprived kittens.

Method

The method is based upon demonstrations [5,6,7] of extremely rapid expression of at least two IEGs, *c-fos* and *NGFIA*, in the extragranular layers of the visual cortex of dark-reared kittens following brief (1-2 hours) exposure to light. Several years ago [7], we demonstrated by use of immunohistochemical methods, expression of Fos in a high proportion of neurons within area 17 of 30 day old dark-reared kittens following 1-2 hours of visual exposure. Fos immunoreactive cells were absent in layer 1, highest in layers 2,3 and 6, and low in layer 5 and lower layer 4. By contrast, Fos immunoreactive cells were extremely low in area 17 of dark-reared control kittens that were not exposed to light but were present in moderate numbers in area 17 of normal light-reared kittens of the same age. A portion of this constitutive Fos expression could represent light-evoked activity as observed following exposure of dark-reared animals to light but a portion might be unrelated to visual activity. With respect to the potential ability to detect neural activity related to *specific* forms of visual stimulation, the constitutive Fos expression represents a relatively high level of background activity which could make such detection very difficult. However, we have established that the level of constitutive activity can be reduced to very low levels by placing the kitten in complete darkness for 24 hrs prior to it receiving a 2 hour period of specific visual exposure. In order to convey the essence of the procedure as applied to visualization of neurons activated by a specific eye, it is necessary first to compare the expected neural activity that would be evoked by monocular visual stimulation in the various cortical layers.

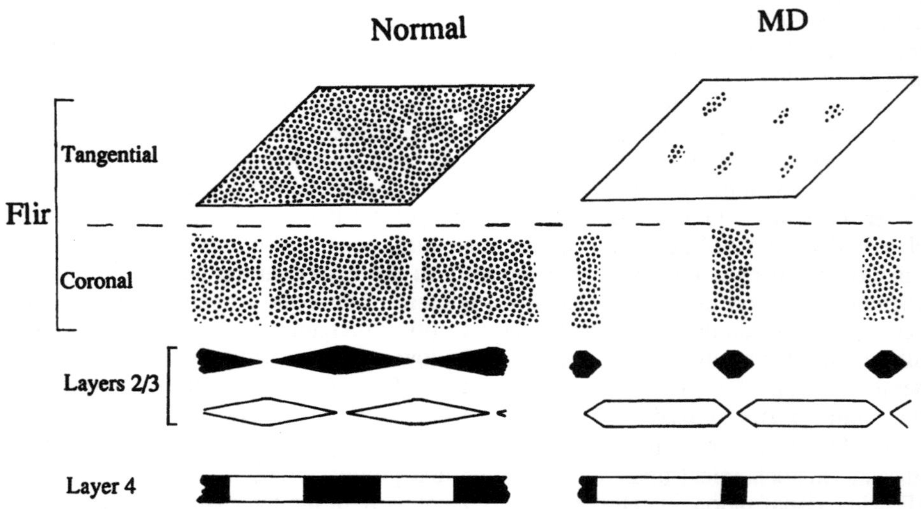

Figure 1. Representation of the different innervation by the two eyes of layer 4 versus layers 2/3 in normal (left) and monocularly deprived (right) kittens. The expected distribution of Fos-like immunoreactivity (Flir) evoked by visual stimulation of one eye (shaded) in coronal and tangential sections through the supragranular layers is illustrated at the top.

Figure 1 is an attempt to illustrate the relative input of the two eyes in layer 4 as well as in the supragranular layers (layers 2/3) of a normal cat (left) and an animal that had been monocularly deprived for several weeks as a young kitten (right). Electrophysiological investigations as well as anatomical methods based on anterograde transport of various tracers, reveal that in normal cats and monkeys the incoming afferents from the two eyes remain completely segregated in layer 4 in so doing providing the anatomical basis for the familiar arrangement of ocular dominance columns in this layer [e.g. 8,9]. On the other hand, electrophysiological investigations conducted in the extragranular layers reveal that the innervation of cortical cells by the two eyes is distributed in a continuous fashion forming the basis of the familiar seven group ocular dominance classification employed in electrophysiological studies. A plausible anatomical substrate for the physiological observations is that the innervation by the two eyes is distributed in the extragranular layers in the graded way illustrated in Figure 1. The two eyes together innervate most of the later al extent of layers 2/3 and only in a small region overlying the center of the ocular dominance column of one eye in layer 4 is innervation from one eye absent. As a consequence of this pattern of innervation, when visual stimulation is provided to one eye, most cells in the extragranular layers will be activated and only in a small region representing the centers of the ocular dominance columns for the non-stimulated eye will cells be not stimulated. Fos immunoreactivity would then be expected to be observed in the majority of cells distributed spatially in the approximate fashion illustrated by the schematic coronal and tangential views shown at the top of Figure 1 (left). Since Fos is located in the nucleus of cells, immunodetection of this protein is revealed by a darkly stained nucleus represented by the dark spots in Figure 1. The small irregularly shaped regions of low immunoreactivity can be recognized among the sea of immunoreactive nuclei only with difficulty at the density levels that are typically encountered.

The very different pattern that would be expected in animals that had been deprived of concordant binocular input in early life is represented by the effects of early monocular deprivation that is depicted on the right of Figure 1. Following early monocular deprivation, the innervation of layer 4 by the nondeprived eye is expanded at the expense of territory originally innervated by the deprived eye. Electrophysiological investigations [1] suggest that the annexation of territory by the nondeprived eye may be enhanced in the extragranular layers. Most cells in these layers can be excited only through the nondeprived eye, a finding that suggests that the innervation of these layers by the nondeprived eye has expanded to an even greater extent than in layer 4. Visual stimulation of the deprived eye would be expected to activate and evoke Fos in only the small group of neurons that represent the centers of the ocular dominance columns of this eye and hence would be manifested as small islands of Fos immunoreactive cells in tangential sections (see top of Figure 1, right). Details of the methodology are provided elsewhere [10].

Results

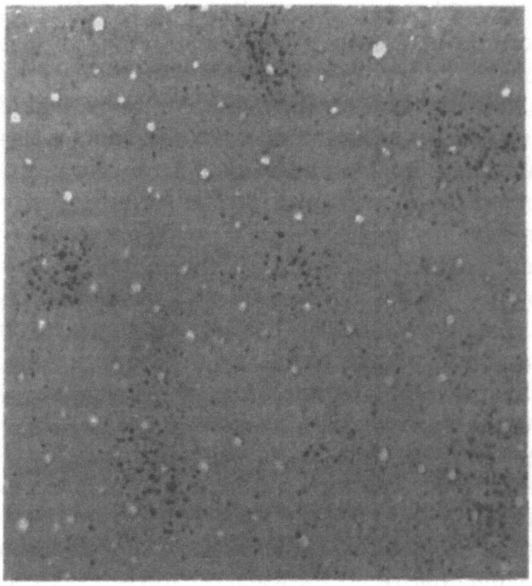

Figure 2. A photomicrograph of a tangential section of area 17 (approx . 0.2 mm from the surface) to show patches of Fos immunoreactive cells evoked by stimulation of the deprived eye of a kitten that was monocularly deprived for 3 days at 4 weeks of age. Scale: 3.6 mm = 100μ.

Preliminary data indicate that the expectations illustrated in Figure 1 for normal and monocularly deprived kittens are indeed met. Figure 2 shows a representative low power photomicrograph of the spatial layout of Fos immunoreactive cells evoked by visual stimulation of the deprived eye of a kitten that had been monocularly deprived for 3 days at 4 weeks of age. Small elongated regions containing large numbers of Fos immunoreactive cells were found surrounded by regions of low immunoreactivity. Several other observations provide even stronger evidence for the view that they represent congregations of neurons that receive input from the stimulated (deprived) eye. One key observation was the columnar nature of the patches of Fos immunoreactive cells which could be followed through the depth of the cortex allowing for the first time, *cellular* resolution of the 3-dimensional arrangement of eye-specific columns. By using one or more blood vessels as referenc points, it is possible to align adjacent sections in order to reconstruct the 3-diemsional appearance of the Fos columns. Another important set of observations concerns the changes in the dimensions of the Fos patches revealed by stimulation of the deprived eye as a function of the length of deprivation as well as their changes during recovery following termination of monocular deprivation. In agreement with the graded magnitude of the shifts of ocular dominance that follow periods of monocular deprivation of increasing duration reported in electrophysiological studies [1], the mean area of the Fos patches evoked by visual stimulation of the deprived eye showed a concomitant decrease. Moreover, following termination of monocular deprivation at 5 weeks of age and the immediate imposition of periods of reverse occlusion, the mean area of the deprived

eye Fos patches increased by a factor of three in just 4 days, a change that qualitatively matches the speed of the reported [1] physiological changes. Future studies will examine the changes in reconstructed eye-related Fos columns during and following monocular deprivation in order to establish the laminae in which the effects of deprivation begin and how these effects vary in magnitude between laminae.

References

1. Mitchell DE, Timney B Postnatal development of function in the mammalian visual system. In: Darian-Smith I, editor. Handbook of physiology. Section I: The nervous system. Vol. 3, Part 1. Sensory Processes. Bethesda: American Physiological Society, 1984: 507-555.
2. Lennerstrand G, von Noorden GK, Campos EC Strabismus and amblyopia. New York: Plenum, 1988.
3. Friauf F Tonotopic order in the adult and developing auditory system of the rat as shown by *c-fos* immunocytochemistry. Eur J Neurosci 1992; 4: 798-812.
4. Chaudhuri A, Matsubara JA, Cynader M Neuronal activity in primate visual cortex assessed by immunostaining for the transcription factor Zif268. Vis Neurosci 1995; 12: 35-50.
5. Mower GD Differences in the induction of Fos protein in cat visual cortex during and after the critical period. Mol Brain Res 1994; 21: 47-54.
6. Rosen KM, McCormack MA, Villa-Komaroff L, Mower GD Brief visual experience induces immediate early gene expression in the cat visual cortex. Proc Natl Acad Sci USA 1992; 89: 5437-5441.
7. Beaver CJ, Mitchell DE, Robertson HA Immunohistochemical study of the pattern of rapid expression of c-Fos protein in the visual cortex of dark-reared kittens following initial exposure to light. J Comp Neurol 1993; 333: 469-484.
8. Shatz CJ, Stryker MP Ocular dominance in layer IV of the cat's visual cortex and the effects of monocular deprivation. J Physiol, 2978; 282: 267-283.
9. Anderson PA, Olavarria J, Van Sluyters RC The overall pattern of ocular dominance bands in cat visual cortex. J Neurosci 1988; 8: 2183-2200.
10. Mitchell DE, Beaver CJ, Ritchie PJ A method to study changes in eye-related columns in the visual cortex of kittens during and following early periods of monocular deprivation. Can J Physiol Pharmacol 1995; 73: 1352-1363.

THE EFFECTS OF BARIUM ON RETINAL FUNCTION IN THE RABBIT

IDO PERLMAN, BO LEI, ESTHER ZEMEL and AVIRAN ITZHAKI
The Bruce Rappaport Faculty of Medicine, Technion-Israel Institute of Technology and the Rappaport Institute, Haifa, ISRAEL.

Abstract

The electroretinogram reflects the light-induced electrical activity in the vertebrate retina. It is highly dependent upon potassium conductances in the neurons of the outer retina. Injecting barium chloride solution into the vitreous of rabbits' eyes induced complex effects on the electroretinogram (ERG). The first marked effect was slight augmentation of the ERG responses and prolongation of the b-wave implicit time. Thereafter, the ERG responses gradually decreased in amplitude until a permanent deficit of about 90% was measured. This permanent ERG reduction was accompanied by a severe structural damage. Barium-induced retinal damage could reflect the inability of the Müller cells to maintain potassium homeostasis due to blockage of their permeability to potassium.

Introduction

The electroretinogram (ERG) is the electrical response of the vertebrate retina elicited by a light stimulus. It is composed of several components originating in different retinal neurons [1, 2]. The a-wave mainly reflects the reduction in the "dark" current of the photoreceptors but is also dependent on Müller cells and the reduction in extracellular potassium in the photoreceptors layer. The b-wave reflects light-evoked electrical activity in the inner nuclear layer (INL). It is believed to be generated by potassium currents across Müller cells' membrane that are associated with transient increases in the concentrations of extracellular potassium in the outer and inner plexiform layers. A common feature of both a- and b-waves is their dependency on potassium ions.

In vitro studies revealed a variety of voltage- and time-dependent potassium channels in all neurons of the outer retina and in Müller cells [3-8]. These include inward rectifiers, delayed rectifier, outward transient current and calcium-dependent conductance. Modulation of either of these potassium conductances is expected to alter visual information processing and to be reflected in the ERG.

Barium ions are commonly used to study the properties of calcium conductances because they are permeable through these channels. However, in low concentrations (< 2 mM), barium ions block most of the known voltage-dependent potassium conductances [7-9]. Therefore, exposing the retina to barium ions is expected to modify drastically retinal function that will be reflected in the ERG responses. Furthermore, potassium homeostasis, a crucial condition for normal retinal function, is maintained by Müller cells through their high permeability to potassium ions [10-12]. Therefore, blocking most of the potassium conductances in Müller cells [7, 8] may prove deleterious to the retina. The goal of this study was to test the above hypothesis.

Material and Methods

Animals: The experiments were performed on 6 adult albino rabbits, weighting 2-3 Kg. The rabbits were housed in separate cages with free access to water and food under 12/12 hrs light/dark cycle. The rabbits were anesthetized by an intramuscular injection of a "cocktail" (0.5 ml/Kg body weight) made up of ketamine (10 mg/ml), acepromazine maleate (10 %) and xylazine (2%) solutions in the following proportions (in ml); 1.0: 0.2: 0.3. The pupils were fully dilated with cyclopentolate hydrochloride 1% and topical anesthesia (benoxinate HCl 0.4%) was administered. Small volumes (0.1 ml) of barium chloride solution and saline were injected into the vitreous of the right and left eyes respectively as described before *[13]*.

Electroretinogram (ERG) [14]: The ERG responses were recorded from both eyes with corneal electrodes (Medical Workshop, Holland). The signals were amplified (X20,000) and filtered (1-100 Hz) by differential preamplifiers (Grass, USA) and then digitized by a Personal Computer equipped with a data acquisition board (Scientific Solutions, USA) at a rate of 2 KHz. Light stimuli were obtained from a Ganzfeld light source (LKC Technologies, USA) with a maximum intensity of 5.76 cd-s/m^2. The amplitude of the a-wave was measured from the baseline to its trough and the amplitude of the b-wave was determined from the trough of the a-wave to the peak of the b-wave. B-wave implicit time was measured from stimulus onset to the peak of the b-wave.

Light microscopy [15]: After enucleation, the eye was soaked for 10 min in 2% paraformaldehyde and 2.5% glutaraldehyde in 0.1 M phosphate buffer (pH 7.4). It was then, slit 2 mm posterior to the limbus to facilitate fixation. After 72 hours, the anterior segment of the eye was removed and the posterior eye cup was bisected at the level of the optic disc. Embedding was done in a JB-4 resin (Bio-Rad, England). Sections of 2 mm thickness were mounted on glass slides and stained with Richardson's stain.

Results

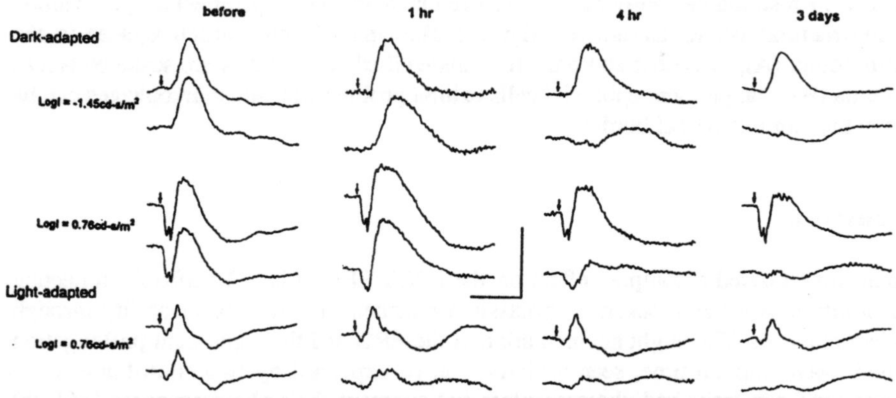

Figure 1: Representative ERG responses of one rabbit, measured before and at different times after injection of saline into the left eye and of barium chloride solution into the right eye (upper and lower traces in each pair of responses). Stimulus onset is marked by arrow. Calibration bars; vertical 200 mV, horizontal 100 ms.

Figure 1 shows representative ERG responses recorded from one rabbit before and at different times after injecting barium chloride solution (vitreal concentration 3.5 mM). In each pair of ERG responses, the control and experimental eyes are compared (upper and lower traces respectively). The first effects of barium ions, observed 1-2 hr after injection, were slight ERG augmentation and prolongation of the b-wave implicit time (2nd column). Thereafter, the ERG of the experimental eye started to decrease in amplitude and to become more delayed (3rd column). At longer time intervals (more than 24 hr), the ERG was reduced by as much as 90% (4th column). No recovery of the ERG responses was seen with continual follow-up of up to two weeks. Similar ERG findings were obtained from a total of 6 rabbits though slight variations in the rate of development of the barium effects were seen. In all 6 rabbits, the ERG responses were severely reduced when measured about 4 days after injection.

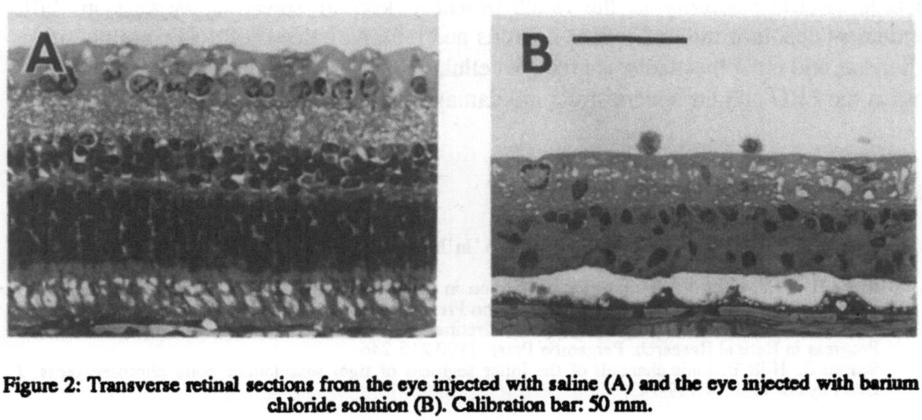

Figure 2: Transverse retinal sections from the eye injected with saline (A) and the eye injected with barium chloride solution (B). Calibration bar: 50 mm.

The severe functional loss (ERG reduction) of the barium-treated retina is also manifest in histological observations. The retina from the experimental eye exhibits severe structural damage as shown in figure 2. The typical layered structure, seen in the control retina (A), is absent and only few unidentified cell bodies are scattered across the retina (B). The pigment epithelial cells exhibit proliferation and macrophages can be seen in the vitreous-retinal border.

Discussion

Barium ions exerted a complex effect on the rabbit ERG (Fig. 1) probably reflecting their multiple roles as blockers of potassium channels and their permeability through calcium channels. The slight augmentation of the ERG and the significant prolongation of the b-wave implicit time, seen initially, can be explained by two contributions. (a) Barium ions depolarize rod photoreceptors and augment their photoresponses [16]. (b) Barium ions permeate through the calcium channels in the pre-synaptic terminals of the photoreceptors. They are more effective than calcium ions in promoting spontaneous asynchronous transmitter release from the pre-synaptic terminals and once they enter the cytoplasm, buffering by intracellular proteins is ineffective [17]. These two contributions are expected to increase the amplitude of the photoresponses in post-synaptic neurons but also to slow down their kinetics leading to the observed effects in the ERG responses.

At longer time intervals after administration of barium chloride solution, the ERG slowly decreased in amplitude to reach a permanent loss of more than 90%. The b-wave and to a lesser extent the a-wave depend on potassium fluxes across the membrane of Müller cells [2]. Since barium blocks most of potassium conductance in Müller cells [7, 8], the potassium fluxes decrease and the amplitude of the ERG waves decrease. Similar findings have been reported for toad ERG [18].

Another, more serious effect of barium-induced block of potassium permeability in Müller cells is the inability of these cells to maintain potassium homeostasis in the retina [10, 19]. The accumulation of extracellular potassium due to ongoing light-induced electrical activity in the retina probably lead to spreading depression [20], permanent depolarization of retinal neurons and massive release of acidic amino acids. All these, and other mechanisms produce cellular death as is evident by the substantial loss in the ERG and the severe structural damage (Fig. 2).

References

1. Berson EL. Electrical phenomena in the retina. In Moses RA editor. Adler's Physiology of the Eye. St. Louis: Mosby, 1981:466-529.
2. Ripps H, Witkovsky P. Neuron-glia interaction in the brain and retina. In Osborne N, Chader G editors. Progress in Retinal Research. Pergamon Press, 1985:181-219.
3. Lasater EM. Membrane properties of distal retinal neurons. In Osborne N, Chader G editors. Progress in Retinal Research. Pergamon Press, 1990:215-246.
4. Barnes S, Hille B. Ionic channels of the inner segment of tiger salamander cone photoreceptors. J Gen Physiol 1989;94:719-743.

5. Maricq AV, Korenbrot JL Inward rectification in the inner segment of single retinal cone photoreceptors. J Neurophysiol 1990;64:1917-1928.
6. Maricq AV, Korenbrot JL Potassium currents in the inner segment of single retinal cone photoreceptors. J Neurophysiol 1990;64:1929-1939.
7. Reichelt W, Pannicke T. Voltage-dependent K^+ currents in guinea pig Müller (glial) cells show different sensitivities to blockade by Ba^{2+}. Neurosci Lett 1993;155:15-18.
8. Newman EA. Potassium conductance block by barium in amphibian Müller cells. Brain Res 1989;498:308-314.
9. Armstrong CM, Swenson Jr RP, Taylor SR. Block of squid axon K channels by internally and externally applied barium ions. J Gen Physiol 1982;80:663-682.
10. Karwoski CJ, Lu H-K, Newman EA. Spatial buffering of light-evoked potassium increases by retinal Müller (glial) cells. Science 1989;217:953-955.
11. Brew H, Gray PTA, Mobbs P, Attwell D. Endfeet of retinal glial cells have higher densities of ion channels that mediate K^+ buffering. Nature 1986;324:466-468.
12. Newman EA. Distribution of potassium conductance in mammalian Müller (glial) cell: A comparative study. J Neurosci 1987;7:2423-2432.
13. Loewenstein A, Zemel E, Lazar M, Perlman I. The effects of depo-medrol preservative (MGP) on the rabbit visual system. Invest Ophthalmol Vis Sci 1991;32:3053-3060.
14. Loewenstein A, Zemel E, Lazar M, Perlman I. Drug-induced retinal toxicity in albino rabbits: Effects of imipenem and aztreonam. Invest Ophthalmol Vis Sci 1994;34:3466-3476.
15. Zemel E, Loewenstein A, Lazar M, Perlman I. The effects of myristyl g-picolinium chloride on the rabbit retina: Morphologic observations. Invest Ophthalmol Vis Sci 1993;34:2360-2366.
16. Fain, GL, Gerschenfeld, HM, Quandt FN. Calcium spikes in rods. J Physiol (Lond) 1980;303:495-513.
17. Silinsky, EM. On the role of barium in supporting the asynchronous release of acetylcholine quanta by motor nerve impulses. J Physiol (Lond) 1978;274:157-171.
18. Wen R, Oakley BI. K^+-evoked Müller cell depolarization generates b-wave of electroretinogram in toad retina. Proc Natl Acad Sci USA 1990;87:2117-2121.
19. Oakley BI, Katz BJ, Xu Z, Zheng J. Spatial buffering of extracellular potassium by Müller (glial) cells in the toad retina. Exp Eye Res 1992;55:539-550.
20. Mori S, Miller WH, Tomita T. Microelectrode study of spreading depression (SD) in frog retina - general observations of field potentials associated with SD. Jap J Physiol 1976;26:203-217.

EXPLORING THE CHARACTERISTICS OF SECRET EYE MOVEMENTS DURING FIXATION: A NEW APPROACH OF CHAOTIC TIME SERIES

RONALD A. SCHUCHARD and JUNG MIN LIM
Eye Foundation of Kansas City, University of Missouri, Kansas City, MO.

Abstract

Unconscious eye movements during fixation exhibit characteristics that are consistent with chaotic behavior. Nonlinear modeling of chaotic time series provides more accurate prediction of eye movements during fixation for computer simulation studies and a better understanding of the parameters affecting fixation with eccentric PRLs.

Introduction

A probabilistic/stochastic model describing small PRL (preferred retinal locus) movements while fixating a stationary target has modeled these eye movements as random movements comprised of drifts interrupted by sudden jerks (microsaccades) followed by drifts or more jerks [1,2]. The drifts and jerks follow a Langevin-like stochastic differential equation with deterministic restoring forces undergoing a diffusion-like process modeled as a Gaussian white noise process. One dimensional (1D) experimental results from a limbus eyetracker concluded that the root mean square of the microsaccade movement was 3 to 7 minutes of arc which agreed well with the 5 minutes of arc microsaccade movement found from the stochastic model. However, a recent study [3] investigated the two dimensional (2D) drift and microsaccadic PRL movements during normal fixation and fixation during perimetry and the results did not agree with the stochastic model. The range of 2D PRL movements during jerks and drifts for foveal PRLs (normally sighted or paracentral scotoma subjects) found by the 2D study were much larger than the results reported in the previous 1D study. Besides the additional dimension, the 2D study also used a more accurate means of determining the PRL movement (scanning laser ophthalmoscope versus limbus eye tracker) which could account for the differences in results.

The failure of the probabilistic/stochastic model to agree with the results of the 2D study has led us to begin developing a new model for PRL movements during fixation. Most eye movements in real world tasks are made consciously to bring a target of interest within the fovea or PRL. However, during fixation all people make small unconscious eye movements (of drifts and jerks/microsaccades) even though we have the impression of keeping our eyes perfectly still. These small eye movements do not appear to be goal-directed; their directions and amplitudes are randomly distributed with respect to the fixation target. Lakshminarayanan et al [4] discovered that during a two point vernier hyperacuity task subjects would unconsciously move their eyes between the two targets when the targets were close to being in-alignment. Low vision researchers have shown that subjects with macular scotomas can make unconscious PRL movements of up to 6 degrees during a fixation task. Thus, while these secret unconscious eye movements often appear random we know that to maintain fixation stability these eye movements have to have some deterministic component. This description of the empirical data agrees with a chaotic system in that apparent randomness in time series data may be due to the chaotic behavior of a nonlinear but deterministic system [5]. This study investigates whether the PRL movements during fixation exhibit chaotic behavior.

Methods

Equipment and Stimuli: The confocal scanning laser ophthalmoscope (SLO) with graphics capabilities was used for assessing PRL movement by determining the retinal location of visual stimuli directly with respect to retinal image characteristics. The SLO with graphics capabilities obtains retinal images continuously with an infrared laser (780 nm) and scans graphics on the retina with a modulated visible red-light laser (633 nm). The stimuli are thus observed by the subject and on the subject's retina by the investigator. Thus, the movement of the visible stimuli on the retina can be monitored continuously and videotaped for further analysis. The SLO provides a 32° x 24° image of the retina (labelled 40° degree field of view) with a resolution of about 3.25 minutes of arc for measurement of the retinal areas and the positioning of targets.

Procedure: The characteristics of the macular scotomas (central or paracentral) were determined by fundus perimetry (macular perimetry with the SLO) with a hybrid perimetry technique. The hybrid perimetry technique combines elements of kinetic and static methods. The stimulus is presented in stationary flashes, as in static perimetry, but successive flashes are moved progressively across the retina to map isopters, as in kinetic perimetry. The retinal illuminance level was set at 50,000 Trolands to determine the dense (possibly absolute) scotoma characteristics.

PRL movement during fixation was found from real-time digitized images of subjects fixating on a one degree cross for at least 30 seconds. A frame-by-frame manual registration determined the two dimensional retinal movement every 30th of a second. The distance (r) of the PRL center movement between each videotape frame with the angle of the motion (Θ) was found except when the retinal image was lost (e.g., blinks). The polar coordinates (R, Φ) give the two dimensional movement of the fixation target relative to the retinal location of the PRL center.

Subjects: Data have been collected from 4 subjects with different diagnosis; normally sighted, drusen, age-related macular degeneration (AMD), and retinitis pigmentosa (RP). The AMD subject had a central scotoma with an eccentric PRL. The RP subject had a small central retinal area (about 6 degrees) with visual function inside extensive visual field loss. The drusen subject had paracentral macular scotomas while the normally sighted subject had no scotomas. The PRL movement data was collected either from both eyes (normal) or from the dominant PRL eye (all others).

Results

Figure 1 shows examples of the subject's PRL movement during fixation.

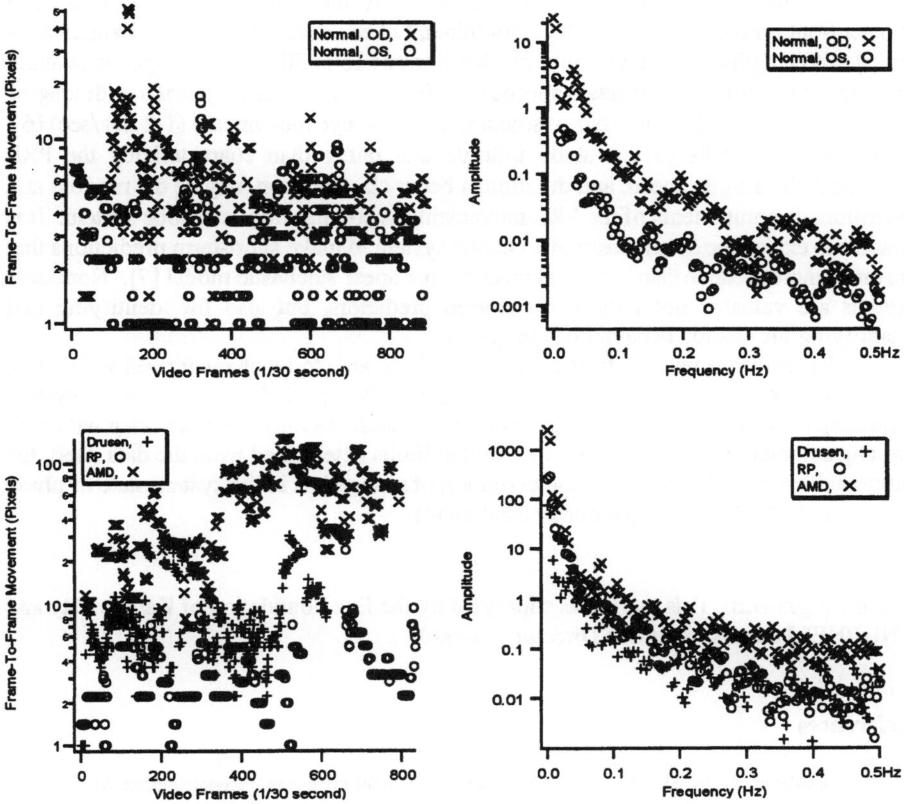

Figure 1. Top panels of normally sighted subject with foveal PRL, bottom panels of low vision subjects with central scotoma and eccentric PRL. The left panels show the PRL movement frame-to-frame while the right panels show the Fourier power spectrum of this time series movement.

Interestingly the power spectrum of the right eye (OD) and left eye (OS) are about a power of ten different in amplitude. Also the power spectrum of the AMD subject (with an eccentric PRL) is also about a power of ten different in amplitude compared to the drusen and RP subjects (with foveal PRLs). This increased amplitude corresponds to a larger PRL size for the left eye compared to the right eye for the normal subject and for the AMD subject compared to the RP and drusen subjects.

Discussion

The broad power spectrum is a first indication of chaotic behavior, though it alone does not characterize chaos. Linear analysis is not well tuned to working with signals with continuous, broad power spectra. These data indicate that the fixation system is a candidate for a chaotic system.

The characteristics of normally sighted PRL movements during fixation (with EOG & other front surface eye trackers) have traditionally been described as: 1) microsaccades (jerks) with lengths as small as 5 minarc, durations of 15 to 30 msec, and speeds as small as 5 deg/sec (normal saccades attain speeds of 400-600 deg/sec) and 2) Drifts with lengths as long as microsaccades, durations of seconds, and slow eye movements (1-2 deg/sec) [6]. However, the results of this study indicate that rather than characterizing the PRL movements by length, speed, and duration, a better classification may be the random and deterministic components of the PRL movements as coming from a chaotic system. It is possible to exploit the determinism of a chaotic system to make short-term predictions that are much more accurate than one could make from a linear stochastic model [7]. Nonlinear models are valuable not only as short-term predictors, but also for identifying and quantifying the chaotic behavior of the system.

We envision that the fixation system will be able to be characterized with a few parameters and we are interested in deducing the characteristics of the chaotic system producing the PRL movement time series (system classification). The next step would be creating a framework in which to predict, within limits determined from the data itself, the future behavior of the system or the evolution of new points in the system state or phase space (model building and parameter estimation).

Acknowledgements: This work was supported by the Eye Foundation of Kansas City and a NIH/NEI James A. Shannon Director's Award.

References

1. Vasudevan R, Phatak AV, Smith JD. A stochastic model for eye movements during fixation on a stationary target. Kybernetik 1972; 11:24-31.
2. Lakshminarayanan V, Vasudevan R. A stochastic model for eye movements. In: Elsner AE, ed. Scanning Laser Ophthalmoscopy, Microscopy, and Tomography. New York: Plenum, 1996.
3. Schuchard RA, Cooper S, Lakshminarayanan V. Time series analysis of PRL movement during fixation. Technical Digest Series. Washington DC: Optical Society of America, 1996; 1:20-23.
4. Lakshminarayanan V, Knowles RA, Enoch JM, Vasudevan R. Measurement of fixational stability while performing a hyperacuity task using a scanning laser ophthalmoscope: preliminary studies. Clin Vis Sci 1992;7:557-563.
5. Abarbanel HDI. The analysis of observed chaotic data in physical systems. Rev. Mod. Phys. 1993; 65:1362-1392.
6. Becker W. Metrics. In: Wurtz RH, Goldberg ME, eds. The Neurobiology of Saccadic Eye Movements. Vol. 3. New York: Elsevier, 1989:13-67.
7. Casdagli M, Jardins DD, Eubank S, Farmer JD, Gibson J, Theiler J. Nonlinear modeling of chaotic time series: Theory and applications. In: Kim JH, Stringer J, eds. Applied Chaos. New York: Wiley, 1992:335-380.

VISUAL IMAGERY AND VIRTUAL REALITY

NEW EVIDENCE SUPPORTING THE SCANPATH THEORY EXPLAINS THE ILLUSION OF COMPLETENESS AND CLARITY

LAWRENCE STARK, YUN CHOI, and YONG YU
School of Optometry, University of California, Berkeley, CA.

Abstract

Virtual Reality (VR) and its technical support drivers is first described; then applications that drive VR are listed together with engineering design features. A basic theme is that normal vision depends upon a set of perceptual visual illusions, such as continuity and 3D-ness of the world, and that these work equally well in virtual environments. An important visual illusion, that of the 'completeness and clarity' of our visual world, must be a 'top-down' perceptual phenomenon and is explicable on the basis of the scanpath theory. This theory states that active looking and perception are controlled by an internal cognitive model. New evidence for this control of the sparse sampling in time and space of the visual world comes from visual imagery experiments; quantitative methods for assessment have been developed. Finally, perceptual philosophical thought is used to situate this new scientific evidence.

Virtual Reality

Virtual reality (VR) is the 'hype' name for virtual environments. VR can be more broadly considered as a man-machine system, a type of human-computer interface. However, hype and public relations alone cannot drive the field of VR; what are the drivers for VR? VR has been boosted by technical developments in other fields as well as being pulled by appetites for applications that it can supply [1,2].

Several important technical drivers deserve immediate consideration ---- computers, displays, especially head-mounted-displays (HMDs), various input/output devices, multisensory surrounds especially 3D audio, and video capture. Computers and displays are essential to very large consumer and industrial activities, and VR receives a "free ride." HMDs have recently attracted commercial development, so that our own laboratory models are falling by the wayside. Some areas of multisensory surrounds, such as haptic and force-feedback information, are still developing technologies in the VR field. The VR-practitioner cottage industry of developing input-output devices may be superseded by "video capture"; a video camera may measure head and limb motion. One may play virtual ping-pong without having special purpose sensors attached.

Among exciting application drivers for VR is the entertainment industry, from video games to movies to theme parks. Industrial applications involve telerobotics, the control of distant robots by human operators sitting in intuitive virtual environments. Training simulators for new aircraft has already moved from the military to cost-effective commercial pilot-training. Of particular interest to ourselves is the use of VR in scientific visualization.

There are three engineering design considerations that work together to gain acceptance of the VR, and enable "suspension of disbelief." If the subject feels immersed in this distant world, if he can interactively participate with hand and head movement to control objects and viewing directions in VR, and if he becomes highly interested in the events of the VR world, be they entertainment or work related, then a feeling of "telepresence" or of actually feeling present in the VR ensues. Interaction, immersion and interest compel telepresence. Intuitive function and engineered information flows can optimize human adaptation to the artificial new world of VR.

Visual Illusions & Experimental Scanpath

Now the question we ask ourselves is: Why do displays work so well? The answer which we propose in this paper is that 'seeing' is an illusion that hides the actual processes of vision and that these illusions apply equally well to the worlds of VR as to the so-called 'real' world [1].

Visual illusions abound in normal vision --- illusions of clarity and completeness, of continuity in time and space, of 3D, of presence and vivacity --- and are part and parcel of the visual world in which we live. Illusions may be defined as the perception of some aspect of the visual world that the actual sensory inputs do not suffice to establish. That visual continuity is an illusion can be realized by considering eye blinking. We are all aware that blinking occurs every few seconds, yet the world does not go blank. Thus, our continuous view of the world must be a mental construction, a picture in the inward eye.

That "clarity and completeness" is an illusion can be realized by considering the richness, color, beauty, detail, and complexity of the world as we look outward onto the scene around us. The rods and cones of the retina, the positioning of the eyes with rapid looking eye movement (EMs), and the visual processing by the brain, cannot possibly handle the overwhelming informational content of the visual scene as we apparently "see" it. Only a sparse sampling of visual information can be obtained by the human visual system, with it high resolution, half to one degree fovea, moved about three times a second from point to point in the visual scene by rapid saccadic EMs. The scanpath theory explains how this bottom-up (BU) sampled visual information is interacted with and partly controlled by the top-down (TD) cognitive model that is what we "see" in the mind's eye [3,4]. An important process in perception is the checking of this BU information against the guessed, expected, or hypothesized loci and elements of the visual scene. Evidence for this includes recent functional MRI pictures of humans viewing projected scenes. Our laboratory has measured sequences of EMs, and we have carefully compared those during viewing of various scenes, objects, ambiguous figures, search fields, and pages of text. Such experiments have led to the scanpath theory, which states that the illusory, wide-field, apparently high-resolution image of a view is generated by an internal cognitive model continually checked by foveations moved by fast EMs.

These experiments by Norton & Stark in 1971 [3], have also defined the scanpath as this alternating sequence of saccades and foveations or fixations, repetitive and idiosyncratic to scene and to viewer. Of course, the internally-directed, high resolution foveal sampling is supplemented by a low resolution, wide peripheral field-of-view, sensitive to motion, binocular disparity, and providing spatial localization for EMs.

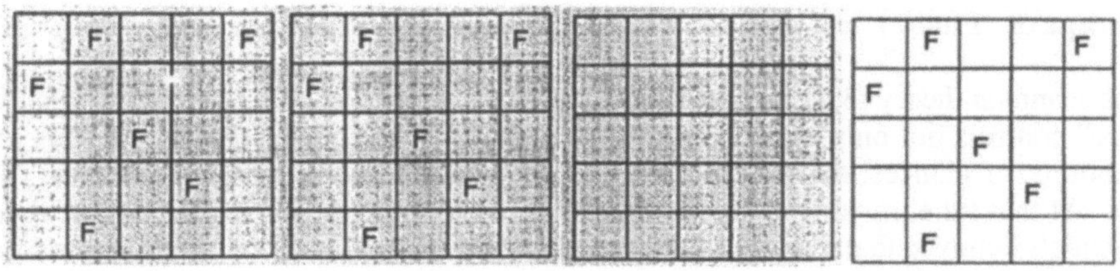

Figure 1. VI Protocol. Experimental protocol indicates two seven second looking presentations of the actual pattern (leftmost and middle left), followed by a third imaging presentation of an empty grid (middle right): then the subject is asked to draw the remembered pattern on a second blank grid (rightmost).

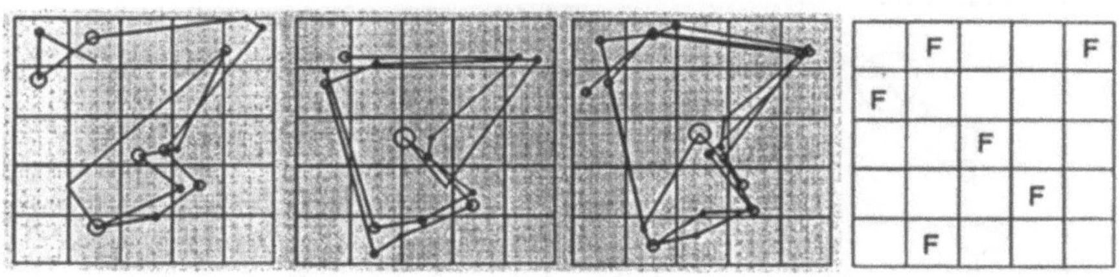

Figure 2. VI Experimental results. Scanpaths of a subject when looking and when imaging. The scanpath under imagery, only viewing a blank grid with NO external world is qualitatively similar to the preceding looking scanpath.

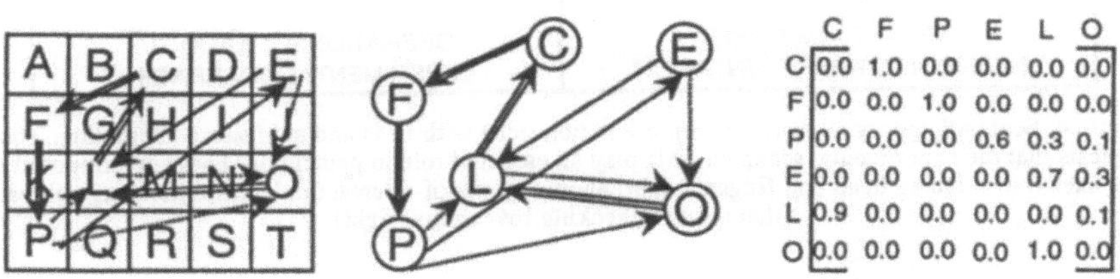

Figure 3. Quantitative analysis methods. Comparing two scanpaths for similarity involves locating sequential fixations on grid pattern (left): grid spaces are labeled by successive letters for use by string editing algorithm. Sequential EM scanpath pattern is shown as a finite state space diagram (middle) and then encapsulated into a Markov model (right): experimental coefficients are somewhat idealized for theoretical Monte Carlo simulations.

Visual Imagery (VI) Experiment

Experimental answers also came from studies of EMs during VI. We will now try to give the flavor of our hard quantitative evidence for the VI experiments, the "Brandt experiment" (Figs 1-3) [5,6]. In this way, the internal memory that controls EMs in looking and viewing, can be demonstrated to be effective when there is no external world, but only the non-iconic internal cognitive model is present to generate the scanpath.

Scanpath Theory of Active Vision

The scanpath theory [3,4] suggests that a top-down internal cognitive model of what we "see" controls not only our vision, but also drives the sequences of rapid EMs and fixations, or glances, that so efficiently travel over a scene or picture of interest (Fig 4.). At that time, most visual neurophysiologists, psychologists, and computer vision scientists believed that events in the external world controlled EMs. We admitted that our internal cognitive model must fairly accurately represent the external world scene or our species would have gone bottom-up like the dinosaurs. How, then, could we have proven our assertion, that an internal model, and not the very similar external world, drives the EMs? The visual imagery experiments described above are a major link in the supportive scientific evidence.

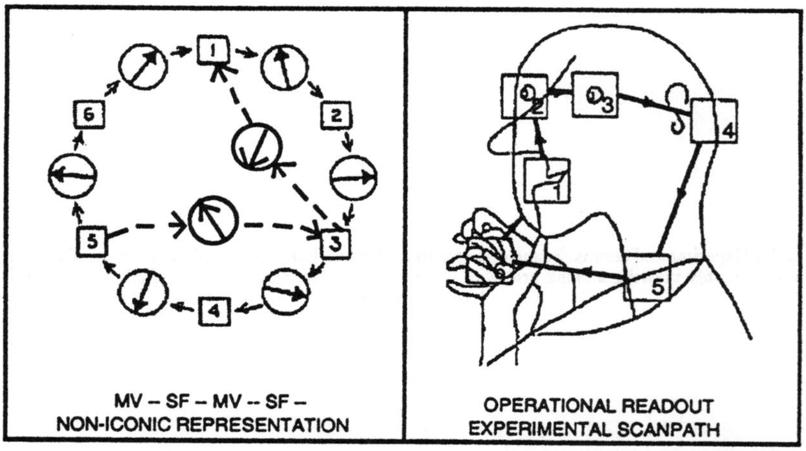

Figure 4. Scanpath theory. Non-iconic representation (left) with EMs and subfeature alternating. Theory suggests that the experimental scanpath EMs play an essential role in perception. EMs superimposed on a Klee sketch of a facing head and fingers (right) show regions-of-interest (as boxes) enclosing subfeatures that require checking foveations (right).

Perception and Philosophy

Philosophers like Plato and Kant have speculated that we "see in our mind's eye", but until the scanpath experiments, little evidence supported this conjecture. Kant divided overall perceptual processes into four stages. The chaotic world of Appearances, "stuff", has energies that impinge on our organs of Sensation, "bottom-up physiology without space and time." Representations, called ideals by Plato and "top-down cognitive models" by us, activate Perception per se to seek for, and interpret, confirm or deny hypothesized models, with the "active looking scanpath as the operational phase of perception per se". Although Kant removed the categories of space and time from BU sensory input, we now know that complex organizational, innate neurophysiological mechanisms add time and space to compute, for example, velocity (Fig. 5).

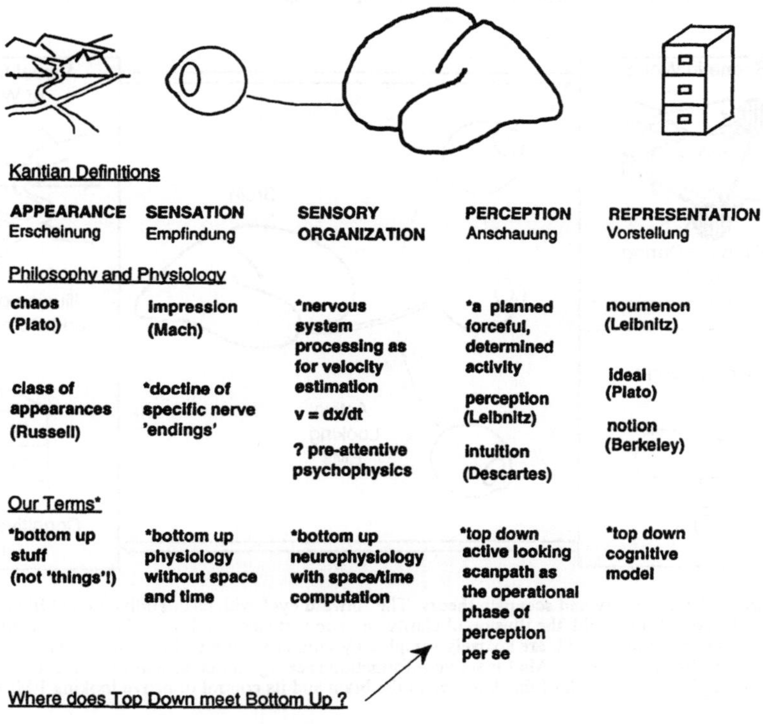

Figure 5. Perceptual processes.

The illusion of vivacity may be a reward for successful guessing by the internal model as judged by agreement of the sampled foveations with the subfeatures of the model. We are left with important neurophysiological questions - where does BU meet TD? Perhaps in the interaction between layers 4 and 6 of visual cortex. Evidence from functional MRI supports the suggested primary visual cortical area [7]. The scanpath is an exciting link connecting scientific studies of vision and these encompassing higher level mental processes (Fig. 6). Finally, we practitioners of crude present-day VR can be grateful for all these visual illusions that make both normal vision and VR "work."

The scientific process and vision are similar. The senior author (LS) once described his scientific approach: "Je vois des modeles partout." (More correct French for "modeles" might be "hypotheses mathematiques.") This turns out to be more valid than even he thought at that time. Scientists dream or imagine a model, theory, or hypothesis to explain a vague phenomenon, and then try to prove or disprove it in the laboratory. Similarly, an object or scene in our visual world is a guessed or hypothesized cognitive model in the visual brain according to the scanpath theory, and is continually checked out by sequential error. Also, when we consider society and its myths in broad contexts, we realize how much of what we here call our cognitive models exist in other forums, themes or theories of consciousness and of religion, permeating our interpretation of events. The scanpath is an exciting link connecting scientific studies of vision and these encompassing higher level mental processes.

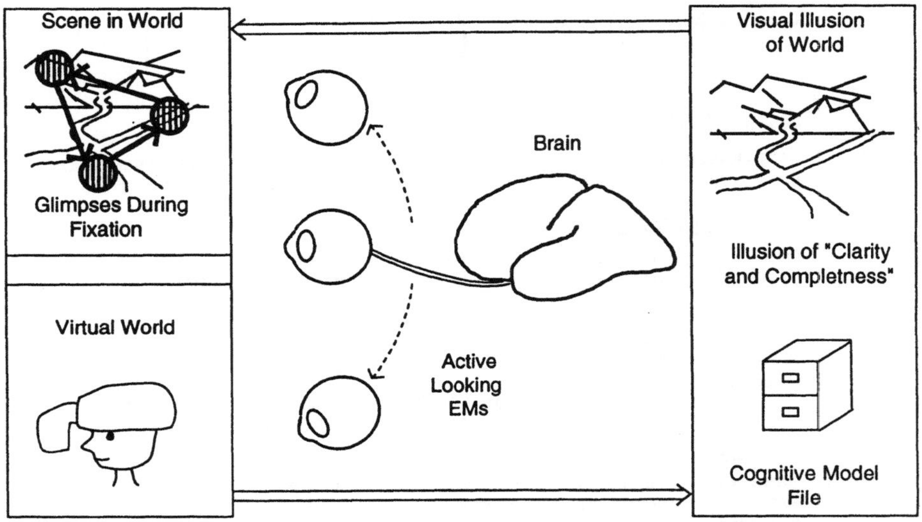

Figure 6. Virtual reality and scanpath theory. The "inward eye" with its cognitive model file provides the visual illusion of the world, the illusion of clarity and completeness (right), while the virtual world, as well as a scene in the real world, are sparsely sampled by glimpses during EM fixations (left). Upper arrow shows top-down control of EMs for active information seeking and bottom arrow indicates feedback for "vivacity". Of course, all of this happens in the brain and its control of active looking EMs (center).

Acknowledgments

We thank J. Stroud, T. Choi and S. Deng for assistance, and T. Blackmon, S. Brandt, S.R. Ellis, C. Freksa, M. Hirose, V.V. Krishnan, R. Welch and W. Zangemeister for discussions about the scanpath and virtual reality, and the NASA-Ames Research Center (NCC-2-949 & NCC-2-757) for partial support. Mr. Yu acknowledges a leave of absence from the Academy of Science Institute for Robotics and Automation, Shenyang, China, and Mr. Choi from Dis. Paru. The senior author would like to dedicate this paper to the memory of Thomas Kuhn, whose *The Structure of Scientific Revolution* so clearly informed him of the nature of science in 1962.

References

1. Stark L. How Virtual Reality Works! The Illusions of Vision in "Real" & Virtual Environments. In: SPIE Proc Symp Electronic Imaging Science & Technology: Bellingham, WA: SPIE ; 1995, 5-10.

2. Hirose M, Taniguchi M, Nakagaki Y, Nihei K. Virtual playground and communication environments for children. Proc IEICE Transactions on Information and Systems 1992;E77-D(12):1330-1334.

3. Norton D, Stark L. Eye Movements of Visual Perception. Sci Am 1971; 224:34-43.

4. Stark L. Top-Down Vision in Humans & Robots. In: SPIE Proc Human Vision, Visual Processing and Digital Display. Bellingham, WA:SPIE, 1993:613-621.

5. Brandt S, Stark L, Hacisalihzade S, Allen J, Tharp G. Experimental Evidence for Scanpath Eye Movements During Visual Imagery. Proc 11th IEEE/EMBS Symp; 1989.

6. Brandt S, Stark L. J Cog Sci 1996 (in press).

7. Kosslyn SM. Image and Mind. Cambridge, MA: Harvard University Press, 1980.

GUIDED SEARCH 3.0

A MODEL OF VISUAL SEARCH CATCHES UP WITH JAY ENOCH 40 YEARS LATER

JEREMY M WOLFE[1] and GREGORY GANCARZ[2]
[1]*Harvard Medical School and Brigham and Women's Hospital*
[2]*Boston University, Boston, MA.*

Abstract

Forty years ago, Enoch reported a central bias in eye movements made during visual search tasks. Here we discuss how our Guided Search 3.0 model incorporates that observation into a general account of visual search behavior.

Visual Search

Vision research has a cyclical component. Important issues fade into the background for a while, only to reappear when a new generation takes them up. In this paper, we present our most recent work on visual search. Some of the core ideas in this work are prefigured in papers written by Jay Enoch some 4 decades ago[1, 2]. Enoch had subjects search for targets in aerial photographs and found that Ss were biased to search the center of the image. Understanding visual search in natural images of this sort has proven to be a difficult topic. Most of the progress in the last generation has been made with more easily analyzed but less realistic stimuli. In these laboratory tasks, the independent variable is the number of items (set size) and one dependent variable is the reaction time (RT) - the time to find the target or to determine that no target is present. Different tasks produce characteristically different results. In feature searches (Fig. 1a), the target is defined by one basic feature (e.g. orientation). RT is roughly independent of set size. Adding more horizontal lines does not slow search. In conjunction searches(1b), the target is defined by a combination of 2 (or more) basic features and RT increases about 5-10 ms for every additional distractor. Targets in serial searches (1c) are defined by the spatial relationship of features. Here each "T" and "L" is composed of a vertical and a horizontal line. Each additional "L" adds 20-30 ms to RT on a target present trial - twice that, 40-60 ms, on a target absent trial. Cases like 1c can be called "serial searches" because the data are consistent with a serial, self terminating search through the items at a rate of 20-25 HZ [3,4].

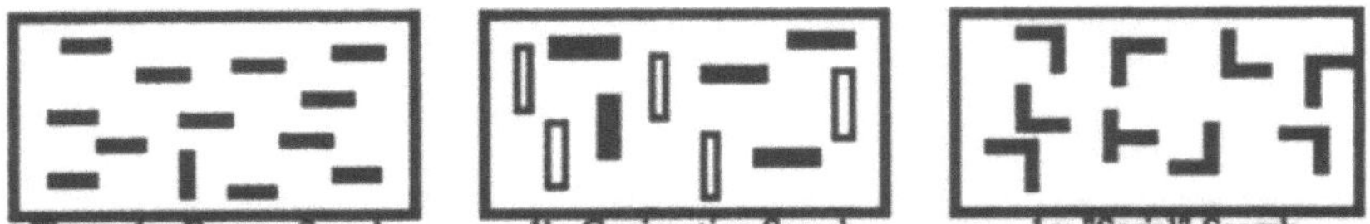

Figure 1a: Feature Search 1b: Conjunction Search 1c: "Serial" Search

Performance on these search tasks can be understood in Neisser's [5] framework. He distinguished between preattentive processes that could perform simple tasks across the entire visual field in parallel and attentive processes that perform more complex tasks only in a limited area at one time. Treisman applied this idea to visual search in her Feature Integration Theory [6]. It held that preattentive feature processes could perform feature searches in parallel, while attention from item to item was required to do all other searches. Subsequent research showed that conjunction searches were too efficient to be explained as purely serial, attentive searches [7]. Wolfe's Guided Search (GS) model accounted for this efficiency by proposing that preattentive feature processes could guide the deployment of attention in conjunction search. The basic idea is shown in Figure 2. No preattentive process can identify black vertical conjunctions but a color process can mark all black items and an orientation process can mark all vertical items. If the output of those two preattentive processes is combined into an attention-guiding *activation map*, attention will be most strongly guided to items that are both black and vertical - the target.

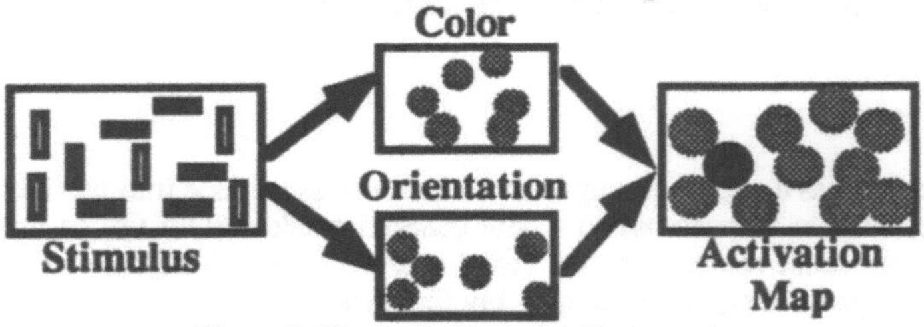

Figure 2: The basic idea of guided search.

Guided Search 3.0

GS (8) and its revision, GS2 (9) successfully modeled a wide range of laboratory search tasks. However, the eventual goal of a model of visual search must be to handle real world images like those that interested Enoch in the 50's. GS had ignored two factors central to Enoch's interests. First, the eyes move during real-world visual search. Most searches involves an interplay of covert attentional movements and overt eye movements. Second, visual processing is much more detailed at the fovea. Presumably, eye movements in search exist to direct the fovea toward regions of interest. Enoch found that viewers spent much more time looking at the center of an image. More recently, it has been shown that visual search targets are found faster and more accurately near fixation than in the periphery [10]. GS3, the newest version of our model (Fig. 3), incorporates eye movements and eccentricity effects as part of an effort to make GS a more realistic model of human search behavior.

The simulation of GS3 starts with a Gray Scale Image as its input. Next the image is processed by an array of On and Off-Center Units, approximating retinal ganglion cell response. These provide input to Preattentive Feature Maps for brightness and orientation. These maps model the representation of the stimulus in V1 by a complex log transform [11]. This realistic overrepresentation of the fovea creates a role for eye movements and a substrate for eccentricity effects in search.

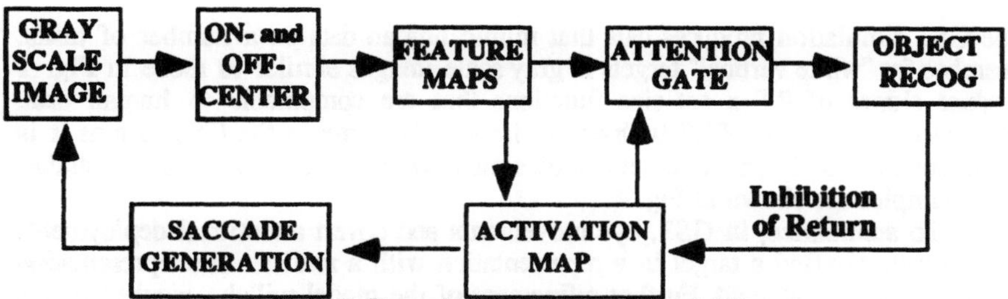

Figure 3: The architecture of Guided Search 3.0

In GS3, attention serves as a gate, allowing feature information from only one object at a time to reach higher processes like object recognition. This attentional gate is under the control of the activation map. Activity in the activation map is a weighted sum of activity in the preattentive feature maps. Thus, if the target is dark and vertical, information from "dark" and "vertical" feature maps is given a large weight. The activation map is a winner-take-all network that converges on a winner about every 50 ms. This allows featural information about new items to pass through to the identification stage at a rate of 20-25 Hz. If the selected item is not the target, feedback from the identification stage to the activation map inhibits that item, permitting a new item to win access to the identification stage. Since the eyes move, this inhibition of return needs to be in head-centered coordinates. Accordingly, the activation map is converted to these coordinates.

In order to move the eyes, a saccade map is created [12]. It is the GS3 analog of the superior colliculus. Activity in this map is a blurred version of activity in the activation map. Every 200-250 ms, the eyes are moved to the point of highest activation in the saccade map. The spatial blurring of this map can cause short latency saccades to be directed to locations between nearby items if the eyes move before the activation map has picked a clear winner. This speed-accuracy trade-off is seen in human eye movement data [13]. The GS3 architecture leads to a cooperative relationship between eye movements and attentional deployments. Because central portions of the visual field are overrepresented in the feature maps, activation tends to be highest for central items. Thus, during a fixation, attention is deployed to 4 or 5 central items. Assuming that these are not targets, their representations are inhibited in the activation map. As a result, when it is time for the eyes to move, they foveate new items. These are then examined by attention and this process repeats until the target is found or a target absent response is made.

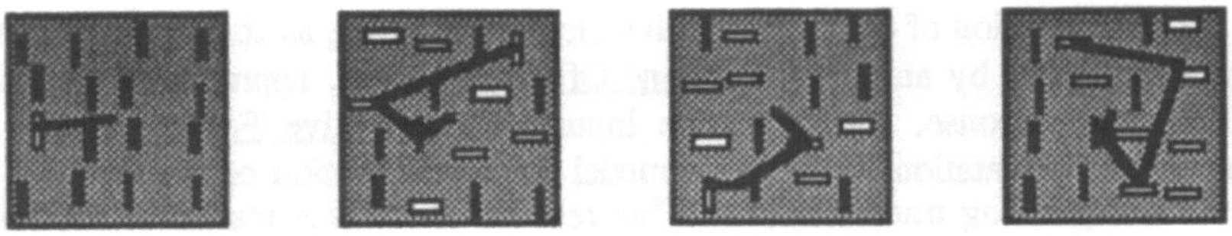

Figure 4: Typical GS3 scan paths for feature and conjunction search tasks.

The GS3 simulation produces data that mimic human data on a number of tasks. Searches for "white vertical" targets in gray scale images similar to those in Fig. 1 produce slopes of RT x set size functions that are comparable to human data. Moreover, the increase of RT with eccentricity is the same in the GS3 data as it is in human data. GS3 eye movements look similar to those recorded in human studies [14]. Samples are shown in Fig. 4.

To summarize, in GS3, eye movements and covert attentional deployments work together to find a target in a representation with a realistic overrepresentation of the central visual field. Further refinement of the model will be required before GS3 can be asked to perform the photointerpretation tasks that Enoch's subjects did in the 50s. However, having moved away from real images and natural tasks for many years, we are heading back toward models of real world visual search tasks.

Acknowledgments

This work was supported by AFOSR 49620-93-1-0407. We thank Todd Horowitz and Sara Bennett for their comments on drafts of this paper.

References

1.Enoch JM. Natural tendencies in visual search of a complex display. Visual Search Techniques 1959;NAS/NRC Pub. 171:187-193.
2. Enoch JM. Effect of the size of a complex display upon visual search. J. Optical. Soc. Am. 1959;March:280-286.
3. Kwak H, Dagenbach D, Egeth H. Further evidence for a time-independent shift of the focus of attention. Perception and Psychophysics 1991;49(5):473-480.
4. Bennett SC, Wolfe JM. Serial search can proceed at 50 msec per item. Investigative Opthalmology and Visual Science. 1996;37(3):S298.
5. Neisser U. Cognitive Psychology. New York: Appleton, Century, Crofts, 1967.
6. Treisman A, Gelade G. A feature-integration theory of attention. Cognitive Psychology 1980;12:97-136.
7. Wolfe JM. Visual search. In: Pashler H, ed. Attention. London, UK: University College London Press, 1996:
8. Wolfe JM, Cave KR, Franzel SL. Guided Search: An alternative to the Feature Integration model for visual search. J. Exp. Psychol. - Human Perception and Perf. 1989;15:419-433.
9. Wolfe JM. Guided Search 2.0: A revised model of visual search. Psychonomic Bulletin and Review 1994;1(2):202-238.
10. Carrasco M, Evert DL, Change I, Katz SM. The eccentricity effect: Target eccentricity affects performance on conjunction searches. Perception and Psychophysics 1995;57(8):1241-1261.
11. Schwartz EL. Spatial mapping in primate sensory projection: analytic structure and relevance to perception. Biological Cybernetics 1977;25:181-194.
12. Sheinberg DK, Zelinsky GJ. A cortico-collicular model of saccadic target selection. In: d'Ydewalle G, Van Rensbergen J, eds. Perception and Cognition. Amsterdam: Elsevier, 1993:333-348.
13. Findlay JM. Visual search: eye movements and peripheral vision. Optometry and Vision Science 1995;72:461-466.
14. Zelinsky GJ, Sheinber DL. Eye movements during parallel / serial visual search. J. Exp. Psychology: Human Perception and Performance 1996;in press.

TREATMENT TRIAL FOR RETINITIS PIGMENTOSA

ELIOT L. BERSON
Berman-Gund Laboratory for the Study of Retinal Degenerations, Harvard Medical School, Massachusetts Eye and Ear Infirmary, Boston MA 02114

Abstract

We conducted a randomized, controlled, double-masked trial to determine whether supplements of vitamin A or vitamin E alone or in combination affect the course of retinitis pigmentosa. We found that the course of retinal degeneration as monitored by the ERG was slower on average among adult patients taking a supplement of 15,000 IU/day of vitamin A in the palmitate form, whereas the course appeared to be hastened by supplementation with 400 IU/day of vitamin E.

Introduction

While studying the course of retinitis pigmentosa with the computer-averaged ERG from 1979 to 1983, we observed that patients self-treating with a separate capsule of vitamin A or vitamin E seemed to be losing less electroretinogram (ERG) amplitude annually than those not on these supplements. Based on food-frequency questionnaires the data suggested that a total daily intake (diet plus supplements) of greater than 16,500 IU of vitamin A or greater than 200 IU of vitamin E or the combination was potentially therapeutic. This preliminary data prompted us to conduct a randomized, controlled, double-masked trial with a four-group design from 1984 to 1991 to determine whether vitamin A or E, alone or in combination, would halt or slow the progression of retinitis pigmentosa as monitored by the computer-averaged ERG. We calculated that 601 patients would be needed to detect a significant treatment effect over 5 years when comparing the two groups receiving a supplement of 15,000 IU per day of vitamin A with the two groups not receiving this dose or when comparing the two groups receiving 400 IU per day of vitamin E with the two groups not receiving this dose. The main outcome variable was the 30 Hertz (Hz) cone flicker ERG. This paper summarizes the results of this trial [1,2].

Methods

In broad outline, patients were evaluated twice over a 6 week interval prior to the institution of vitamin supplementation. The screening visit was used to determine eligibility and the baseline visit to determine intervisit variability. The average of screening and baseline was used to provide pretreatment measures of visual function.

The procedure for randomization took into account the estimated dietary intake of vitamins A and E as well as the genetic type recorded at the screening examination. ERGs were monitored annually. Visual field areas and visual acuities were also followed as additional measures of function, although we had no expectation that we could detect significant treatment effects with these measures over the course of this study. We followed elaborate masking protocols. Staff members in contact with patients did not know the results of the study until its end. The patients agreed not to know exactly what they were being given, as this would scientifically compromise the study. An outside Data Safety and Monitoring Committee selected by the National Eye Institute met with us prior to the onset of the trial and annually thereafter and the recommendations resulting from this trial were the unanimous recommendations of that Committee.

Results

We found that mean annual rates of decline of remaining ERG amplitude were slowest for the group taking 15,000 IU per day of vitamin A and fastest for the group taking 400 IU per day of vitamin E. These rates were observed among all randomized patients as well as among a subgroup of 354 with slightly higher initial ERG amplitudes who could be followed more reliably and whom we designated as "the higher amplitude cohort." Mean annual rates of decline of remaining 30 Hz ERG amplitude among this cohort were as follows: Group A, 8.3%; Group Trace, 10%; Group A+E, 8.8%; and Group E, 11.8%. Rates of decline for visual field area showed similar trends, although the differences were not statistically significant. No significant differences were observed among groups with respect to rates of decline of visual acuity. These results are summarized in Table 1.

Table 1: Mean Rates of Decline in Visual Function by Treatment Group

	All Randomized Patients				Higher Amplitude Cohort			
Test	A	Trace	A+E	E	A	Trace	A+E	E
30 Hz*	6.1	7.1	6.3	7.9	8.3	10.0	8.8	11.8
0.5 Hz*	8.7	9.6	9.1	10.6	8.1	9.4	8.4	10.9
Field Area*	5.6	5.9	6.2	6.3	6.3	7.2	7.3	7.8
Visual Acuity†	1.1	0.9	0.7	0.9	0.8	0.8	0.7	0.7

* Percent decline in remaining function per year
† Letters lost per year

Modified from: Berson EL, Rosner B, Sandberg MA et al, Arch Ophthalmol 1993; 111:761–772; copyright 1993, American Medical Association

We also performed survival analyses on the higher amplitude cohort. The two groups receiving 15,000 IU of vitamin A were 32% less likely to have a decline in cone ERG amplitude of 50% or more from baseline in a given year than those not receiving this dose and this was significant ($p = 0.01$). The two groups receiving 400 IU of vitamin E were 42% more likely to have a decline in cone ERG amplitude of 50% or more from baseline in a given year than those not receiving this dose and this was also significant ($p = 0.03$).

The effects of these treatments by year for the higher amplitude cohort are plotted in Figure 1. The mean decline in 30 Hz cone ERG amplitude from baseline values was least for the group on vitamin A in 5 of the 6 years of follow-up and greatest for the group on vitamin E for all 6 years. The greatest separation among treatment groups occurred at years 5 and 6.

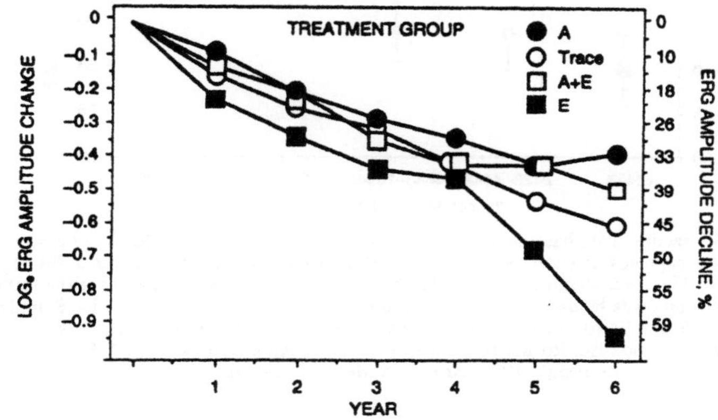

Figure 1: Mean change from baseline over 6 years in 30 Hz electroretinogram amplitude in the higher-amplitude cohort by treatment group. Sample sizes for years 1 through 6, respectively, were 83, 82, 83, 82, 62, and 27 for group A; 88, 90, 84, 85, 64, and 35 for group Trace; 88, 85, 85, 82, 61, and 32 for group A+E; and 90, 92, 88, 86, 61, and 29 for group E. From: Berson EL, Rosner B, Sandberg MA et al, Arch Ophthalmol 1993; 111:761–772; copyright 1993, American Medical Association

Mean change analyses revealed patients receiving 15,000 IU of vitamin A per day had, on average, significantly smaller declines from baseline than those not receiving this dose at years 1, 2, 5 and 6 ($p < 0.01$ in each of these years) while patients receiving vitamin E at 400 IU per day had, on average, significantly greater declines in retinal function than those not on this dose at years 1, 3, and 6 ($p < 0.03$ in each of these years). The mean declines from baseline in 30 Hz cone ERG amplitude were related to the total vitamin A intake (i.e., diet+supplement) irrespective of randomization assignment. The average decline in amplitude in the higher amplitude cohort was greatest for those with a daily vitamin A intake lower than 2428 IU, intermediate for those between 2428 and 16,946, and least for those with intake of 16,947 IU or greater (Figure 2); a significant difference was found among these subgroups. These data confirmed our preliminary impression that the optimal total intake of vitamin A appeared to be ~18,000 IU per day; that is, a supplement of 15,000 IU plus a regular diet of ~3,500 IU of vitamin A per day resulted in the smallest ERG decline. Intake greater than 18,380 IU provided no greater benefit. Doses of 25,000 IU or greater over the long term are considered potentially toxic. With respect to compliance, 95% of eligible patients completed this trial. At least 94% of capsules were consumed in any given year, and 88% of patients reported taking capsules more than 90% of the time.

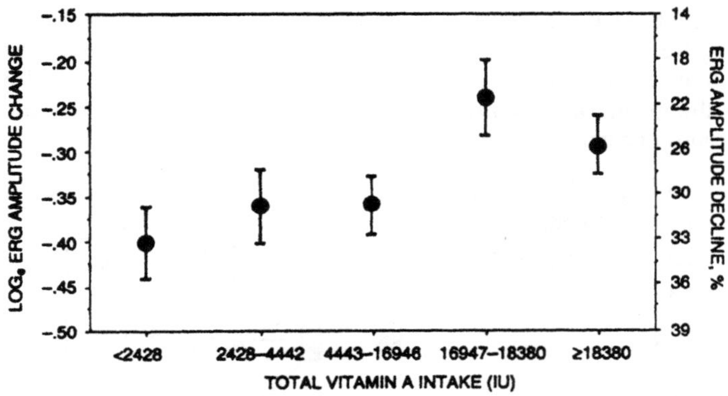

Figure 2: Mean±SE decline from baseline in 30Hz electroretinogram (ERG) amplitude by total vitamin A intake (diet plus capsules) irrespective of randomization assignment for all patients in the higher amplitude cohort. The mean decline was calculated as the mean of screening and baseline minus the mean of all follow up visits by quintile of total vitamin A intake averaged over all visits. Sample sizes were 69, 72, 74, 65, and 74 for the lowest to highest quintiles of total vitamin A intake. Vertical bars indicate SEs. From: Berson EL, Rosner B, Sandberg MA et al, Arch Ophthalmol 1993; 111:761–772; copyright 1993, American Medical Association

Discussion

These data support the hypothesis that a 15,000 IU/day supplement of vitamin A will slow the progression of retinitis pigmentosa as monitored by the ERG. The findings also suggest that a 400 IU/day supplement of vitamin E may have an adverse effect. With respect to rates of decline of remaining 30 Hz ERG amplitude, the beneficial effect of vitamin A was shown for all randomized patients ($p = 0.01$) and for the higher amplitude cohort ($p < 0.001$). The possible adverse effect of vitamin E was shown for the higher amplitude cohort.

Based on these ERG results, it is recommended that most adults with the common forms of retinitis pigmentosa should take 15,000 IU of vitamin A daily under medical supervision and avoid high dose supplements of vitamin E such as the 400 IU daily used in this trial. It is also recommended that patients continue on a regular diet without specifically selecting foods containing high levels of preformed vitamin A. As a precaution patients are advised to have a pretreatment assessment of fasting serum vitamin A and liver function and annual evaluations thereafter. Because of the potential for birth defects, women who are pregnant or planning to become pregnant are advised not to take this dose of vitamin A. Since patients under age 18 were not evaluated, no formal recommendation for such patients can be made.

We observed no toxic side effects attributable to this vitamin A supplement over 4-6 years. Furthermore, we know of no reported case of toxicity in adults in good general health on this dose. We have recommended the palmitate form of vitamin A as this was the form used in this study. Other forms might be suitable, but some are probably not, for example beta-carotene, which is not predictably converted to vitamin A from one patient to another.

Assuming that the rates of decline observed during the course of this study are sustained over the long-term, vitamin A supplementation can be estimated to provide 7 additional years of useful vision for the average patient in this trial. Although not a cure, for some patients with retinitis pigmentosa with larger pretreatment ERGs, vitamin A supplementation may make the difference whereby these patients retain some vision for their entire lives.

Acknowledgments

Supported by NEI grant EY02014 and in part by the Foundation Fighting Blindness.

References

1. Berson EL, Rosner B, Sandberg MA, et al. A randomized trial of vitamin A and vitamin E supplementation for retinitis pigmentosa. Arch Ophthalmol 1993;111:761–772.
2. Berson EL, Rosner B, Sandberg MA, et al. Vitamin A supplementation for retinitis pigmentosa. Correspondence, Arch Ophthalmol 1993;111:1456–1457.

EVALUATION OF LYMPHOCYTE PROLIFERATION ASSAY TO PURIFIED PROTEIN DERIVATIVE, ENZYME LINKED IMMUNOSORBANT ASSAY, AND TUBERCULIN HYPERSENSITIVITY IN EALES' DISEASE

JOYTIRMAY BISWAS, SHISHIR NARAIN, SARA ROY,
HAJIB N. MADHAVAN
Medical and Vision Research Foundations, 18 College Road, Madras 600006, INDIA.

Abstract

We investigated the immunological responses against mycobacterial antigens in Eales' disease. Fifty six patients with Eales' disease and fifty age-and-sex matched healthy volunteers with normal fundus findings taken as controls, were subjected to Mantoux test using 2 TU/0.1 ml of purified protein derivative (PPD). Lymphocyte proliferation assay did not differ significantly in the two groups suggesting a similar cellular immune response. The number of individuals with recent exposure/reexposure to tuberculosis (IgM^+) was significantly higher among patients. However, the number of people with past exposure (IgM^-IgG^+) was significantly higher among controls. Our study indicates that there are no statistically significant differences in the humoral and cellular immune responses to Mycobacterial antigens between the patients with Eales' disease and controls, except for a significantly higher IgM positivity among the patients.

Introduction

Eales' disease is primarily retinal vasculitis of unknown etiology occurring in otherwise health adults, mostly men, between the ages of 15 and 40 and is mostly seen in India, Pakistan and Afghanistan [1]. Among the several infectious etiologies, tuberculosis has been implicated by Axenfold and Stock and supported by several other workers [2]. In one series, only 1.3% of patients had Eales' disease[3]. In our earlier studies none of the 1005 cases with active pulmonary or extrapulmonary tuberculosis, or the 110 cases with healed tuberculosis had Eales' disease. The high incidence of positive Mantoux positivity [6-8] had led some to believe in the possible role of an allergic reaction to tuberculoprotein, but its validity is doubtful in population with high endemicity of tuberculosis [8].

We evaluated the role of tuberculosis in Eales' disease by comparing humoral immune response to Mycobacterial A-60 antigen, lymphocyte proliferation assay and cutaneous response to purified protein derivative (PPD) in 56 patients with Eales' disease and 50 healthy, age-and-sex matched controls.

Materials and Methods

Subjects: All unrelated new patients of either sex, between 15 and 40 years attending the out-patient department of a major referral eye center in Madras, who presented with at least one of the three inclusion criteria: (1) Peripheral retinal periphlebitis in any eye, (2) Neovascular or fibrovascular proliferation at the level of retina, or elevated into the vitreous cavity with or without tractional retinal detachment with periphlebitis in the same and/or other eye, and (3) vitreous hemorrhage with periphelbitis in the same or other eye, scrutinized to rule out conditions mimicking Eales' disease. For this purpose, a battery of laboratory tests comprising of a haemogram, electrophoresis for sickly cell trait, rheumatoid factor, antinuclear antibodies, LE cell phenomenon, venereal disease research laboratory test (VDRL), Treponema pallidum heme-agglutination test (TPHA), serum angiotension converting enzyme, Mantoux test, chest x-ray, and a postprandial blood sugar was performed. Patients with periphlebitis due to secondary causes such as syphilis, sarcoidosis, collagen disorders or sickly cell retinopathy were excluded.

Patients with active or healed choroiditis, diabetes mellitus, central or branch vein occlusion without periphlebitis and those who had undergone a photocoagulation, cryotherapy or a vitreous surgery prior to presentation, were excluded. Fifty six consecutive patients with Eales' disease and 50 age-and-sex matched controls were enrolled. The controls also underwent a complete ocular examination and investigations to rule out intraocular inflammation, perivasculitis or lesions mimicking Eales' disease.

ELISA Technique: ELISA was done by a standard protocol for detection of IgM and IgG antibodies against Mycobacterial A-60 antigen using a commercially available ELISA kit obtained from Anda Biologicals, France.

Mantoux Test: Mantoux test (MT) was done by injecting 2 TU/0.1ml of tuberculin PPD supplied by BCG Laboratories, Madras. The results were read after 48 hours. An induration of more than or equal to 10 mm was considered as positive.

Lymphocyte Proliferation Assay: This test was carried out as described by Maluish and Strong [9].

Statistical analysis was done using the chi-square test.

Results

The results of the ELISA for IgM and IgG antibodies against the Mycobacterial A-60 antigen showed that the number of individuals with positive IgM antibodies was significantly higher (29.16%) among the patients than among the controls (12.5%; $p=0.04$). There was no statistically significant difference in the positivity for the IgG antibodies in the two populations. ELISA results were further analyzed by dividing into four classes depending upon the detection of one or both the IgM and IgG antibodies. The number of individuals who showed negative results for both the antibodies was 16 (33.34%) and 10 among the controls (20.83%). Five patients (10.41%) and three controls (6.25%) had only IgM antibodies. Nine patients (18.75%) and three controls (6.25%) were positive for both the antibodies. The difference in the number of people belonging to these three classes was not statistically significant. However, the number of individuals belonging to IgM^-, IgG^+ class was significantly higher (32; 66.67%) among the controls than among the patients (18; 37.50%). Overall seropositivity rates, based on detection of atleast one of the two antibodies were 66.67% (32 patients) and 79.16% (38 controls). The difference was insignificant ($p=0.17$).

The results of the Mantoux test were statistically not significant in the two groups with 89.28% patients and 75% controls positive ($p=0.055$). Similarly, the numbers of individuals in the two classes with positive lymphocyte proliferation assay, i.e., with a stimulation index of one or more, were similar (71.42% of patients and 74% of controls).

The correlation between Mantoux test and lymphocyte proliferation assay was studied. The various permutations had similar frequencies in both the populations. The difference in the results among the groups were not significant. Finally, we studied the correlation between the results of ELISA, Mantoux test and lymphocyte proliferation assay. There was no statistically significant difference in this analysis also. The detailed results will be reported elsewhere (paper in preparation).

Discussion

Our study shows no statistically significant difference in the humoral and cellular immune responses to Mycobacterial antigens between the patients with Eales' disease and controls, except for a significantly higher IgM positivity among the patients.

At this stage, there is no evidence except for a statistically significant difference in the IgM positivity rates, to believe that tuberculosis is an etiological factor for Eales' disease. Any association with tuberculosis may merely be incidental as may have been several other associations with non-tubercular entities such as thoromboangitis obliterans, multiple sclerosis, coagulation disorders and parasitic infections studied in the past.

References

1. Gieser SC. Murphy RP. Eales' disease. In: Ryan S, Ed. Retinal Disease. Vol 2. St. Louis: CV Mosby, 1989: 535-539.
2. Axenfold KT and Stock D. XI Int Cong Ophthalmol 1909;Naples:367.
3. Awasthi P, Mehrotra ML, Srivastava SN. Ocular conditions in pulmonary tuberculosis patients in India. Acta XX Concilium Ophthalmologicum 1966:1025.
4. Biswas J, Badrinath SS. Ocular morbidity in patients with active systemic tuberculosis. Int Ophthalmol. 1996 (in press).
5. Biswas J. Ocular morbidity in patients with healed systemic tuberculosis. Nethralaya Insight 1988;4:7-8.
6. Elliot AJ. Recurrent intraocular haemorrhage in young adults (Eales' disease). A report of 31 cases. Trans Am Ophthalmol Soc 1954;52:811-875.
7. Donders PC. Eales' disease. Doc Ophthalmol 1958;12:1-105.
8. Raj N, Krishnamurthy MS, Ananthararaman DS. Prevalence of non-specific sensitivity in some parts of India. Ind J Med Res 1975;63:1098-1109.
9. Maluish AE, Strong DM. Lymphocyte proliferation. In: Rose NR, Friedman H, Fabey JL, eds. Manual of clinical Laboratory Immunology. 3rd edn. Washington DC: American Society for Microbiology,1986.

REFRACTIVE SURGERY IN FLUX

THOMAS J. CAMPEN, RENEE BOVELLE and
HERBERT E. KAUFMAN
LSU Eye Center, Louisiana State University, New Orleans, LA.

Introduction

For many years, ophthalmic professionals have pursued the correction of ametropia without spectacles or contact lenses. This has led to the burgeoning field of refractive surgery, a significant portion of which is directed toward modification of the cornea. This review will briefly discuss some of the more widely used modalities, their strengths and weaknesses, as well as developmental trends, with emphasis on current studies of the use of phakic intraocular lenses (IOLs) for correction of ametropia.

Radial Keratotomy

Radial keratotomy (RK) is now the most frequently performed procedure for myopia of less than 6 diopters (D). In this technique, metal or diamond blades are used to make radially oriented incisions of approximately 90% corneal depth in the paracentral and peripheral cornea. This causes bulging of the sides of the corneal dome with peripheral steepening and central flattening, which provides the myopic correction. Nomograms are used to guide the surgeon regarding incision length, number, and optical zone diameter in relation to patient age and the desired correction. In good hands, with enhancement operations, approximately 90% of patients have 20/40 or better vision after RK [1,2].

The long-term results of RK have been studied extensively and show that this procedure is effective in decreasing myopia, most predictably for small degrees of refractive error. Serious complications are rare, but refractive instability can occur in 15-30% of patients [2]. Undercorrection is relatively common after RK, compared with other keratorefractive procedures, as is cyclical fluctuation of central corneal curvature and, therefore, refraction. Regression toward hyperopia occurs in approximately 25% of patients years after RK and 5-10% of patients have a lasting regression toward myopia [2]. Newer techniques with shorter and fewer cuts may reduce or eliminate this problem, but the long-term results are uncertain. It should also be noted that after RK, it may be difficult or impossible to acceptably fit contact lenses due to the alterations in corneal shape and almost all patients experience some glare, especially at night.

Astigmatic Keratotomy

Astigmatic keratotomy (AK) refers to incisional techniques that can be performed alone or in conjunction with RK to correct idiopathic and postoperative astigmatic errors. Depending on the cause of the astigmatism, straight or arcuate incisions of varying number and location may be made to attempt refractive correction, based on nomograms in the case of idiopathic astigmatism, or intraoperative keratoscopy in the case of postoperative astigmatism. In the latter context, predictability is less satisfactory. Many of the postoperative complications of AK are similar to those of RK.

Synthetic Implants

Synthetic intracorneal implants are also being used for the correction of ametropia. Polysulfone and hydrogel implants can be placed intrastromally in the visual axis after lamellar dissection. This approach offers certain theoretical advantages, including lack of reliance on adequate donor material, a high degree of quality control possible through prefabrication, and absence of intraoperative thermal tissue damage and/or perturbation of the more anterior corneal layers. Hydrogel implants are currently being studied in the United States for correction of myopia and aphakia. Their permeability characteristics are especially favorable, allowing essential nutrients to diffuse into anterior cornea, but they require that the anterior layers of the cornea be completely detached with a microkeratome, so that the cornea can assume a new anterior curvature. Polysulfone achieves refractive correction by means of its higher refractive index rather than by reshaping the cornea, so severing the anterior corneal layers is not required. The material, however, is impermeable to metabolites, which may cause late abnormalities of the overlying stroma. Polymethyl methacrylate (PMMA) rings can be placed intrastromally either fully or partially surrounding the visual axis to create central corneal flattening. Both polysulfone and PMMA implants produce predictable and stable correction of low degrees of myopia. Advantages of the ring include absence of permanent structural alterations of the optical zone, reversibility, and the potential for adjustment; however, predictability of effect may be a problem.

Epikeratophakia

Epikeratophakia is a refractive procedure developed by Kaufman [3,4] which evolved from Barraquer's lamellar techniques of keratomileusis and keratophakia. In this technique, corneal tissue is implanted onto the intact Bowman's membrane of the recipient cornea. Donor tissue is frozen and lathed to the proper correction and lyophilized for storage and shipping. The resulting tissue lens is then sent to the surgeon, rehydrated and the edges are sewn into a shallow peripheral annular keratotomy. This procedure is safer, simpler, and more easily reversible than previously developed lamellar procedures, in that Bowman's layer and stroma in the visual axis are not disturbed and a microkeratome is not required. Moreover, the tissue lens is relatively easily removed. Undercorrection, as well as regression after high myopic epikeratophakia, occurs in about 20% of patients, but infants and children with monocular cataracts and some cases of keratoconus can be treated effectively.

Laser Surgery

A great deal of current keratorefractive effort is centered on excimer laser-based systems. This technology is based on the generation of excited dimer molecules of rare gases and halides. Upon return of these dimers to a lower energy state, ultraviolet light is released, which can be used to remove minute amounts of corneal tissue with extreme accuracy in a process called ablative photodecomposition. The area of residual acute damage in the wound bed is much less with excimer laser ablation than with mechanical or other laser-based techniques.

Photorefractive keratectomy (PRK) refers to the use of this modality to perform a large area ablation in the visual axis to achieve the desired refractive effect. In the case of myopic PRK, the ablation is deepest centrally in the visual axis and shallows peripherally to the edge of the desired optical zone. For hyperopia, the deepest area of ablation is in the mid-periphery. Various delivery systems are available, including laser beam paths with a varying diaphragmatic aperture, a scanning slit, a rotating wheel with apertures of increasing size, and ablatable polymer masks. Regular astigmatism can also be treated using a scanning laser slit beam or an ablatable toric mask. The FDA has recently approved the use of PRK for correction of myopia up to 6 D with an optical zone of 6 mm. Side effects of this modality in the treatment of myopia include regression of refractive error and the appearance of subepithelial haze, which may reduce best-corrected visual acuity. These problems appear to be greater as higher degrees of myopia are treated. Start-up and maintenance costs are substantial for these systems.

To better address some of the limitations of PRK, physicians abroad and now in the United States are using a combination of excimer laser photoablation and lamellar dissection called LASIK (laser in-situ keratomileusis). In this procedure, the automated microtome is used to dissect a lamellar flap beneath Bowman's layer, proceeding temporally to nasally and leaving a hinge on the nasal side. Ablation is then performed in the lamellar bed and the cap is replaced. Advantages of LASIK over PRK include more predictable treatment of higher degrees of myopia, absence of subepithelial haze, and faster visual rehabilitation. Disadvantages include the technical difficulty of the lamellar portion of the procedure, which, if not performed optimally, may lead to serious difficulties ranging from irregular astigmatism to loss of the corneal cap. Although definitive data are not available, LASIK appears to offer superior results for higher degrees of myopia. In that PRK provides 94% of patients with 20/40 or better visual acuity [5], however, the use of LASIK in patients with low to moderate myopia is questionable.

Correction of Hyperopia

With so many alternatives for myopic correction now available, research into hyperopic correction is beginning to increase. Holmium YAG laser thermal keratoplasty has been investigated internationally with promising results for low hyperopia (< +3 D). Concerns include stability of refraction, the possibility of inducing irregular astigmatism, and poor wound healing. For moderate hyperopia (+3D to +7D), research is now being con-ducted with hyperopic PRK, LASIK, and intrastromal rings, gels, and lenses. To date, clear lens extraction remains the only surgical choice for hyperopia greater than 7D.

Phakic Intraocular Lens Implantation for Myopia

Refractive surgery is patient-driven because patients want to be free of the need for contact lenses and spectacles and are willing to accept the risks associated with surgery for this benefit. Incisional and laser modalities can accomplish this goal, but the various complications noted above may be encountered. In addition, the quality and sharpness of vision may be diminished, in part due to the iatrogenic abnormalities created in the cornea to achieve the refractive correction.

It should be reemphasized that, from the surgeon's perspective, certain disadvantages of the incisional and laser techniques are especially worrisome, namely unpredictable healing, prolonged visual recovery time, and unstable vision. Moreover, most of the procedures are not reversible if the patient is dissatisfied with the outcome. Additionally, the expense of the instrumentation and the ease or difficulty of the technique must also be taken into consideration.

The phakic IOL eliminates many of these liabilities, because it involves a simple and safe procedure that has been performed for more than 40 years. It requires only minor adaptations to a familiar technique that ophthalmologists already perform routinely. The patients see well the next day; visual recovery time is short and the resulting vision is exquisite.

The only clinical trial of phakic IOLS conducted in the United States was done at the LSU Eye Center in New Orleans [6,7]. The lens used was the ZB5M, which is a convex anterior chamber lens made of PMMA and manufactured by Domilens in France. The study was conducted under strict FDA protocol.

Five women (ages 37-43 years) were enrolled in the investigation. All patients were contact lens-intolerant high myopes, with refractions ranging from -8.00 to -10.50 D. Preoperative examination included central, midperipheral and far peripheral endothelial cell counts, as well as measurement of intraocular pressure. The patients were told that if the ZB5M lens proved successful in the first eye, an implant could be done in the second eye after approximately 1 year if they desired. In fact all of the patients requested and underwent the second implantation. Therefore for purposes of analysis, the data from both eyes of all five patients were combined, yielding a total of 10 eyes in the trial. The first surgery was done 4 years ago; all of the first eyes have had at least 2 years of follow up and all of the second eyes at least 1 year of follow up.

On postoperative day 1, seven of the 10 eyes had an uncorrected visual acuity of 20/40 or better and after 1 month, eight of the 10 eyes had a visual acuity of 20/40 or better. (The two eyes with uncorrected visual acuity of 20/40 or worse after 1 month were from the same patient, who had more than 3 D of with-the-rule astigmatism in each eye. After neutralization of the astigmatism by astigmatic keratotomy, uncorrected visual acuity improved to 20/40 or better in both eyes.) The nylon sutures used for wound closure remained in place for 4 weeks after which they were removed. Since then the wounds have remained stable with little or no induction of astigmatism. The refraction also remained stable, and except for the onset of presbyopia in two of the five patients, no optical changes have been noted. Statistical analysis revealed no significant difference between preoperative and postoperative endothelial cell counts in any eye at any time 2 or more years after implantation. Elliptical pupils developed in three eyes of two patients: the second operated eye in one patient and both eyes in a second patient. Examination revealed that the foot plates of the IOL and the iris root had been displaced posteriorly, which stretched the iris in the direction of the haptics resulting in an elliptical pupil. These patients were not disturbed by the cosmetic appearance of the pupil and, sur-prisingly, had no symptoms of glare or halos at night.

The only consistently voiced complaint was that of glare and halos in dimly lit environments, noted by three of the five patients. This characteristically manifested itself at night while the patients were driving. However the problem appeared to be minor, and all three of these patients elected to have the implantation surgery in the other eye. Four tests examining glare and contrast sensitivity were used to compare the degree of glare disability in the ZB5M patients with the typical amount of glare experienced by high myopes wearing contact lenses or spectacles. The tools applied were the MCT-8000 for daylight and night-time contrast sensitivity and glare, the Regan low contrast acuity test, the Pelli-Robson contrast sensitivity test, and the B-VAT II-SG video acuity tester. The results of the B-VAT, Pelli-Robson, and Regan contrast sensitivity tests showed no significant differences between the ZB5M IOL group and a group of myopic patients who wore rigid gas-permeable contact lenses, soft contact lenses, or spectacles. However the MCT-8000 test revealed a significant decrease in contrast sensitivity in the ZB5M IOL group, compared with the soft contact lens-wearing myopes when they were tested with spectacle correction. Furthermore, the MCT-8000 night time glare test revealed a significant increase in glare in the ZB5M lens group, compared with all of the other groups. Thus, the results of this night time glare test provided a objective measure of the subjective visual complaints from the ZB5M IOL group in relation to nighttime driving and other activities conducted in low-light environments. The results of the extensive glare testing on these patients led to a halt in further implantation of the current ZB5M phakic anterior chamber implants in the United States. It should be noted, however, that although no psychometric tests measuring patient satisfaction and complaints concerning this implant were formally administered, the patients' informal opinion of the lens was quite favorable.

Although the ZB5M lens appears to be safe in that it did not cause endothelial damage, glaucoma, cataracts, or chronic inflammation, three problems must be addressed. First, haptic design must be improved, the foot plates must be modified and anterior chamber measurements must be made more accurately to prevent the development of an elliptically shaped pupil caused by inserting a lens that is too long and not adequately supported in the angle. Second, the need to reduce glare may be dealt with, in part, by modification of the lens surface with an anti-glare coating. Third, the sharp discontinuity of the surface curve at the periphery of the optic appears to contribute to the glare and decreased contrast sensitivity. By blending the peripheral edge of the lens, a smoother curvature may be obtained. It may also be possible to increase the diameter of the optic without increasing the risk of endothelial damage in the midperipheral cornea. These proposed changes in optic design should help to minimize glare, improve contrast sensitivity, and reduce pupillary distortion caused by the anterior chamber placement of this intraocular lens. Worst [8] has used an anterior chamber "lobster claw" lens that required iris to be inserted into plastic "claws." This lens is more difficult to insert but shows promise. Fechner and others [9] have developed a foldable lens, sometimes called a contact lens, that is inserted under the iris, vaulting in front of the patient's lens as it rests in the ciliary sulcus. Uncertain biocompatibility of the materials, which may touch the iris and lens, and reports of lens opacities make careful future evaluation necessary.

References

1. Werblin TP, Stafford GM. The Casebeer system for predictable keratorefractive surgery. One-year evaluation of 205 consecutive eyes. Ophthalmology 1993;100:1095-1102.
2. Talamo JH, Steinert RF. Keratorefractive surgery. Chapter 20. In: Albert DM, Jakobiec FA, editors. Principles and practice of ophthalmology: clinical practice. Volume 1. Philadelphia: WB Saunders, 1994:342-361.
3. McDonald MB, Morgan KS: Epikeratophakia for aphakia and myopia. Chapter 32. In: Kaufman HE, Barron BA, McDonald MB, Waltman SR, editors. New York: Churchill Livingstone, 1988:823-847.
4. McDonald MB. Onlay lamellar keratoplasty. Chapter 26. In: Kaufman HE, Barron BA, McDonald MB, Waltman SR, editors. New York: Churchill Livingstone, 1988:697-711.
5. VISX, Inc. Food and Drug Administration Approval Application, March, 1996.
6. Kaufman HE. United States experience with anterior chamber phakic lenses. Presented at the Symposium on Cataract, IOL, and Refractive Surgery. Congress on Ophthalmic Practice Management. American Society of Cataract and Refractive Surgery, Seattle, Washington, June 1-5, 1996.
7. Kaufman SC, Kaufman HE. Phakic IOLs and clear lens extraction for high myopia: counterpoint. In: Elander R, Rich L, Robin J, editors. Textbook of refractive surgery. Philadelphia: WB Saunders, in press, 1996.
8. Fechner PU, Strobel J, Wichmann W. Correction of myopia by implantation of a concave Worst-iris claw lens into phakic eyes. Refract Corneal Surg 1991;7:286-288.
9. Fechner PU, Haigis W, Wichmann W. Posterior chamber myopia lenses in phakic eyes. J Cataract Refract Surg 1996;22:178-182.

VISUAL FUNCTION FAVOURS AGE-RELATED MACULAR DEGENERATION? A TENTATIVE HYPOTHESIS

EMILIO C. CAMPOS, COSTANTINO SCHIAVI, ALESSANDRA BALDI
Clinica Oculistica Ia, Università di Bologna
via Massarenti 9 - 40138 Bologna, ITALY.

Abstract

In five patients with documented amblyopia with excentric fixation, age-related macular degeneration (ARMD) developed in the non-amblyopic eye. Over a five year period of observation, there was no evidence of ARMD in the amblyopic eye. In a control group of five patients with ARMD and with normal binocular vision, the disease affected the second eye in a relatively short period of time. It is postulated that a misuse of the foveal region has a protective effect on the macular area. These differences could be looked for in the dopaminergic system of the inner retina.

Introduction

A peculiar occasional observation prompted our attention some years ago on the relationship between age-related macular degeneration (ARMD) and amblyopia. A 75 years old gentleman, family friend of one of us (ECC) for decades, developed an hemorragic type of ARMD in his sound eye. The fellow eye had a severe strabismic amblyopia, with excentric fixation and a visual acuity not better than 6/30. Initial fluorangiographic retinal changes were present in this eye as well. Over an eight period no functional deterioration took place in the amblyopic eye, eith only light perception present in the sound eye. We therefore undertook a prospective study for evaluating the time course of a possible symmetrization of ARMD in patients with strabismic amblyopia in the eye not affected by ARMD.

Material and methods

Ten patients with ARMD took part in this study. Five had normal binocular vision and five had an esotropia with deep amblyopia of the deviated eye. Pertinent data on age, sex, best corrected visual acuity and presence or absence of strabismus are summarized in Table One. The amblyopic patients were selected on the basis of the presence of an ARMD in the sound eye. In the five patients with strabismic amblyopia the angle of strabismus was measured with the Krimsky test and fixation examined with the visuscope. These data are summarized in Table Two. In all patients a retinal fluorescein angiography (RFA) was performed in both eyes. Visual acuity testing and RFA was repeated every six months. All patients were followed for a five year period.

Results

Visual acuity of the eye with ARMD in the patients with strabismic amblyopia deteriorated rapidly to levels lower than that one of the amblyopic eye (between 2 and 8 months from the initial observation). In the amblyopic eye, there was no change in the visual acuity over the six years period. The RFA of the eyes with ARMD deteriorated from an hemorragic to a cicatricial stage in all five patients in between 2 and 12 months. The RFA of the amblyopic eye showed initial changes between 6 and 48 months form the beginning of the study. These data are summarized in Table Three.

Visual acuity testing in both eyes of the five patients without strabismus showed a progressive although slow deterioration in both the originally affected eye and the fellow eye. An initial deterioration of visual acuity in the fellow eye could be observed between 12 and 38 months from the beginning of the study. Visual acuity in the two eyes tended to be equal at the end of the observation period of six years. Initial RFA changes in the non-affected eye were present between 8 and 24 months after the beginning of the study. The data from this group of patients are summarized in Table Four.

Discussion and conclusions

Our data suggest a different natural history of ARMD in patients with normal binocular vision and in patients with strabismic amblyopia of the non-affected eye. In the patients without amblyopia, ARMD became clinically evident relatively early in time. Functional deterioration, in terms of visual acuity reduction, was preceeded by RFA changes. On the other hand, in the amblyopic eye of patients with ARMD of the sound eye, initial RFA changes were not followed by a significant decay in visual acuity of the amblyopic eye.

It is well known that ARMD is a tendentially symmetrical desease. There is a tendency towards an involvement of the second eye in a relatively short period of time. Interestingly, no conclusive data exist in the Literature on the time course of this phenomenon. It is often simply stated that ARMD more or less invariably affects both eyes, even if not with an absolutely parallel pattern of behaviour [1].

This symmetrical pattern was not followed in the group of patients with ARMD and strabismic amblyopia in the originally non-affected eye. Here, RFA changes were not followed by a significant decay in visual acuity.

The original visual acuity of the amblyopic eye was extremely low. For this reason, it is impossible to record possible initial reductions, which could have been documented if the visual acuity was higher. On the other hand, our data show that visual acuity in the group of non-strabismics deteriorated in the second eye to levels lower than those found in the amblyopes. All amblyopes were able to maintain fixation with the amblyopic eye for teh six year observation period and have a useful vision. It has to be noted that they all exibited localization problems, attributable to the fact that the now fixing eye had excentric fixation. Diplopia was often a disturbing element. We have no elements for stating that ARMD would not become clinically relevant beyond the six year observation period. We can postulate that amblyopia is probably able to at leat delay the occurence of ARMD.

It is also obviously possible to see patients in which ARMD affects first the amblyopic eye. These were purposely excluded from this study, because we were not interested in analysing the opposite effect. This element needs further evaluation. More patients and for longer periods of time need to be followed in order to substantiate our initial findings. It is extemely difficult for a strabismologist to see patients with ARMD. It is equally difficult to find reliable patient's histories relative to amblyopia in a retinal service. Prospective studies, as ours, are therefore necessary, on a larger scale.

Very little is known on the potentially favouring elements of ARMD. Great weight has been given to the effect of light. Protective glasses are often prescribed to ARMD patients, with the hope of delaying the natural course of the disease [2]. In the patients with amblyopia, there is a relevant asymmetry in the clinical manifestation of ARMD. Nevertheless, the same amount of light enters the two eyes. One could argue on the fact that the light reaches the foveal area of the deviated eye with a different angle as related to the sound eye. Moreover, in an esotropic eye the quantity of light entering the eyeball may be different from that one reaching the sound eye [3]. These factors need certainly further analysis, but do not appear to us as significant.

The image of the amblyopic eye is suppressed cortically. There is a misuse of the macular region of the amblyopic eye. The inner retinal methabolism is changed as a consequence of a long-standing inhibition [4]. There are alterations in retinal receptive field properties. Neurotransmitters involved in inner retinal methabolism as dopamine are probably implied in this process. If indeed one could postulate that ARMD has a delayed manifestation in the second eye if this one is amblyopic, then an explanation could be thought in the different retinal methabolism present in amblyopia. This hypothesis is tempting, but needs obviously substantiating findings. From the practical point of view, a modulation of the inner methabolism could protect against ARMD.

References

1. Bressler BM. ARMD. Focal points American Academy of Ophthalmology 1995;XIII:2
2. Taylor HR, West S, Munoz B et al. The long term effects of visible light on the eye. Arch Ophthalmol 1992;110:99-104.
3. West S, Rosenthal FS, Bressler NM et al. Exposure to sunlight and other risk factorsassociatedwithARMD. Arch Ophthalmol 1989;107:875-9.
4. Campos EC. Amblyopia. Surv Ophthalmol 1995;40:23-39.

COMPARISON OF GOLDMANN TONOMETRY MEASUREMENTS USING CREAMER VS FLUORESCEIN IN CYNOMOLGUS MONKEYS

MARY ANN CROFT, JULIE KILAND, STEPHEN J. GANGE, AMIR AREF, CHRISTOPHER D. PELZEK, PAUL L. KAUFMAN
Dep't of Ophthal. and Vis. Sci., Univ. of Wisconsin Medical School, 600 Highland Ave., Madison WI 53792-3220

Abstract

Fluorescein cannot be used to measure intraocular pressure (IOP) repeatedly at short intervals, or during fluorophotometric determination of aqueous flow. Therefore, we compared minified Goldmann tonometer measurements of IOP obtained using commercial fluorescein vs dairy or non-dairy creamer to highlight the mires. In ocular normotensive monkeys, measurements using fluorescein averaged 1.94±0.49 mmHg higher than with creamer ($p<0.001$), and fluorescein- vs creamer- measured IOP ratios averaged 1.17±0.05 ($p<0.005$). However, when IOP was manometrically controlled from 15-60 mmHg, the mean difference between fluorescein and creamer readings was only 0.49 ± 0.94 mmHg and the fluorescein/creamer IOP ratio averaged 1.01 ± 0.032. This essential identity held from 15-60 mmHg IOP, the difference increasing by only 0.013±0.055 mmHg/ mmHg manometric pressure. Coffee creamer is an alternative to fluorescein to measure IOP.

Introduction

Fluorescein provides bright mires and a distinct end-point for Goldmann applanation tonometry. However, an alternative indicator is needed during concurrent measurement of aqueous flow by fluorophotometry (so as not to interfere with corneal and anterior chamber fluorescence decay), during repetitive tonometry or when the corneal epithelium is disrupted (since fluorescein can accumulate in the epithelium and stroma and render the mires indistinct). Cream has been used as an alternative to fluorescein, and while providing a less distinct endpoint, does not interfere with fluorophotometric readings or accumulate in the cornea. We compared Goldmann tonometry measurements with dairy or non-dairy creamer vs commercial fluorescein-Na ophthalmic strips or solution in living monkeys.

Materials and Methods

Animals and Anesthesia. Juvenile and adult ocular normotensive cynomolgus monkeys

(*Macaca fascicularis*) were anesthetized with ketamine (10mg/kg i.m. initially, 5mg/kg at ~45 min intervals when needed) and placed prone in a head-holder, with the eyes elevated 4-8 cm above the heart. All IOP measurements were performed with a minified Goldmann tonometer (MGAT, 4.5 mm tip diameter),[1] calibrated and mounted on a Zeiss slit lamp.

Protocols:

Spontaneous IOP. A) IOP of eight monkeys was measured bilaterally using Coffee Rich® non-dairy creamer (Rich Products, Buffalo NY, ingredients: water, corn syrup, partially hydrogenated soybean oil) in one eye and commercial fluorescein-impregnated paper strips (Fluor-I-Strip®) in the contralateral eye. Right and left eyes were assigned randomly. One observer looked through the eye piece and adjusted the tension knob without viewing the scale; a second observer read and recorded the measurement without revealing it. B) Fluorescein (Fluor-I-Strip®) was administered to the right eye of 4 monkeys, IOP measured, the eye rinsed with balanced salt solution, Borden's Half and Half® dairy creamer (Borden Inc. Columbus OH, ingredients: milk, cream, disodium phosphate, sodium citrate) applied to the same eye, and IOP again measured. The protocol was repeated in the left eye of the same 4 monkeys, but using creamer first and fluorescein second. C) IOP was measured in both eyes of 6 monkeys using Half and Half®, and the eyes rinsed with balanced salt solution. Ten minutes later, IOP was measured in both eyes using 0.25% fluorescein sodium/0.4% benoxinate HCl solution (Fluress®). In 6 different monkeys, the protocol was repeated using fluorescein first and creamer second. D) Four monkeys were divided into 2 groups of 2. In the first group IOP was measured in both eyes using fluorescein, the eyes rinsed, and IOP then measured using Half and Half®. In the second group, creamer was applied first and then fluorescein.

Manometrically Set IOP. In 3 monkeys, the anterior chamber of each eye was cannulated with a branched 26 gauge needle, one arm of which was connected to a reservoir of degassed Bárány's solution[2], the other arm to a pressure transducer. The manometric IOP of each eye was recorded. IOP was measured with the MGAT using fluorescein in one eye and Half and Half® creamer in the opposite eye in masked fashion as in A. A single drop of fluorescein or creamer was placed on the tonometer tip, minimizing delivery to the eye. The manometric pressure of each eye was then raised at ~ 5 mmHg increments between baseline IOP and 60 mm Hg, with MGAT IOP measurements taken at each level after 60 sec of stabilization, using flourescein and creamer for the respective eyes. Both eyes and the tonometer were rinsed thoroughly between IOP readings. The reservoir was open to the eye throughout.

Viscosity and Surface Tension. The viscosity of Half and Half® (dairy) and Coffee Rich® (non-dairy) creamers, and of saline, 0.0625% fluorescein, and 0.5% fluorescein, was measured at 24°C with a Haake model RV12, spindle cup NV. The fluorescein concentrations were chosen assuming that 1/4 of the applied concentration was achieved in the tear film. Surface tension was measured at 24°C using the Wilhelmy Plate method. The osmolarity of Half and Half®, Coffee Rich®, 0.0625% fluorescein, and 0.5% fluorescein was measured using a Wescor 5500 Vapor Pressure Osmometer. The lipid content was obtained from Borden (Half and Half®) and Rich.

Statistical Analysis. In experiments where fluorescein or creamer was administered bilaterally, average IOP of the 2 eyes was used for each indicator. Thus, in all protocols each monkey contributed 1 fluorescein and 1 creamer measurement. Mean differences and ratios of fluorescein and creamer spontaneous IOPs were compared to 0.0 and 1.0 respectively using the 2-tailed paired t-test. Intercepts and slopes from linear regression models were used to test for systematic differences and trends in fluorescein or creamer MGAT IOPs, and paired MGAT IOP, as a function of manometric IOP. Group data are reported as mean ± SEM. Computations used SAS statistical software.

Results

Spontaneous IOP (Table 1). Measurements of IOP in the normotensive range using fluorescein were consistently 1-3 mmHg (8% to 25%) higher than measurements using either creamer. The differences were significant only for protocol C where fluorescein- vs. creamer differences averaged 2.65±0.92mmHg ($p<0.02$) and fluorescein- vs. creamer ratios averaged 1.25±0.10 ($p<0.05$), and for pooled data from all protocols (A-D) where the difference was 1.94±0.49mmHg ($p<0.001$) and the ratio averaged 1.17±0.05 ($p<0.005$).

Table1. Intraocular pressure measurement using fluorescein and creamers.

Protocol	n	Fluorescein	Creamer	Fluorescein - Creamer	Fluorescein / Creamer	Creamer & Fluorescein Used
A	7	15.47±1.40	14.29±0.91	1.19±0.69	1.08±0.05	Coffee Rich®, Fluor-I-Strip®
B	4	16.19±0.90	14.81±0.84	1.38±0.81	1.10±0.06	Half and Half®, Fluor-I-Strip®
C	12	16.21±0.98	13.58±1.21	2.65±0.92[b]	1.25±0.10[a]	Half and Half®, Fluress®
D	4	16.09±1.11	14.31±0.86	1.78±1.17	1.13±0.09	Half and Half®, Fluor-I-Strip®
A-D	27	16.00±0.58	14.06±0.60	1.94±0.49[d]	1.17±0.05[c]	

IOP data are mean±S.E.M. (mmHg; applanation reading) using fluorescein or creamer in ketamine-anesthetized cynomolgus monkeys; ratios are unitless. Each monkey contributes one fluorescein and one creamer reading. Significantly different from 0.0 (difference) or 1.0 (ratio) by the 2-tailed paired t-test: [a]$p<0.05$; [b]$p<0.02$; [c]$p<0.005$; [d]$p<0.001$.

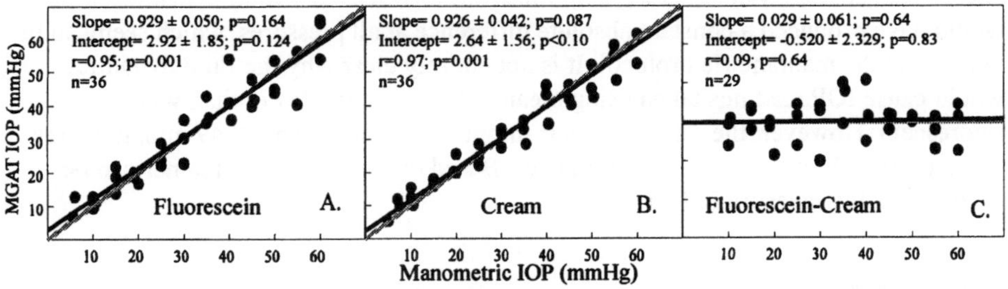

Figure 1. MGAT IOP measurements with fluorescein (A), creamer (B), or fluorescein-creamer difference (C) vs manometric IOP measurements in monkeys. Black line = least squares regression of fluorescein, creamer or fluorescein-creamer IOP measurements on manometrically measured IOP, gray line = identity. r= correlation coefficient. In A and B, p=probability that slope = 1.0, intercept = 0.0, r=0.0. For plot C, p=probability that slope = 0.0, intercept = 0.0, r=0.0. Data in Panel C includes only those monkeys where manometric pressure was equal in both eyes.

Manometrically Set IOP. The slopes and the intercepts of the regression equations for the fluorescein (Figure 1A)- or cream (Figure 1B)- measured IOP vs manometric IOP did not differ significantly from 1.0 and 0.0, respectively. The slope and intercept of the regression equation for the difference between fluorescein- or cream-measured IOP vs manometric IOP did not differ significantly from 0.0 (Figure 1C). Where manometric IOP was equal in both the cream and fluorescein measured eyes (n=29), IOP measurements taken using fluorescein were 0.49±0.94 mmHg higher than measurements taken using creamer ($p<0.61$), and fluorescein- vs. creamer measured IOP ratios averaged 1.01 ± 0.03 ($p<0.66$).

Viscosity and Surface Tension (Table 2). Both creamers exhibited higher viscosity and lower surface tension values than did the fluorescein solutions. The fluorescein solutions and Half and Half® were isotonic, while the Coffee Rich® was hypertonic. The creamers contained calcium, the fluorescein solutions did not.

Table 2. Viscosity, surface tension, osmolarity, fat content and calcium concentration values for Borden's Half and Half®, Rich's Coffee Rich®, 0.0625% Fluorescein and 0.5% Fluorescein.

	Viscosity (cps)	Surface Tension at 30 sec (dynes/cm)	Osmolarity (mOsm)	Fat Content (% w/v)	[Ca++] (mg/g)
Half and Half®	4.88	46.5	298.6	15	0.7
Coffee Rich®	3.08	36.2	500.0	10	0.0348
0.0625% Fluorescein-Na	1.6	72.2	300.3	0	0
0.5% Fluorescein-Na	1.4	72.0	313.8	0	0

Discussion

Overall, IOP measurements taken using creamer were comparable to those using fluorescein. The weak tendency toward slightly lower readings with creamer could theoretically relate to differences in optical sharpness of the mires, or in viscosity and surface tension of the fluids compared to the tear film + fluorescein solutions. The lower surface tension and consequently lower capillary attractive force of the creamers would necessitate more tonometer force and, consequently, higher tonometric readings. It is not immediately apparent that the differences observed in viscosity or calcium content would have any effect. It may be that the differences relate to lower contrast of the mires with the creamers. We would have predicted that an optical effect would increase with increasing IOP, which did not occur. Any fluid dynamics effects would have produced a constant absolute difference at all pressures, which seems to be the case in the manometric protocol. It is not entirely clear why the fluid dynamics would cause IOP readings taken using creamer to be slightly lower than with fluorescein. However, the difference was minimal, averaging only 0.49 mmHg where manometric IOP was the same in both eyes. Based on these results, creamer can be used to reliably measure IOP.

Acknowledgments

Supported by grants from the NEI (EY02698) and Research to Prevent Blindness. We are grateful to Dr. Robinson and his staff for determining viscosity, surface tension, osmolarity, and calcium concentration.

References

1. Kaufman PL, Davis GE. Minified Goldmann applanating prism for tonometry in monkeys and humans. Arch Ophthalmol 1980;98:542-46.
2. Bárány EH. Simultaneous measurements of changing intraocular pressure and outflow facility in the vervet monkey by constant pressure infusion. Invest Ophthalmol 1964;3:135-43.

WAVELENGTH DEPENDENT LENS TRANSMISSION PROPERTIES IN DIABETICS AND NON-DIABETICS

CHRIS A JOHNSON, JACQUELINE M NELSON-QUIGG,
LAWRENCE S MORSE
Optics and Visual Assessment Laboratory (OVAL),
Dept of Ophthalmology, University of California, Davis, CA.

Abstract

The lens transmission properties of Type I and Type II diabetics were compared to those of non-diabetics, using the Lens Absorption Monitor (LAM), a procedure that provides a rapid objective assessment of lens density by measuring the intensity of the 4th Purkinje image for different wavelengths. Because previous research has shown that lens density varies with pupil size, each patient's pupil size was determined during LAM measures, and all data was normalized to 3 mm. Approximately 25% of the Type I diabetics were outside the lens density limits for non-diabetics, whereas only one Type II diabetic exceeded the limits. In contrast to the results of a prior study which reported greater lens yellowing at an accelerated rate in nearly all Type I diabetics, our findings indicated that only a small portion of diabetics showed this effect. Differences between the two investigations may be related to the effects of pupil size.

Introduction

Lutze and Bresnick [1] recently reported that the lenses of diabetics "yellow" at an accelerated rate, with the results of young and middle-aged Type I diabetics resembling the greater lens transmission loss often reported for older normal individuals over the age of 60. [2] However, long-standing diabetics tend to have smaller, less reactive pupils than non-diabetics, and Mellerio [3,4] has shown that lens density measures are higher when pupils sizes are small and lower when pupils sizes are large. This is due to the fact that the absorbing pigment is located in the nucleus of the lens, which has a biconvex shape that is similar to the whole lens. With a small pupil, light passes only through the central thick portion of the nucleus, resulting in a greater average path length through the absorbing pigment. With a large pupil, light also passes through the thinner peripheral portions of the lens nucleus, resulting in a smaller average path length through the pigmented region. Weale [5] has published a comprehensive series of curves that show the effect of pupil size on lens density for different age groups. Thus, it is

possible that Lutze and Bresnick's results were confounded by different pupil sizes that may have been present for diabetics and normal observers.

The purpose of the present study was to evaluate the lens transmission properties of diabetics and non-diabetics using both Type I and Type II diabetics, a larger sample of both diabetics and non-diabetics, an objective method of measuring lens transmission, and accounting for variations in pupil size for both diabetics and non-diabetics.

Methods

Measurements of lens transmission properties were obtained with the Lens Absorption Monitor (LAM), which is based on the procedure originally described by Said and Weale. [6] This procedure consists of measuring the intensity of the specular reflection from the back surface of the lens (the 4th Purkinje image) for different wavelengths of light. In their original study, Said and Weale exposed photographic plates and performed densitometric readings of the 3rd (front surface of the lens) and 4th (back surface of the lens) Purkinje images and a calibration strip containing different densities for a series of different wavelengths. By taking the ratio of intensities of the 3rd and 4th Purkinje images for each wavelength, they were able to derive the amount of lens absorption as a function of wavelength. Numerous measures were required, because small changes in eye position dramatically affect the intensity of the Purkinje images.

We sought to overcome some of the difficulties of the Said and Weale procedure by automating the process. Details of the LAM device, as well as the results of a validation study we conducted, have been previously published. [7] The LAM procedure is non-invasive, provides a direct, objective measure of lens transmission, requires only a few seconds to perform, and has considerably better test-retest reliability than other methods. Basically, the LAM consists of a quartz-Halogen light source, two relay lenses, a rotating filter wheel (placed in the collimated beam between the relay lenses) containing 8 interference filters (10-12 nm bandwidth) with peak transmission at 410, 420, 430, 450 470, 500, 530 and 550 nm, and an intensified charge-coupled device (ICCD) video camera with a close-up lens system. The entire assembly is mounted on a slit lamp table. The filter wheel is synchronized to the frame rate of the video camera, and 16 measures are obtained for each wavelength in about 2 seconds. In addition, measurements of the scatter profile above and below the 4th Purkinje image are obtained with each measure to provide a scattered light correction. The results are compared to intensities for reflections of a calibrated glass bead standard. A software artifact rejection procedure is used to eliminate "outliers" that represent measures during eye movements.

We tested a total of 314 eyes of non-diabetics between the ages of 13 and 82 who had elevated intraocular pressure (ocular hypertensives) but an otherwise normal eye examination, and no evidence of diabetes. Previous studies have reported no differences in lens transmission properties among ocular hypertensives and normal subjects. [8,9] Sixty six eyes of Type I diabetics and fifty nine eyes of Type II diabetics were measured for comparison. Pupil size was recorded at the time the lens transmission measures were obtained, and all data was normalized to a 3 mm diameter pupil by applying the pupil size correction values reported by Weale. [5]

Results

Figure 1 presents the log relative lens density for 430 nm (relative to 550 nm) as a function of age for non-diabetic ocular hypertensive and normal patients (open circles), type I diabetics (filled triangles) and type II diabetics (filled squares). The solid line indicates the best-fitting least-squares linear regression of the non-diabetic data. We also performed various nonlinear curve fits as well as a two segment bilinear fit to the data, but were unable to obtain a fit that was clearly superior to a linear fit of the data. The two dashed lines indicate the 95% confidence intervals for the data from the 314 non-diabetic eyes. The upper confidence limit was used as the basis for comparison with the diabetic eye lens density measures. All data has been normalized to the values for a 3 mm diameter pupil.

Observation of Figure 1 reveals that most of the lens density values for the diabetic eyes fall within the confidence limits for non-diabetic eyes. Only one eye of a Type II diabetic patient fell outside of the confidence limits. Approximately 25% of the Type I diabetic eyes had lens density measures that were higher than those obtained for the non-diabetic eyes. All of the Type I diabetic patients whose lens density values exceeded the non-diabetic confidence limits had a long history of poor diabetic control. Other than this, we found no clinical or other factors that were common to these patients.

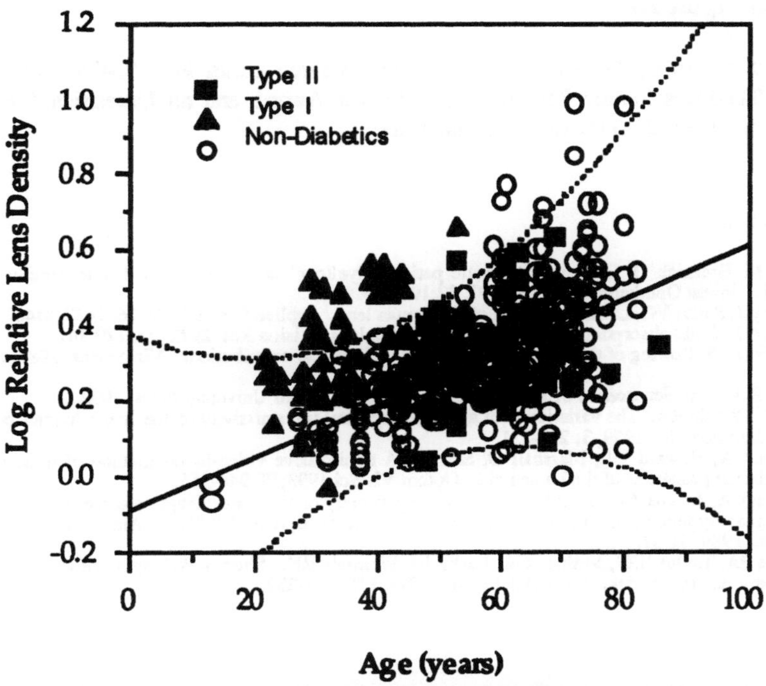

Figure 1 - Log relative lens density as a function of age for non-diabetics (open circles), type I diabetics (filled triangles) and type II diabetics (filled squares).

Discussion

Our findings indicate that approximately 25% of the Type I diabetics had lower transmission of short wavelength light than non-diabetics of the same age. Only one Type II diabetic exhibited lens transmission properties that were outside the limits for non-diabetics. This is considerably lower than that reported previously by Lutze and Bresnick. [1] In addition, our results indicate that most diabetics do not exhibit an accelerated lens yellowing, and even the data for diabetics outside normal limits do not clearly reveal an accelerated amount of lens yellowing. Our current findings thus suggest that at least part of the accelerated lens yellowing that has been previously reported for Type I diabetics may be accounted for by pupil size. In general, diabetics tend to have smaller pupils, which results in a greater average path length through the central portion of the lens nucleus and subsequently produces higher estimates of lens density.

Our lens density measures for non-diabetics are well-fit by a single linear function. This suggests that some of the accelerated lens yellowing that has been reported for normal observers over the age of 60 might also be accounted for on the basis of pupil size, which also becomes smaller with age in normal, non-diabetic individuals. Future investigations will be necessary to explore this possibility.

Acknowledgments

Supported in part by National Eye Institute Research Grant #EY-03424a Research to Prevent Blindness Senior Scientific Investigator Award, and an Unrestricted Research Grant from Research to Prevent Blindness, Inc.

References

1. Lutze M, Bresnick G. Lenses of diabetic patients "yellow" at an accelerated rate similar to older normals. Invest Ophthalmol Vis Sci 1991, 32:194-199.
2. Pokorny J, Smith VC, Lutze M. Aging of the human lens. Applied Optics 1987, 26: 1437-1440.
3. Mellerio J. Light absorption and scatter in the human lens. Vision Res 2972, 22: 129-141.
4. Mellerio J. Yellowing of the human lens: nuclear and cortical contributions. Vision Res 1987, 27: 1581-1587.
5. Weale RA. The Senescence of Human Vision. Oxford: Oxford Universiy Press, 1992.
6. Said FS, Weale RA. The variation with age of the spectral transmissivity of the living human crystalline lens. Gerontologica 1959, 3: 213-231.
7. Johnson CA, Howard DL, Marshall D, Shu H. A noninvasive video-based method of measuring lens transmission properties of the human eye. Optom Vis Sci 1993, 70:944-955.
8. Johnson CA, Adams AJ, Lewis RA. Automated perimetry of short-wavelength mechanisms in glaucoma and ocular hypertension. In Heijl, A, Editor. Perimetry Update 1988/89. Amsterdam: Kugler and Ghedini, 1989: 31-37.
9. Sample PA, Taylor JDN, Mrtinez GA, Lusky M, Weinreb RN. Short-wavelength color visual fields in glaucoma suspects at risk. Am J Ophthalmol 1993, 115: 225-233.

PHOTOTOXIC CONSEQUENCES OF THE CORNEAL DOME

L. STEPHEN KWOK
Department of Optometry and Vision Science
The University of Auckland, Auckland, NEW ZEALAND

Abstract

The cornea's transparency is essential to human vision. However, other components of sunlight such as near ultraviolet irradiation can also impinge upon the ocular tissues. Limbal light focusing may provide an explanation for some of the ophthalmohelioses such as pterygium and senile cataract. We confirm previous results which show that the posterior nasal limbus is the catchment area for focused light from the temporal limbus. Exposure of the eyes to sunlight, over a period of many years, may lead to a derangement of cell growth in the anterior segment. The principal mechanism for pterygium formation may be the same mechanism for the development of many cases of cortical lens cataract.

Introduction

The cornea gives an important service to clear vision by contributing two-thirds of the eye's optical power while acting as a stable, transparent portal to the retina. The cornea's light transmittance and absorbing properties are well known. [1,2] Indeed, the self-evident importance of the ocular media to human vision merited its inclusion in Stiles' 1967 book *Color Science* with Wyszecki.

Less well known is the ability of the corneal dome to direct light upon itself and surrounding tissue. [3,4] This paradox is a consequence of the geometry of the corneal dome and the anterior eye upon which it sits. More importantly, this phenomenon may have profound phototoxic consequences as discussed below.

Coroneo and co-workers [3,4] pointed out that the geometric prominence of the corneal dome exposes the corneal limbus to tangential irradiation from the environment. The protrusion of the cornea from the scleral shell imparts sufficient clearance for the limbus to realize its potential to act as a convex lens, where near-tangential light rays incident at the temporal limbus are converged across the anterior chamber to a focus at the nasal limbus.[3-5]

Maloof, Ho, and Coroneo [6] were the first to quantify the limbal light focusing effect. Using various model corneal domes, they used ray tracing to locate convergence points within the nasal limbus for light rays incident at the temporal limbus at near-tangential angles. However, they assumed a first-order drop off in light intensity within each medium. This assumption will affect the estimated positions of maximum light amplification in the nasal limbus, as absorbing media usually impose an exponential decrease in the intensity of penetrating irradiation.[7]

Limbal light focusing has been proposed as the fundamental mechanism which governs the formation of actinic diseases such as pterygium. [8] The present work aims to re-examine the penetration of light focusing into the limbus, when an exponential absorbance of the medium is included.

Methods

The attenuation of a monochromatic irradiant beam which passes through an absorbing medium can be calculated from the Bouguer-Lambert-Beer exponential law of absorption. [7] For absorptivity α, and optical path length x; the ratio of emergent and incident irradiance is called the transmittance $T = I/I_0 = exp(-\alpha x)$. The absorbance A is calculated from $A = \log(1/T)$, and total absorbance is the sum of the parts if a series of different media are encountered in the path length. The present calculations for the peripheral cornea assume $T = 0.5$, which for $x = 1$ mm yields $\alpha \cong 700\ m^{-1}$.

The effect of exponential absorption by the limbal tissue was estimated by multiplying the point peak-intensities at limbal distance x (Fig. 8 of Maloof, Ho, and Coroneo [6]) by the factor $exp(-\alpha x)$. Positive limbal distance x extends from the aqueous humour ($x = 0$) to the tears, and is parallel to a vector which is normal to the peripheral corneal surface and is approximately sagittal. Six angles of incidence were used previously: 95, 100, 102, 104, 106, 108 degrees [6] where 0 degrees is the sagittal plane containing the visual axis.

Maloof et al. [6] only allowed for three adjustable parameters: anterior and posterior corneal radius, and anterior surface shape. The shape factor for a rotationally symmetric cornea can be defined as $p = 1 - e^2$, where e is the eccentricity of the corneal dome. The average human p value is 0.74-0.85 and the p values assumed for high, standard, and low shape factors are 1.00, 0.75, and 0.50 respectively. The corresponding radii are given in Table 1 of Maloof et al. [6]

Results

The results agree with those of Maloof, Ho, and Coroneo [6] and show that the greatest focusing effect occurs at the posterior limbus, near to the aqueous humour (Fig. 1). Corneas with a lower shape factor $p \rightarrow 0.5$ have peak intensities which locate in pronounced posterior sites. Among the intensity peaks calculated for the standard cornea, the ratio of the largest value to the smallest is about 9.5:1. The direct corneal route ("sclerotic scatter") where light is internally reflected to the opposite limbus entails such a significant path length that the terminal irradiance is much smaller.

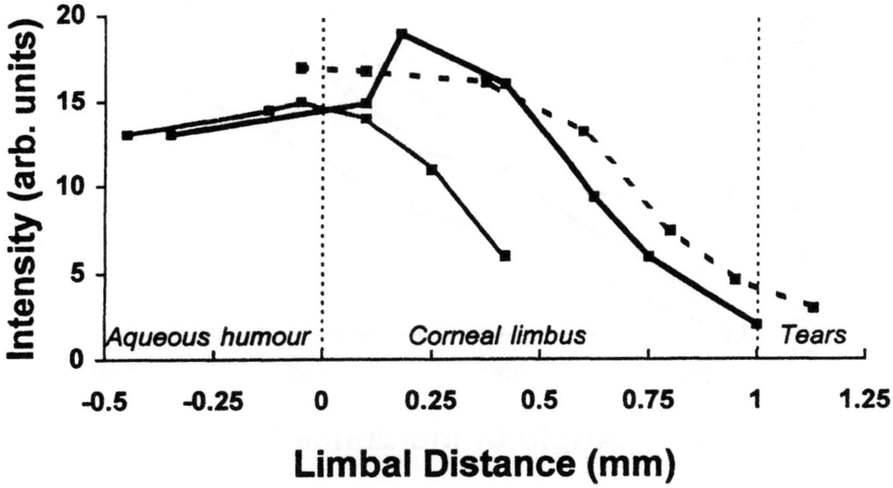

FIGURE 1. Position of peak intensity of focusing effect calculated for standard cornea (*solid line*), high shape factor (*broken line*), and low shape factor (*grey line*). Six angles of incidence are assumed for each cornea, from 95 deg (left) to 108 deg (right). The anteriormost point (tear/cornea interface, *right*) in the curves for the standard and high shape factor corneas is extrapolated from Fig. 8 of Maloof et al.[6]

The effect of angle of incidence is shown in Fig. 2. An increase in the angle of incidence has two effects: (1) the peak focusing location moves more anteriorly; (2) the magnitude of the amplification *falls* (see Fig. 1). Lowering the corneal shape factor shows the same general relationship between angle of incidence and peak focusing location, except that the sites are more posterior than for the standard cornea.

Discussion

The present results indicate that peripheral light focusing "action" sites (of peak intensity) are located in the posterior nasal limbus. This confirms our previous conclusions which assumed first-order light absorption within the medium. [6] The incorporation of exponential absorption has reemphasized the importance of the posterior nasal limbus. I did not replicate the previous procedure, but the present assumptions are unlikely to have a significant effect on the results (A. Ho, personal communication).

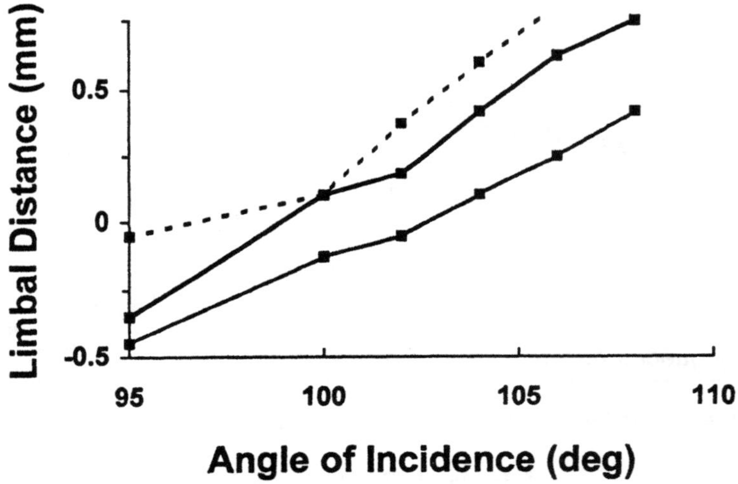

FIGURE 2. Variation of peak intensity position as the angle of incidence varies. The lines have the same meaning as in Fig. 1. The zero limbal position corresponds to the aqueous humour interface with the cornea, while the anterior cornea/tear surface occurs at a *y*-value of +1 mm (not shown). Angle of incidence is the field angle, wherein the sagittal plane (visual axis) is taken as zero degrees, and the tangential plane is 90 degrees. At each angle, the relative intensity is not the same (see Fig. 1) because of the additional path length associated with larger angles. For example, in the standard cornea (solid line), the highest value of 19 occurs at 102 deg, and the lowest of 6 occurs at 108 deg.

The posterior limbus is believed to be the site of stem cells for the cornea and conjunctival epithelium [see ref. 9]. Kwok and Coroneo have proposed that aberrant stem cell development due to long-term stimulation by a light focusing effect could lead to pterygium development. [8] This would explain the biomedical enigma of primary pterygia which show a mysterious anatomic predilection for the nasal limbus. The same mechanism could also explain [9] the preponderance of cortical lenticular cataracts in the inferior nasal region of the human lens.[10]

These results have important implications for the pathogenesis of the ophthalmohelioses such as pterygium, pinguecula, and "senile" cataract. The mechanism(s) mediating changes in cell function is unknown. However, exposure to sunlight is a well-known risk factor for diseases such as pterygium and age-associated cataract. [5,10] The ocular tissues in the putative light path (conjunctiva, cornea, and aqueous humour) are able to transmit measurable levels of UVA and some UVB. We assumed that the irradiance had a transmittance of ~0.50, which corresponds to near ultraviolet (UVA, 320-400 nm) wavelengths. [1,2] Ocular epithelial cells are known to be susceptible to UVA and UVB radiation but the cytotoxicity of 365 nm wavelength radiation is only 0.05% that of 297 nm radiation. [11] Nevertheless, it is possible that many years of regular exposure to UVA-containing sunlight could elicit biologic effects in the limbus and anterior segment tissues. Phototoxicity could arise from UVA generated free radicals in cornea, lens, and retina [12,13] as well as the amplification effect which can reach a maximum of 10-20 times.[4] In support of this argument is the finding that pterygia cells demonstrate changes in cell surface antigens. [14] The susceptibility of limbal stem cells to chronic UV irradiation is yet to be detailed.

Acknowledgments

Arthur Ho, PhD is thanked for helpful discussions. Financial support from the Auckland Medical Research Foundation is gratefully acknowledged.

References

1. Beems EM, van Best JA. Light transmission of the cornea in whole human eyes. Exp Eye Res 1990; 50: 393-395.
2. van den Berg TJTP, Tan KEWP. Light transmittance of the human corneal from 320 to 700 nm for different ages. Vis Res 1994; 34: 1453-1456.
3. Coroneo MT. Albedo concentration in the anterior eye: a phenomenon that locates some solar diseases. Ophthalmic Surg 1990; 21: 60-65.
4. Coroneo MT, Muller-Stolzenburg NW, Ho A. Peripheral light focusing by the anterior eye and the ophthalmohelioses. Ophthal Surg 1991; 22: 705-711.
5. Narayanan P, Merriam JC, Vazquez ME, Dillon J. Experimental model of light focusing of the peripheral cornea. Invest Ophthalmol Vis Sci 1996; 37: 37-41.
6. Maloof AJ, Ho A, Coroneo MT. Influence of corneal shape on limbal light focusing. Invest Ophthalmol Vis Sci 1994; 35: 2592-2598.
7. Meyer-Arendt JR. Introduction to classical and modern optics. Englewood Cliffs: Prentice Hall:, 1972: 390-395.
8. Kwok LS, Coroneo MT. A model for pterygium formation. Cornea 1994; 13: 219-224.
9. Coroneo MT. Pterygium as an early indicator of ultraviolet insolation: a hypothesis. Br J Ophthalmol 1993; 77: 734-739.
10. Schein OD, West S, Munoz B, Vitale S, Maguire M, Taylor H, Bressler NM. Cortical lenticular opacification: distribution and location in a longitudinal study. Invest Ophthal Vis Sci 1994; 35: 363-366.
11. Andley UP, Lewis RM, Reddan JR, Kochevar IE. Action spectrum for cytotoxicity in the UVA- and UVB-wavelength region in cultured lens epithelial cells. Invest Ophthalmol Vis Sci 1994; 35: 367-373.
12. Yamanashi BS, Hacker H, Klintworth GK. Wavelength dependence and kinetics of UV-induced free radical formation in the human cornea and lens. Photochem Photobiol 1979; 30: 391-395.
13. Rózanowska M., Jarvis-Evans J, Korytowski W, Boulton ME, Burke JM, Sarna T. Blue light-induced reactivity of retinal age pigment. *In vitro* generation of oxygen-reactive species. J Biol Chem 1995; 270: 1825-1830.
14. Dushku N, Reid TW. Immunohistochemical evidence that human pterygia originate from an invasion of vimentin-expressing altered limbal epithileal basal cell. Curr Eye Res 1994;13: 473-481.

TOPOGRAPHY OF ROD AND CONE SENSITIVITY LOSS IN RETINITIS PIGMENTOSA

STEVEN NUSINOWITZ[1] and DAVID G. BIRCH[2].
[1]Jules Stein Eye Institute, Los Angeles, CA. and [2]Retina Foundation of the Southwest, Dallas, TX.

Abstract

Using static threshold perimetry and stimuli designed to isolate rod- and cone- mediated function, we show that rod and cone sensitivity loss in patients with retinitis pigmentosa (RP) share similar topographical patterns.

Introduction

In patients with RP, previous studies have documented the progressive loss of rod and cone function both in the electroretinogram (ERG) and in rod- and cone- mediated visual fields [1-3]. The end result of this disease is widespread loss of both rod and cone function. Less well understood is the relationship between *patterns* of rod and cone functional loss in RP. Mid-peripheral scotomas in cone visual fields are common [4,5]. Similarly, rod sensitivity losses are typically greatest in the mid-peripheral retina with relative sparing of the far periphery [6]. To explore this relationship further, we compare rod- and cone- mediated visual fields in a group of patients diagnosed with RP who are in relatively early stages of the disease.

Method and Procedure

Subjects. Rod and cone visual fields were measured in twenty patients who had been diagnosed with RP. Patients were selected from a larger group because they retained detectable rod and cone ERGs and had measurable rod and cone thresholds throughout large areas of the visual field. The control group consisted of twenty subjects with normal ophthalmic exams. Informed consent was obtained from each participant after the procedures, goals, and potential risks and benefits of the study were explained.

Visual Fields. All testing was conducted with pupil dilation (1% tropicamide and 2.5% phenylephrine hydrochloride). Static parametric thresholds were measured at 76 locations (grid spacing of 15°) using an Octopus automated perimeter (Interzeag, Schlieren,

Switzerland). One test location fell on the blind spot and was used as a measure of fixation compliance. A second point fell on the fovea. Both the blind spot and the fovea were excluded from further analysis. Stimulus size was constant at 0.43° (corresponding to Goldmann III), stimulus duration was 100 msec, and stimulus location was randomly ordered. Rod visual fields were obtained following 40 minutes of dark-adaptation using a blue stimulus (Kodak Wratten 47A, λ_{max}=450 nm, half-bandwidth=55 nm). Prior research has indicated that dark-adapted responses to blue stimuli are rod-mediated in normal subjects[6]. As a validity check in nine patients, thresholds were also obtained using a red stimulus (Kodak Wratten 26, $\lambda_{50\%}$ cut-on, 605 nm). A comparison of blue and red fields supported the view that virtually all tested locations (except the fovea) measured with the blue stimuli were rod-mediated in this subgroup of patients. Cone visual fields were obtained with the standard background (2.2 log scot td) of the Octopus perimeter and an orange stimulus (Tiffen, λ_{max}=588 nm) to enhance detection by cones. All other procedures were the same as for the dark-adapted rod visual fields.

Results

Departures from mean normal sensitivity were calculated for each of the 74 locations in the rod and cone fields to provide a distribution of difference scores. For each patient, the difference scores were averaged to give an index of overall average sensitivity loss for rods and separately for cones. Pairwise comparisons of rod and cone sensitivity showed significantly greater losses for rods than for cones ($t=4.56$, $df=19$, $P<0.001$). On average, rods were 13.6 ($\pm$ 5.6) dB less sensitive than normal and cones 8.4 ($\pm$ 3.1) dB less sensitive than normal. Across all patients, average rod sensitivity loss was moderately correlated with average cone sensitivity loss ($r = 0.56$, $df = 20$, $P = 0.013$).

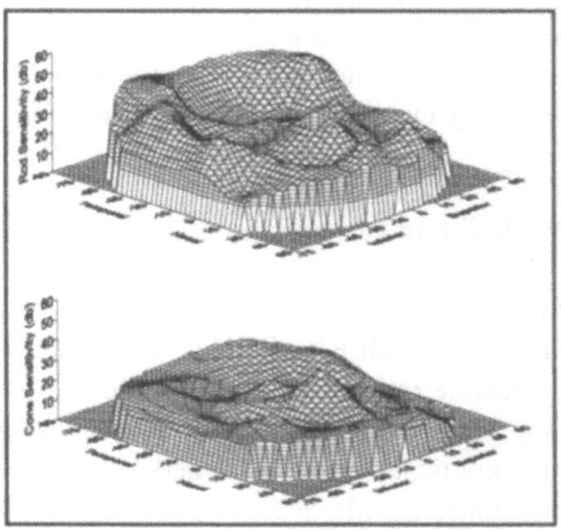

Figure 1. Rod (top) and cone (bottom) field topographies for a representative RP patient.

Rod and cone visual fields for a representative patient with autosomal dominant RP are shown in Figure 1. Sensitivity losses for both rods (top) and cones (bottom) appear greatest in a ring extending from about 15° to 40° eccentricity, with relative preservation of the far periphery. Except for a small region in the central retina, the majority of locations with near-normal rod and cone sensitivity are located in a ring at an eccentricity of >50°. The similarity in field topographies is indexed by a Spearman correlation coefficient (r_s) relating rod and cone sensitivity across the field. For the patient shown, r_s=0.62, $P<0.01$. The overall average r_s ($\pm$ 1 sd) across all patients was 0.60 ($\pm$0.17). (All but two coefficients had Ps<0.0001; the exceptions had Ps < 0.05.)

Patterns of sensitivity loss. The pattern of rod and cone sensitivity loss is shown in Figures 2 and 3. Figure 2 shows the proportion of the field where sensitivity losses fell within three ranges: 0.3 log unit of normal (bottom panel), between 0.3 and 1.0 log units of normal (middle panel), and more than 1.0 log units (top panel). These ranges of sensitivity loss can be characterized as: normal to near normal, sick, and marginally-functional, respectively [7]. The figure illustrates that the area of retina with near normal function (bottom panel) is similar for rods and cones. Of the remaining retina that functions abnormally, cones are less affected than rods. In this area, significantly more cones than rods were down between 0.3 and 1.0 log units (middle panel), whereas rod sensitivity losses in this area were more frequently greater than 1.0 log unit (top panel).

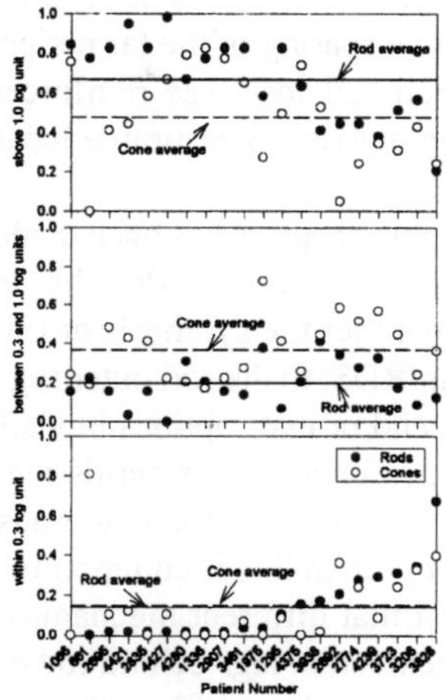

Figure 2. The proportion of rod (filled circles) and cone (open circles) fields with difference scores within each of three ranges.

Average departures from normal sensitivity were calculated for each of the three regions: 15°-45° from fixation, 45°-60° eccentricity, and >60°. The results are plotted in Figure 3. The results indicate a significant main effect of region (F=11.62, df=2/38, P<0.001). For both rods and cones, the greatest losses occurred in the region from 15°-45° from fixation and the smallest losses occurred in the periphery. The interaction between the receptor type and region was not significant (F=0.06, df=2/40, P>0.10) consistent with a similar pattern of regional sensitivity loss for rods and cones.

Discussion

This study was designed to gain a better understanding of the relationship between topographical patterns of rod and cone sensitivity loss in retinitis pigmentosa. Three overall trends emerged from a comparison of the rod and cone fields in these patients. First, with few exceptions, overall rod sensitivity loss was greater than cone sensitivity loss. Second, the area of the retina with normal or near-normal sensitivity was similar for rods and cones. Regions of the retina that were relatively sick showed greater

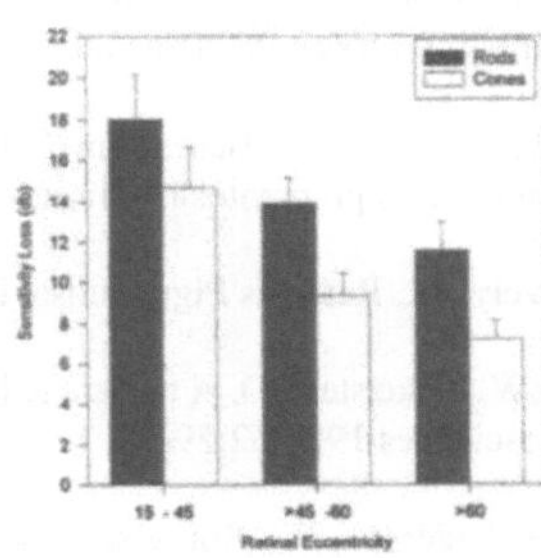

Figure 3. Rod and cone sensitivity losses as a function of retinal eccentricity.

rod sensitivity losses than cone sensitivity losses. Third, both rods and cones showed the greatest sensitivity losses in central and mid-peripheral regions (excluding the macula), with relative sparing of the far periphery. This overall similarity in topography of rod and cone functional loss was reinforced by more sensitive comparisons of rod and cone sensitivity at every measurable location throughout the visual field.

Considerable progress has been made in identifying specific gene mutations that ultimately lead to rod cell death. Possible mechanisms affected by these mutant genes include defects in either the synthesis or transport of membrane proteins, such as rhodopsin and peripherin/RDS, to the rod outer segment, disruptions in the maintenance of the rod outer segment, and/or interruptions in vital metabolic pathways. The underlying mechanism(s) of cone dysfunction in retinitis pigmentosa is less well understood. One possibility in some forms of retinitis pigmentosa is that a mutant gene produces a defect in a structurally important protein that is common to both rods and cones. This hypothesis would require the caveat that different mechanisms trigger the start of the degenerative process, since cone degeneration lags behind rod degeneration, or that the effects of the defective protein manifest themselves differently in rods and cones. In addition, some mechanism would be required to regionally constrain the effects of the defective protein to account for the topographical similarity of rod and cone sensitivity loss seen in this study. An alternative possibility that is more parsimonious with this study, places cone cell death secondary to rod cell death. Degenerating rod photoreceptors are known to have shortened and disorganized outer segments and eventually die leaving gaps in the receptor mosaic. Cone dysfunction might occur because of a disorganization of cone photoreceptors as a result of rod photoreceptor cell death and the structural support that they may provide, or by the toxic by-products of rod cell death.

References

1. Berson, EL, Sandberg, MA, Rosner, B, Birch, DG, Hanson, AH. Natural course of retinitis pigmentosa over a three year interval. American Journal of Ophthalmology 1985;99:240-51.

2. Birch, DG. Hood, DC. Abnormal rod photoreceptor function in retinitis pigmentosa. In Anderson, R., Hollyfield, J. LaVail, M. (Eds.). Degenerative Diseases of the Retina. New York: Plenum, 1995:359-69.

3. Massof, RW, Dagnelie, G, Benzschawel, T, Palmer, RW, Finkelstein, D. First order dynamics of visual field loss in retinitis pigmentosa. Clinical Vision Science 1990;5:1-26.

4. Heckenlively, JR. Retinitis Pigmentosa. Philadelphia: Lippincott, 1988.

5. Massof, RW, Finkelstein, D. A two-stage hypothesis for the natural course of retinitis pigmentosa. Advances in Biosciences 1987:62;29-58.

6. Birch, DG, Anderson, JL. Rod visual fields in cone-rod degeneration: Comparison to retinitis pigmentosa. Investigative Ophthalmology and Visual Science 1990; 31:2288-99.

7. Hood, DC, Shady, S., Birch, DG. Heterogeneity in retinal disease and the computational model of the human rod response. Journal of the Optical Society of America - A 1993; 10:1624-30.

RESIDUAL PSYCHOPHYSICAL DEFICITS FOLLOWING RECOVERY FROM THE CUBAN EPIDEMIC OF OPTIC NEUROPATHY

ALFREDO SADUN and RICHARD RUBIN
Doheny Eye Institute, University of Southern California, Los Angeles, CA.

Abstract

From the Spring of 1992 until the middle of 1993, an epidemic of blindness swept across Cuba. Men between the ages of 25 and 64 presented with complaints of bilateral symmetrical visual loss and dyschromatopsia often associated with peripheral neuropathy. Patients were noted to have a wedge-shaped defect of their optic disk and papillo-macular bundle. In contrast to Leber's Hereditary Optic Neuropathy, there was an absence of mitochondrial DNA defects. Risk factors included a high rate of smoking, of missing meals, and of heavy drinking, especially home brewed rum. It was concluded that there was a combined set of insults to the mitochondria due largely to folic acid and vitamin B-12 insufficiency, aggravated in some patients by cyanide from smoking and in others by low grade chronic consumption of methanol from home brewed rum. Four months following implementation of vitamin therapy, we found improvement of visual acuity, color vision and contrast sensitivity at low and mid spatial frequencies. Initial large central and centrocecal scotomas improved to small central scotomas. Finally, saccadic smooth pursuit eye movements completely resolved. We hypothesize that compromise of mitochondrial function due to acquired metabolic disease led to a viscious cycle which caused a severe disruption of the axonal transport system. Contrast sensitivity at the high spatial frequencies subserved by P cells and their smaller axons was lost. Upon vitamin therapy and resumption of a healthier diet, the larger caliber axons and M cell function were able to recover providing a dramatic subtotal improvement of visual acuity. In conclusion, we believe that this process provided a model for the selective loss of P cells in the human retina.

Introduction

From the Spring of 1992 until the middle of 1993, an epidemic of blindness due to an optic neuropathy swept across Cuba challenging the social and medical infrastructure of that island as well as investigators from around the world. In general, men between the ages of 25 and 64 were presenting in ever increasing numbers with complaints of visual loss often associated with peripheral neuropathy. There were a number of systemic findings as well, most commonly malaise, fatigue, weight loss and polyuria as well as ataxia and hearing loss [1]. Initially, the diagnosis of tobacco-alcohol amblyopia was made. However, as the epidemic grew to staggering proportions, most of the scientists placed by the Cuban government on a special task force to investigate this illness concluded that there was possibly a viral etiology. Coxacci virus was cultured out of many cerebral spinal fluid samples. This later proved to be a laboratory error [1].

Initial Findings

In May of 1993, by which time about 50,000 cases of optic and peripheral neuropathy had been identified by the Cuban health system, the Cuban Ministry of Public Health made an appeal to the international community which led to a visit to the island by at least four teams of clinicians and scientists. Dr. Sadun led one team of clinicians from the combined groups of Project Orbis International and the Pan American Health Organization [1]. The team found a substantial number of patients had no organic basis for their complaints putting into doubt the findings of all previous epidemiological investigations. Fortunately, the team was able to establish an objective element found in all cases of the optic form of this epidemic, a wedge-shaped defect of the optic disk and papillo-macular bundle which in every way resembled Leber's Hereditary Optic Neuropathy [1]. The typical patient was found to be in a general state of malaise and fatigue and had lost about twenty pounds of weight in the preceding two or three months. Ataxia, hearing loss and polyuria were also often found.

The patients generally complained of rapidly progressing bilateral symmetrical visual loss characterized primarily as dyschromatopsia and central scotomas. Visual acuities were approximately 20/400 OU and they could on average only make out 2/8 of the American Optical (AO) color test plates. Pupil reactions were sluggish to light but brisk to near and contrast sensitivity function losses were seen across all spatial frequencies. Naturally, there were profound losses in the central field as established by tangent field, Amsler grid or threshold Amsler grid testing. There were always central or centrocecal scotomas with occasionally peripheral field constriction as well. Additionally ocular motility was remarkable for saccadic smooth pursuits. The fundus examination on newly diagnosed cases demonstrated a fairly normal appearing optic nerve, but there was a wedge-shaped loss of the papillo-macular nerve fiber layer bundle. Moreover, the nerve fiber layer above and below this bundle was often markedly swollen.

The team was struck by the similarity between these cases in Cuba and Leber's hereditary optic neuropathy which is known to be due to one or more mitochondrial DNA defects. However, unlikely that such large numbers of individuals would suddenly demonstrate mutations, DNA studies were performed and mitochondrial DNA defects in the Cuban patients were not common [2,3]. The team was also quite sure that a viral etiology did not apply especially in so far as none of of the patients had family contacts and the epidemic relatively spared women and men over the age of 65 and absolutely spared children under the age of 15. Moreover, there was never any pleocytosis of the cerebral spinal fluid nor were there other signs of CNS infection.

The resemblance to Leber's hereditary optic neuropathy suggested that the pathophysiology of the epidemic was also at the level of the mitochondria. An acquired mitochondrial injury most likely would come from nutritional and/or toxic etiologies. An evaluation of risk factors found that there was a high rate of smoking, of missing meals, of weight loss, and of heavy drinking, especially home brewed rum. There was probably a combined set of insults to the mitochondria due largely to vitamin insufficiency (particularly of folic acid and B-12) aggravated in some patients by cyanide (from smoking) and in others by low grade chronic consumption of methanol (from home brewed rum).

There are a variety of mechanisms by which oxidative phosphorylization in the mitochondria can be compromised. In particular, low levels of folic acid not only directly interfere with oxidate phosphorylization but permit the accumulation of formate (a metabolic product of methanol) that requires folic acid for detoxification. This collection of factors would interfere with mitochondrial respiration and the availability of ATP necessary for axonal transport. The longest axons (hence, the peripheral neuropathy) and the axons of the smallest caliber (hence, the papillo-macular bundle) would be most vulnerable to such compromise of axoplasmic transport.

Treatment and Results

Recommendations made to the Cuban government included a new case definition of the disease which emphasized the observation by red-free direct ophthalmoscopy of the wedge-shaped defect in the papillo-macular bundle. Vitamin therapy was implemented to the patients as well as vitamin prophylaxis to all the citizens of Cuba.

Within a few months the epidemic was said to have halted. On the teams return to Cuba in September of 1993, they had an opportunity to reassess many of the same patients previously seen in May 1993. They found an impressive but incomplete recovery of visual acuity from an average of 20/400 to an average of 20/50. There was a more impressive improvement in color vision. The patients who could initially see on average only 2 out of 8 AO color test plates had improved to see on average 7 of 8 of the same plates. Naturally, the loss of the papillo-macular bundle was permanent; however, it was ophthalmologically less obvious since the adjacent swellings of nerve fiber had receded. Finally, while many patients initially had not demonstrated any optic disk changes per se, four months later temporal pallor was now noted in all patients.

Further psychophysical evaluations were most interesting. Whereas initially, there were decreases in contrast sensitivity across all spatial frequencies, subsequent evaluation of those patients who had recovered demonstrated that they had regained contrast sensitivity functions at low and mid spatial frequencies but maintained profound losses of the high spatial frequencies. Although initially large central and centrocecal scotomas with sharp borders were found as established by tangent field, Amsler, and threshold Amsler grid testing; upon recovery very small central scotomas with very shallow borders were found. Finally, the cogwheeling (or saccadic) smooth pursuit eye movements had completely resolved to normal eye movements.

Discussion

The resolution of signs and symptoms, and in particular the residual psychophysical impairments suggested an anatomical distinction between those fibers which underwent degeneration as a consequence of the epidemic of optic neuropathy and those that only suffered temporary injury. The papillo-macular bundle is composed primarily of P cells whose somas are small and whose axons are of small caliber. Their function is primarily to subserve visual acuity, color vision and high contrast at high spatial frequencies [4]. In contradistinction, M cells are larger, have axons of larger diameter and are more uniformly distributed across the human retina. They largely subserve low contrast sensitivity at low and midspatial frequencies and movement detection [4].

It was hypothesized that compromise of mitochondrial function due to acquired metabolic disease during the Cuban epidemic led to a viscious cycle of depletion of ATP, resulting in slowed axonal transport, leading to delayed mitochondrial transport causing further depletions of ATP. The viscious cycle created a severe disruption of the axonal transport system that manifested itself first and foremost in the smallest fibers (whose surface area to volume ratio is highest) leading to axonal degeneration. However, in the larger caliber fibers the blockage in axonal transport led to cellular and physiological dysfunction but not to the point of cellular death. Hence, upon vitamin therapy and resumption of a healthier diet, the larger caliber axons were able to recover their function. In other words, there was a selective loss of P cells. Recovery of M cell function provided a dramatic but subtotal improvement of visual acuity but left a residual loss of contrast sensitivity at the high spatial frequencies subserved by P cells. It should be noted that the abnormality in ocular motility (cogwheeling smooth pursuits), which likely was based on M cell dysfunction, resolved upon recovery of the M cells.

The one psychophysical finding which does not conform to this hypothesis is that of an improvement in color vision. However, while it is true that M cells are color ignorant and P cells are required for color discrimination, all P cells are not of equal size and caliber. As one moves away from the fovea, the P cells, while still much smaller than the M cells, are larger than the foveal P cells. Therefore, it is likely that the larger more eccentric P cells along with the M cells survived, permitting at least some color vision.

In conclusion, we believe that impairment of mitochondria in this epidemic affected the smallest caliber axons and hence provided a model for the selective loss of P cells in the human retina.

References

1. Sadun AA, Martone JF, Muci-Mendoza R, et al. Epidemic optic neuropathy in Cuba: Eye Findings. Arch Ophthalmol 1994;112:691-699.
2. Johns DR, Sadun AA. Cuban epidemic optic neuropathy: Mitochondrial DNA analysis. J Neuro-ophthalmol 1994;14:130-134.
3. Newman NJ, Torroni A, Brown MD, Lott MT, Fernandez MM, Wallace DC. Epidemic neuropathy in Cuba not associated with mitochondrial DNA mutations found in Leber's hereditary optic neuropathy patients. Cuba Neuropathy Field Investigation Team. Am J Ophthalmol 1994;118:158-168.
4. Livingston MS, Hubel DH. Psychophysical evidence for seperate channels for the perception of form, color, movment and depth. J Neurosci 1987;7:3416-3468.

IN VIVO CELLULAR CHARACTERIZATION OF RETINAL PATHOLOGY IN A SMALL EYE ANIMAL MODEL

H. ZWICK, R. ELLIOTT, S.T. SCHUSCHEREBA, D.J. LUND, and B.E. STUCK
US Army Medical Research Detachment
Walter Reed Army Institute of Research
San Antonio, TX 78235

Abstract

We have used confocal scanning laser ophthalmoscopy (CSLO) to evaluate acute laser injury to the retina in a small eye animal model. The snake eye is optically unique, combining a high numerical aperture with a clear non-turbid ocular media. These optical qualities optimize image resolution in the spatial and depth dimension. We demonstrate that acute laser exposures capable of damaging the photoreceptor matrix may also alter the blood flow imaged at more interior levels of the retina. At lower levels of exposure more photoreceptors survive but turn highly reflective and are better detected with non-visible (780 nm) than visible (633 nm) imaging laser sources.

Introduction

Recent studies of laser-induced retinal pathology suggest a role of retinal blood flow in the progression of photic pathology induced in the photoreceptor retinal pigment epithelial (RPE) complex of the outer retina. Damage to the photoreceptor RPE complex can release inflammatory mediators into the blood having both negative and positive effects on retinal neural cells distant from the actual injury site [1]. In this paper we demonstrate an ability to image cellular detail in the retina of the snake at posterior and anterior retinal sites. Such imaging capability depends in part on the snake's optics - its high spatial resolution and high numerical aperture or short focal length eye [2,3,4].

Methods

Images of the Checkered Garter snake (*Thamnophis m. marcianus*) and the Great Plains Rat Snake (*Elaphe guttata emoryi)* retinas were recorded and digitized from a Rodenstock confocal scanning laser ophthalmoscope (CSLO). The dioptic powers of these eyes are 445 and 370 diopters, respectively; a 0.1 diopter change in these eyes corresponds to a 0.5 and 0.7 micron shift, respectively, in focal depth which is transitioned from the posterior to the anterior retina with the CSLO [4]. An air-cooled Argon laser (488 and 515 nm) provided acute laser exposures ranging from 1000 to 152 μjoules Total Intraocular Energy (TIE) for 10-20 msec pulse widths. Retinal spot size was about 35 microns. Anesthesia was achieved with a combination of Ketamine and Xylazine in a ratio of 3.5:1.

Results

Figure 1A is a CSLO view of the Checkered Garter snake retina imaged at the photoreceptor matrix showing large, small single, and small secondary cones [5]. Figure 1B is a similar view from the Great Plains Rat snake showing similar cone types. In both images, large cones show possible receptor mode structure [6].

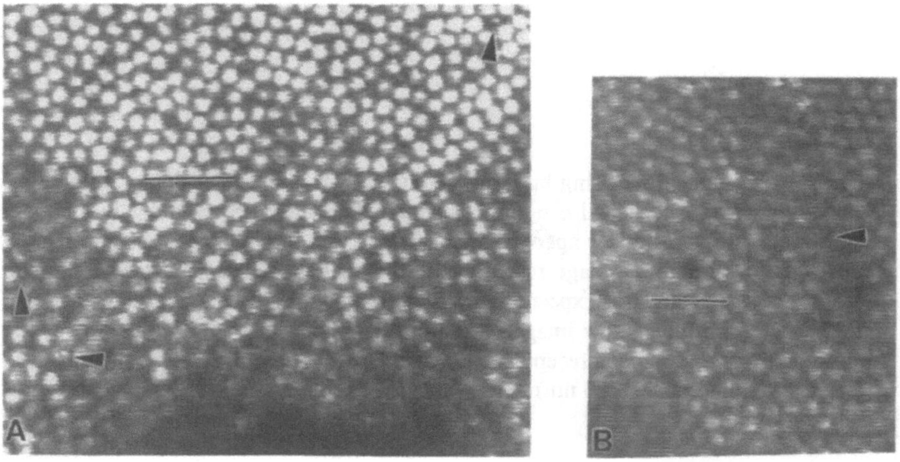

Figure 1. (A) The Checkered Garter snake's photoreceptor layer with vertical arrows indicating small single and double cones, large cones showing receptor mode structure. Great Plains Rat snake photoreceptor layer (B) with arrows indicating a group of large cones with possible mode structure (bars = 50 microns).

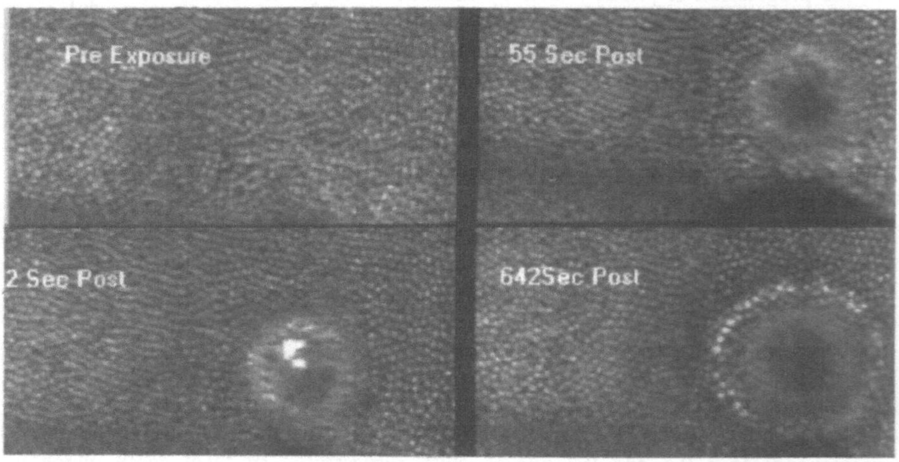

Figure 2. Temporal course of laser-induced retinal photoreceptor damage imaged in vivo over a 10.8 min post exposure period.

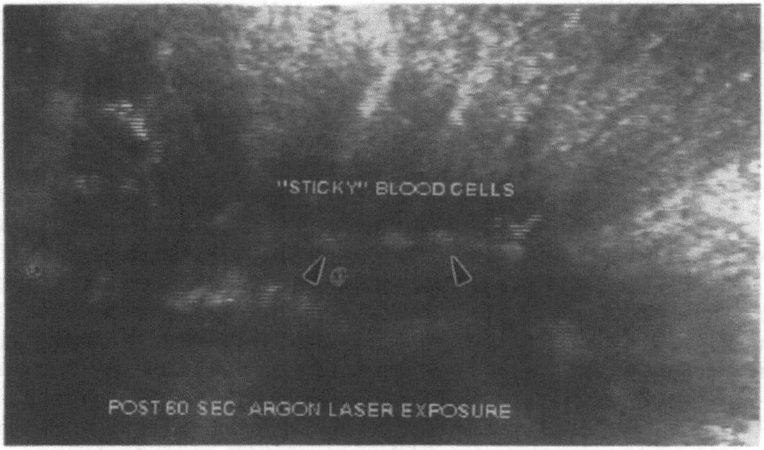

Figure 3. Sticky blood cells imaged at 60 sec post 1000 μjoule, 10 msec Argon laser exposure.

Figure 2 shows the alteration in the photoreceptor layer of the Checkered Garter snake induced by a single 1000 μjoule, 10 msec pulse over a 10.7 min post exposure period. Initially, a thermal gas bubble forms transitioning to a central gray area devoid of photoreceptors. At 60 sec, this gray area is surrounded by an annulus of highly reflective photoreceptors. At the end of 10 min, the affected area has doubled in size with an outer ring of highly reflective, slightly swollen photoreceptors. An intermediate area exists with low contrast enlarged photoreceptors apparent at the outer edge of this area adjacent to the highly reflective photoreceptors. In lower level exposures, the affected photoreceptor areas remain populated with highly reflective and slightly swollen photoreceptors (see Figure 4).

In Figure 3, the confocal image plane is at the anterior vascular system of the Checkered Garter snake, imaging a large vessel superior to the *conus papillaris*. The arrows indicate blood cells, about twice the size of photoreceptors (14-18 microns), morphologically consistent with blood cell types found in the snake [7], that have stopped flowing, appearing stuck within the vessel wall. Cell "sticking" begins about

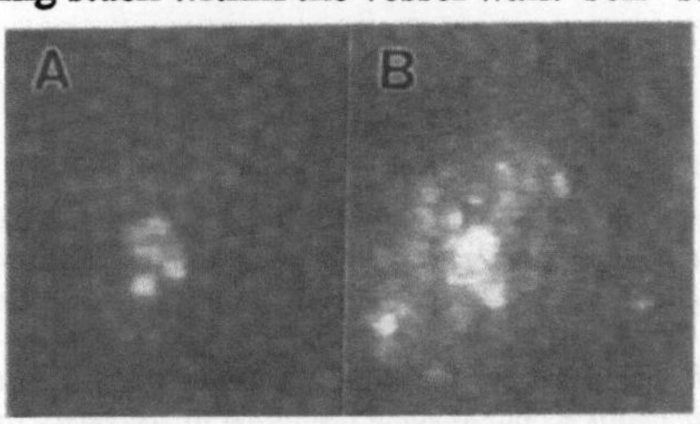

Figure 4. The same laser exposure site is imaged at 633 (4A) and at 780 (4b) nm.

20 sec post exposure and may last several minutes with frequent recurrence at the same site with some cells appearing to enter adjacent intraretinal space. This cellular behavior is characteristic of leukocytes in response to tissue injury [1].

Figure 4 shows a low level (152 μjoules) exposure imaged at 633 (A) and 780 nm (B). More reflective photoreceptors are observed at 780 nm than at 633nm.

Discussion

We have demonstrated an enhanced capability to image *in vivo* laser-induced retinal cellular pathology in both the posterior and anterior retina by combining the high numerical aperture and high spatial resolution of the snake eye with the CSLO's ability to traverse retinal depth. At the posterior retina, laser induced photoreceptor damage varies with exposure dose. At high doses, photoreceptors in the lesion center degenerate within several sec, but survive at the lesion edges, becoming highly reflective, slightly swollen with minimal visible receptor mode structure [6]. At lower levels, such altered photoreceptors survive over the entire lesion area. Imaging in the near IR (780 nm) reveals a higher number of altered photoreceptors than with visible sources (633 nm), suggesting that labile and nonlabile retinal pigments mask structural damage in the visible to a greater extent than in the near IR where their absorption is minimal.

On the other hand, immediate damage to the retinal cone photoreceptors, impacts on the anterior vascular blood cell flow within 10 to 20 sec. Blood cell "stickiness" first appears 20 sec post laser exposure. Induction of blood cell "sticking" may depend on the initial insult itself or the release of neurotrophic factors associated with laser induced photoreceptor damage [1].

Acknowledgments

In conducting this research, the investigators adhered to the "Guide for the Care and Use of Laboratory Animals," as promulgated by the Committee on Revision of the Guide for Laboratory Animal Facilities and Care, Institute of Laboratory Animal Resources, National Academy of Sciences - National Research Council. Opinions or assertions contained herein are the private views of the authors and are not to be construed as official or as reflecting the views of the Department of the Army or the Department of Defense.

References

1. Humphrey MF, Chu Yi, Sharp C, Moore S, Mann K, Rakoczy P, and Constable I. Proceedings SPIE: Laser Eye Injuries. Glial reactions to argon laser photocoagulation injury in rabbit and rat retinas. 1996;2674: 98-106.
2. Land MF and Snyder AW. Cone mosaic observed directly through natural pupil of live vertebrate. Vis Res, 1985: 25; 1519-1523.
3. Zwick H, Lund JD, Stuck BE, Zuclich JA, Elliott R, Schuschereba ST, Gagliano DA, Belkin M, Glickman RD. Confocal scanning laser ophthalmoscopic imaging resolution of secondary retinal effects induced by laser radiation. Proceedings Coherence Domain Optics, SPIE: (Special Series), 1996: 2732; 187-198.
4. Zwick H, Lund JD, Elliott R, and Schuschereba ST. Proceedings of SPIE: Ophthalmic Technologies V. Confocal spectral ophthalmoscopic imaging of retinal laser damage in small vertebrate eyes. 1995; 2393: 182-188.
5. Wong ROL. Morphology and distribution of neurons in the retina of the American Garter snake *Thamnophis sirtalis*. J of Comp Neurol, 1989; 283: 587-601.
6. Enoch JM, and Tobey Jr FL.Waveguide properties of retinal receptors: techniques and observations. In: Enoch JM and Tobey Jr, FL, editors. Vertebrate photoreceptor optics. New York, Berlin, Heidelberg: Springer - Verlag, 1981: 169-216.
7. Marie-Charlette Saint Girons. Morphology of the circulating blood cells. In Gans C and Parsons TS, editors. Biology of the reptilia. New York: Academic Press, 1970:73-91. c

OUTSIDE-IN PROCESSING AND THE GLOBAL PRECEDENCE EFFECT

GHOLAMALI AMIRKHIABANI
Faculty of Arts, Central Queensland University, Rockhampton, QLD4702, AUSTRALIA

Abstract

The outside-in hypothesis was investigated by considering the effect of size on the speed of processing to outside and inside figures. The results showed that when the size of the compound pattern was large the outside figure was responded to more slowly than the inside figure, whereas with small patterns the speed of processing of the outer figure was faster than the inner one. It seems that outside precedence is not inevitable and depends on a number of factors including size. It has been suggested that outside-in processing may be related to the global-local relationship.

Introduction

Earhard and Walker [1] and Earhard [2] examined the discriminability of line elements as a function of inner and outer locations. Line drawings of forms such as octagons, crosses, and sets of small and large forms of rectangles and diamonds were used as the stimuli. The task was to detect the location of the target line, which was thinner than the other lines of the form, either at inner or outer location. The results of these studies indicated that outer lines were discriminated more accurately than inner lines. Meanwhile, from the presence of outline advantage in a divided attention and not in a selective attention condition, Earhard and Walker concluded that more accurate discrimination of outer details of a visual object is organized by an attentional strategy and is not a process originating from a retinally tied, peripheral-to-central scanning.

Outside advantage may be related to the global precedence effect. Local components of an object are always surrounded by the outer contours of the global configuration. Therefore any global advantage may be associated with a dominance in the processing of the lines located in the outer side of the image. Navon [3] suggested that processing of global elements was given temporal precedence over processing of local elements. Kinchla and Wolfe [4] however, suggested that the temporal order of processing is not always from global to local but varies according to the size of the compound pattern. Experiments 1 and 2 have been targeted to examine the role of size of the stimulus on the temporal processing of the outside and inside figures in divided and selective attention conditions, respectively.

Experiment 1

Method:: Twenty-one undergraduate students at Central Queensland University served as subjects. All had normal or corrected to normal vision. The stimuli were programmed and generated by an IBM AH compatible computer. All stimuli were white on a black background. The stimulus was two concentric circles one of which, either the inside or the outside one, had an opening of 20 degrees facing either to the right or to the left. There were two types of stimuli that differed in visual angle size. In the small visual angle condition, the diameters of the inside and outside circles measured 14 mm (1 degree) and 58 mm (4.15 degrees), respectively. In the large visual angle condition, the diameters of the inside and outside circles subtended 58 mm (4.15 degrees) and 175 mm (12.34 degrees), respectively. Thus, the outside figure of the small visual angle condition was the same size as the inside figure of the large visual angle condition.

The stimulus was presented to the subject for 50 msec. The task was to indicate whether the property of direction of the opening, either at the outside or inside level, was to the right or to the left. Two specially marked keys were assigned for the left and right opening. To indicate the direction of the opening, subjects had to divide their attention between the two levels. Each experimental session consisted of a tutoring tour, two practice and four experimental blocks. The order of experimental blocks was counter balanced across the subjects. There were 20 trials in each practice and 40 trials in each experimental block. A trial started with the presentation of a '+' sign in the middle of the screen as the fixation point. Then the test stimulus was presented, which was replaced by a mask consisting of randomly located slashes and back slashes. The mask disappeared after a correct response, or after a time-out of 2 seconds. The next trial began with the appearance of the fixation stimulus 2000 msec after the previous response or the disappearance of the mask. The subjects were required to respond as fast as possible but to avoid errors. Reaction times and accuracies were recorded.

Results: The RT data were analysed by a two factor repeated measures analysis of variance (ANOVA). The factors were target level (inside or outside) and visual angle condition (large or small). The analysis indicated a significant main effect of visual angle size, $F(1,20) = 16.66$, $p < 0.0006$. Although the main effect of target level was not significant, the interaction of target level and visual angle size, $F(1,20) = 45.21$, $p < 0.0001$, was significant. Further analysis indicated that the outside figures were identified faster than the inside ones (Figure 1a) when the visual angle of the stimulus was small, $F(1,20) = 20.88$, $p < 0.0002$. However when the visual angle of the stimulus was large, the property of opening on the inside figure was identified faster than when it was on the outside figure, $F(1,20) = 24.18$, $p < 0.0001$.

Experiment 2

Most of the details of the method of this experiment were similar to the corresponding ones in Experiment 1 except for the following. Twenty subjects from the same pool used in the previous experiment participated in this experiment. None of them had participated in Experiment 1. Unlike Experiment 1, both inside and outside figures had opening either to the right or to the left. Therefore before each experimental block, subjects were advised whether they had to respond to the outside or inside figure while ignoring the other level.

Results: Reaction times were analyzed using a repeated measures analysis of variance with target level (inside or outside), consistency (consistent versus inconsistent), and visual angle size (large versus small). The only significant main effect was consistency, $F(1,19) = 56.00$, $p < 0.0001$. This indicated that the attended level was identified faster when it was consistent with the unattended level. The significant interaction of target level and visual angle size, $F(1,19) = 93.02$, $p < 0.0001$, indicated that the speed of processing of the outside and inside figures varied due to the visual angle of the stimulus. More detailed analysis revealed that in the small visual angle condition outside figures were identified faster than the inside ones in both consistent, $F(1,19) = 19.78$, $p < 0.0003$; and inconsistent, $F(1,19) = 56.67$, $p < 0.0001$ conditions. In contrast, in the large visual angle condition the inside figures were recognized faster than the outside ones in both consistent, $F(1,19) = 16.70$, $p < 0.0006$; and inconsistent, $F(1,19) = 38.99$, $p < 0.0001$; conditions (Figure 1b). The results of the accuracy analyses of both experiments did not indicate any speed-accuracy trade-off.

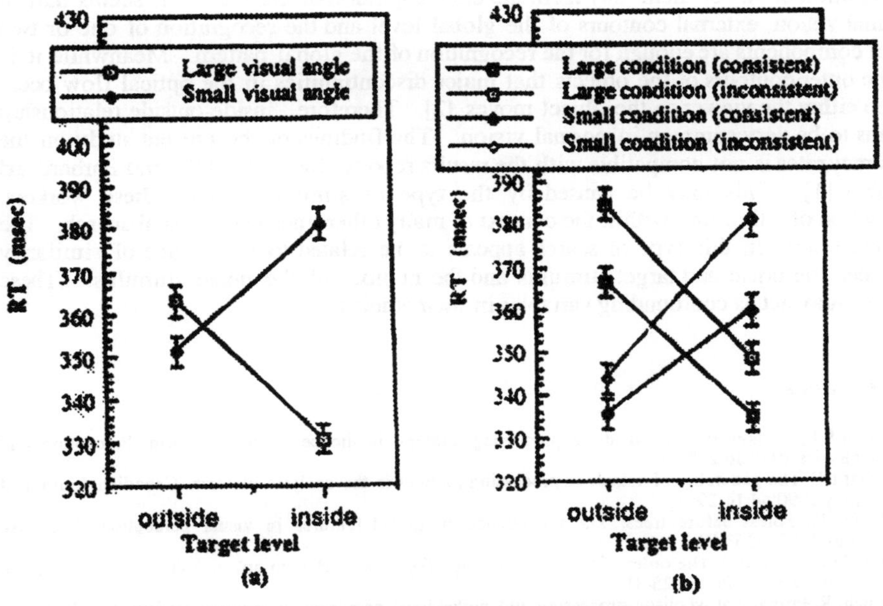

Figure 1. (a) Mean RTs as a function of target level and visual angle in Experiment 1; (b) mean RTs as a function of target level, visual angle and consistency in Experiment 2.

General Discussion

In Experiment 1, the response latencies to the outside and inside figures were studied in a selective attention condition. The results demonstrated an outside advantage in the small visual angle condition and an inside advantage in the large visual angle condition. These findings were replicated in Experiment 2, where there was a Stroop-type semantic relationship between the two levels of the stimulus. These findings are compatible with Kinchla and Wolfe's [4] finding about the existence of a turning point in reaction times to the global and local levels of a compound pattern in which global configuration is made of the spatial arrangement of the local elements. The results also indicated that speed of processing of the outside and inside levels was not determined by the experimental presentation conditions (selective versus divided).

The concepts of global and local, and the attributed relationship between these two vary among different studies [5,6]. In the crudest sense global and local may refer to the outer and inner features of a visual object. That means the most distinct aspect of the global and local relationship is that contours of the global configuration surround the local shape(s). In this type of relationship the local level does not constitute the global configuration in a sense that a special arrangement of some small letters forms a large letter. For example, a map of France is a figure located within the map of Europe. France is a part of Europe, but in order to identify Europe it does not seem to be necessary to identify France or the other European countries or vice versa, although the recognition of any of them may facilitate the recognition of the other. It seems that in normal vision, external contours of the global level and the recognition of one or two local components are enough for the recognition of the global pattern. Meanwhile it is at the outer contours of the objects that major discontinuities in the optical flow occur when either the viewer or the object moves [2]. Therefore, inside-outside relationship seems to be very common in normal vision. The findings of the present study on the accuracy rates is not compatible with the results reported by Earhard [2] and Earhard and Walker [1]. This may be caused by the type of stimuli used by these workers. Detection of a thin line within the context of many other lines needs visual search. The response time in this type of search appears to be related to the degree of similarity between the noise and target stimulus and the number of the noise stimulus. These factors may act as confounding variables in their studies.

References

1. Earhard B, Walker H. An outside-in processing strategy in the perception of form. Perception and Psychophysics 1985;36:285-95.
2. Earhard B. The generality of outside-in processing routines in the analysis of form. Canadian Journal of Psychology 1990;44:14-29.
3. Navon D. Forest before trees: The precedence of global features in visual perception. Cognitive Psychology 1977;9:353-83.
4. Kinchla RA, Wolfe J. The order of visual processing: 'Top down', 'Bottom up', or 'middle out'. Perception and Psychophysics 1979;25:225-31.
5. Kimchi R. Primacy of wholistic processing and global/local paradigm: A critical review. Psychological Bulletin 1992;112:24-38.
6. Lasaga MI. Gestalts and their components: Nature of information-precedence. In:Shepp B, Ballesteros S, editors. Object perception: Structure and process. NJ: Erlbaum, 1989: 53-89.

VISUAL FIELDS AND FUNCTIONALITY

IAN L. BAILEY
School of Optometry, University of California,
Berkeley, CA 94720-2020

Abstract

Many different issues have to be taken into consideration when measuring visual fields for functional purposes. These issues are discussed.

Introduction

The choice of method and stimulus parameters used for visual field testing should depend on the purpose of the measurement. Most commonly, visual fields are measured for screening, diagnosis, or monitoring of eye disease. In the clinical assessment and treatment of low vision patients, the usual purpose of visual field testing is to obtain measurements of visual field that will be relevant to predicting the patient's ability to perform visually-guided functional tasks. Typically, the presence of scotomas is known and the clinician's primary objective becomes to determine the extent of absolute scotomas. Relative scotomas are of less immediate importance.

Clinical Procedures

Most modern clinical field-testing procedures present static targets at fixed locations within a bowl perimeter. Kinetic techniques are preferred for identifying the location and shape of absolute scotomas of low vision patients. The test targets are moved over a tangent screen or bowl perimeter while the patient reports whether the target is visible or not. Arc perimeters and confrontation methods, while less controlled than testing in a bowl perimeter, are alternative procedures often used in assessing peripheral fields in low vision patients.

Target motion

When the general location of the scotoma is known, it is common practice to move the target steadily from within the blind region into the seeing region, asking the patient to report when the target becomes visible. This strategy encourages steady eye positioning. If the target is moved from seeing to non-seeing areas, the patient is aware of the direction of motion and has a reasonable estimate of the location of the target after it has entered the blind area. There is a strong tendency for the patient, possibly out of habit, to make quick eye movements to check on the presence of objects of interest when they fall within a scotomatous region. Another technique important for the efficient and reliable determination of scotoma borders is to make the direction of target motion approximately orthogonal to the presumed border of the scotoma. This provides crisper and easier responses from the patient. In contrast, moving the target along the border of the scotoma has the patient in a state of uncertainty and responses become unreliable.

The first step in evaluating of visual fields usually is to identify the location of the physiological blind spot. Doing this verifies that the patient can make appropriate responses and provides information about reliability of responsiveness and eye steadiness. A displaced blind spot can indicate the magnitude of eccentric viewing if the patient uses a non-foveal point in order to fixate the central fixation marker and it can also indicate systematic changes of the field due to the effect of spectacle lenses. In patients with nystagmus or other pronounced unsteadiness of the eyes, it is often not possible to confirm the presence or location of the physiological blind spot. This informs the clinician that the visual field measurements will be gross and that only major defects such as substantial constriction, quadrantic and hemianopic defects are likely to be identifiable.

Fixation control

Central scotomas or nystagmus are commonly present in low vision patients. Problems arise with maintaining fixation. For central scotomas, it is common to use a large fixation cross to help the patient maintain steady fixation. Sometimes the patient is encourage to use "foveal" fixation even though the central scotoma might cause the fixation target to disappear. The patient is advised to direct the gaze towards the center of the cross. Peripheral and para-central retina can see the cross and its configuration is recognized so that the patient is aware of the direction in which the eye should be pointed. An alternative method for the patient with a central scotoma is to use eccentric viewing. It is well established that many with central scotomas develop a preferred retinal locus (PRL) for use for inspection or close attention tasks. When using eccentric viewing, the patient maintains a view of the fixation target with a preferred retinal locus that is not the fovea. It is believed the fixation cross helps in the control of such deliberate eccentric viewing behavior.

Stimulus parameters

Targets should be of high visibility for evaluating functional visual fields. White targets of 10, 25, and 50 millimeters are often used against a black tangent screen. On projection bowl perimeters (such as the Goldmann), larger and brighter targets are used on darker backgrounds when testing low vision patients. In the Low Vision Clinic at the School of Optometry at UC Berkeley, we usually use a flashing diode wand for tangent screen and confrontation evaluation of visual fields. This device has an LED of variable luminance flashing at about 4 Hz mounted on the end of a black wand. This is a stimulus of high visibility. The flashing provides a redundant cue that reduces uncertainly about the presence of the target when it is at or close to threshold. Patients are less inclined to "sneak a peak" when this target is used. This device has a suppress button which allows the target to be turned off silently. This effectively allows a static technique to be used and this is useful for patients who, despite instructions, make eye movements to follow the movement of the target or the wand that carries it. Holding this LED target steady and presenting brief exposures means there is less reward for the patient making an eye movement.

The Amsler Grid Test

The Amsler Grid test is often used in the functional assessment of central visual fields. When patients report that parts of the grid appear to be absent, faint or distorted, it provides information that is useful for predicting performance difficulties of visual tasks such as reading. However, many patients with well established central scotomas will report no apparent abnormalities in the appearance of the grid even though it may be demonstrated that there are scotomatous regions.

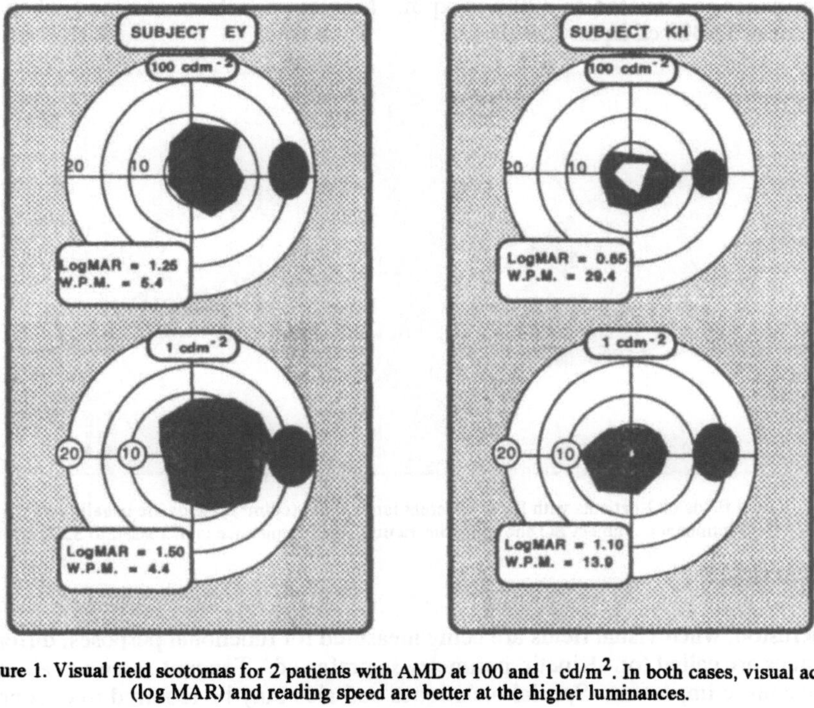

Figure 1. Visual field scotomas for 2 patients with AMD at 100 and 1 cd/m^2. In both cases, visual acuity (log MAR) and reading speed are better at the higher luminances.

Effect of Field Luminance

Scotomas size can be substantially dependent on the field luminance. At the Low Vision Clinic at the UC Berkeley School of Optometry, we commonly measure visual field using tangent screen techniques where a light-box (75 cm) provides a light background on which a black target is presented. A black fixation cross is created by stretching black plastic cord from corner to corner. The black target (typically 25 mm) is mounted at the tip of a clear Plexiglas wand. A variac allows the luminance of the white field to be varied from 1 to 1,000 cd/sq m.

Figure 1 shows field results for two different patients with central scotomas. The scotomas change size substantially with luminance. Visual acuity and reading speed also show related changes with changing field luminance. For patient KM, a small foveal region of vision is present at high luminance but it disappears at low luminance. There is a corresponding substantial reduction in visual acuity and in reading efficiency. In patients who show substantial changes in central scotomas with changing field luminance, there is often a change in the responses on Panel D-15 color vision test.

Retinitis pigmentosa patients often show substantially greater visual field constriction at lower luminance levels. Figure 2 presents two examples of visual fields from two different patients with restricted fields due to retinitis pigmentosa. It is interesting to note that for patient E.O., the visual field becomes restricted again when the luminance is elevated to 3200 cd/sq m. Maximum field is obtained when the luminance is 32-320 cd/sq m.

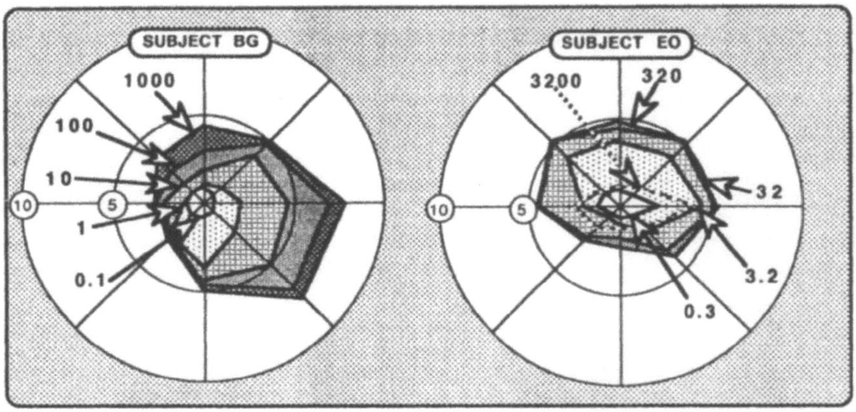

Figure 2. Visual fields of 2 patients with RP at different luminances (cd/m^2). Fields are usually larger with increased field luminance. Subject EO shows a constriction when luminance is increased to 3200 cd/m^2.

Conclusions

In conclusion, when visual fields are being measured for functional purposes, different techniques are called for. Kinetic perimetry is preferred. Tangent screen evaluation becomes more important. Special techniques and aids may be required to encourage steady fixation. Stimulus conditions are changed in order to provide high visibility for the test target. Target motion should be controlled using strategies to maximize reliability of measurement. Field luminance has functional significance in many patients and there is value in modifying test procedures to allow a broad range of field luminances to be presented.

ASSESSING READING ABILITY IN NORMAL AND LOW VISION USING THE MNREAD READING ACUITY CHART: PRELIMINARY RESULTS

JAMES E. BAILEY[1] and VASUDEVAN LAKSHMINARYANAN[2]
[1]*Southern California College of Optometry, Fullerton, CA.*
[2]*University of Missouri-St. Louis, St. Louis, MO.*

Abstract

Clinicians and vision scientists are increasingly interested in reading ability as a psychophysical measure. A new test, MNREAD reading acuity, appears to offer potential. The range of print sizes accommodate the large variation in acuities found in normal and low vision(1.3 to -0.5 LogMAR in 0.1 Log MAR steps). We report MNREAD data on normal(n=50) and low vision(n=10) subjects with diverse pathology. For comparison and control, subjects' letter acuity also was tested with the Lighthouse Near Visual Acuity Test(LNVAT). Corrrelations between both reading and letter acuity and reading acuity and smallest print size for maximum reading speed are high(r>0.9). Although the minimum print size for optimal reading speed for normal and low vision patients was 1.5-3x the size at the reading acuity limit, neither letter or reading acuity were adequate predictors of reading speed in low vision.

Introduction

Reading ability is a measure of visual function that can be of great value in the treatment and care of patients with low vision, or prescribing optical corrections for patients with normal vision. The MNREAD acuity charts are continuous-text reading acuity charts with a series of sentences divided onto four lines, and printed in high contrast, fixed-width typeface(courier-bold) on both sides of an 11 inch x 16 inch card[1]. There are two versions of the chart, matched for mean word length and word frequency. The time to read each sentence can, in principle, be converted to words per minute(wpm) reading speed. Here we report data on the black text with white background version of the new chart, and its relationship to letter acuity measured with the Lighthouse Near Visual Acuity Test(2nd edition). Subjects were nonselectively recruited and participated in accordance with informed consent.

The following questions were addressed in this study: 1) What is the relationship between MNREAD and LNVAT acuities? 2) How does reading and letter acuity relate to the smallest print size for maximum reading speed? 3)How is reading speed in low vision patients related to their letter and reading acuity?

Methods

We studied 50 adults with normal vision and 10 with low vision[macular degeneration(3), nystagmus(3), retinitis pimentosa(1), rod-cone dystrophy(1), diabetes/glaucoma(1), optic nerve hypoplasia(1)]. All subjects were tested binocularly with their normal near correction. Illumination was approximately 650 lux (185cd/ m^2). The order of measuring letter and reading acuities was randomized. Subjects read down the charts until they were unable to make out any of the test targets. An occluding white card prevented previewing subsequent sentences. Reading times were measured with a stopwatch to the nearest tenth of a second. The *critical print size for reading* was taken as the size at which reading time began to increase as the subject approached the reading acuity limit.

Results

MNREAD reading acuity was better than letter acuity by approximately 1 step in print size(0.09$\pm$0.1) for both normal and low vision patients. These acuities were highly correlated (r= 0.98). We found the critical print size to be 2x larger (0.3 Log $\pm$0.1) than the smallest print size normal and low vision patients could read with few or no errors. These measures also were highly correlated(r=0.91).

Figure 1 shows measurements of reading rate as a function of print size for normal and selected low vision patients. For normal patients average maximum reading rate was 200wpm and critical print size was 0.0-0.1 LogMAR. The range of maximum reading speeds in the low vision patients was 35-270 wpm with corresponding critical print sizes in the range 1.0-0.7 LogMAR. Reading speed was only moderately correlated with letter chart(r= -0.57) and reading(r= -0.61) acuities. Reading acuity on versions A and B of the MNREAD test differed by approximately 1/2 sentence; critical print size differed by approximately 1.5 sentences on average but did not depend on order of presentation or chart version.

As print size is increased from the reading limit, the gain in reading speed is different for different low vision patients. It appears that three types of reading speed functions characterize the normal subjects and low vision patients. Type I is an increase(variable) in reading speed to a maximum that is maintained with still larger print size. Examples of this type are normal vision(panel A), macular degeneration(ARMD I; panel B), rod-cone dystrophy(panel D), and nystagmus/albinism(panel C). Type II is a flat function: maximum reading speed is achieved at or near the reading acuity limit. Examples of Type II are ARMD II(panel B) and nystagmus/congenital(panel C). Type III is a peaked or tuned function: reading speed increases to a maximum , then decreases for larger print sizes. An example of this type is the retinitis pigmentosa patient(RP; panel D).

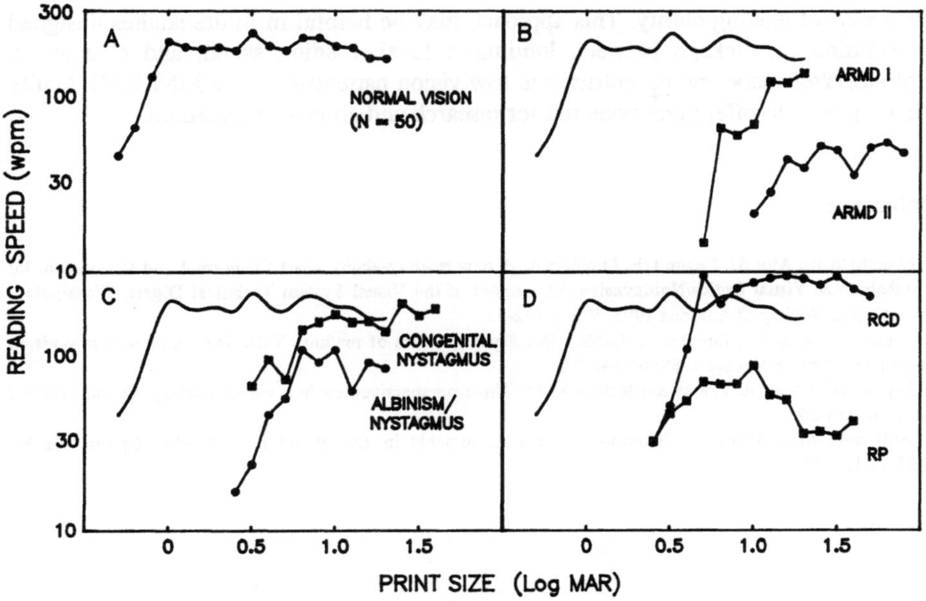

Figure 1. The effect of MNREAD print size on reading speed for normal and low vision subjects. The upper curve without symbols in panels B-D is the average of 50 normal subjects(panel A). Log MAR print sizes are corrected for each low vision subject's reading distance.

Discussion

Letter acuity(LNVAT chart) in normal and low vision subjects, although highly correlated with MNREAD reading acuity, slightly underestimates reading acuity. The difference in these measurements of acuity may be due to context effects of reading charts, different scoring criteria used for letter and reading acuity, or both.

A reading-speed vs. print size function can be defined by timing patients as they read text samples. Print substantialy larger than the reading(letter) acuity limit is required for maximum reading speed. In agreement with previous reports[2,3], MNREAD results show considerable variation in the way the low vision patients approached the reading limit, and their maximum reading speed was only moderately correlated with letter or reading acuity. We also show that such individual variation in MNREAD-measured reading speed functions can be used to classify different categories of reading ability. This approach may be helpful in future studies designed to examine the linkage between luminance level, reading speed, and changes in scotoma size, shape and eccentricity in low vision patients[4]. The MNREAD Acuity Chart appears to offer great potential for research and clinical applications.

References

1. Mansfield JS, Ahn SJ, Legge GE, Luebker A. A new reading-acuity chart for normal and low vision. In: Ophthalmic & Visual Optics/Noninvasive Assessment of the Visual System Technical Digest, Washington, D.C.: Optical Society of America 1993, Vol.3, 232-35.

2. Legge GE, Ross JA, Luebker A, LaMay JM. Psychophysics of reading. VIII. The Minnesota low-vision reading test. Optom Vis Sci 1989; 66:843-53.

3. Legge GE. Glenn A. Fry award lecture 1990: Three perspectives on low vision reading. Optom Vis Sci 1991; 68:763-69.

4. Bullimore MA, Bailey IL. Reading and eye movements in age-related maculopathy. Optom Vis Sci 1995;72:125-38.

SENSORY DEFICITS IN IDIOPATHIC CONGENITAL NYSTAGMUS

HAROLD E. BEDELL and MICHAEL T. UKWADE
College of Optometry, University of Houston, Houston, TX.

Abstract

In some subjects with idiopathic congenital nystagmus (CN), letter and Vernier acuities are worse than normal observers, despite comparable conditions of retinal image motion. Visual performance in these subjects with CN is degraded by a sensory deficit, as well as by the more-or-less constant motion of the retinal image.

Introduction

Persons with congenital nystagmus (CN) make incessant rhythmic eye movements, predominantly in the horizontal plane, which are accompanied by corresponding motions of the retinal image. Abnormalities of the afferent visual system clearly exist in some individuals with CN, for example, those who are albinos or rod monochromats [1]. However, many persons with CN appear to have what Cogan [1] called motor nystagmus, and what we refer to as idiopathic CN, in which no detectable abnormalities exist in the eye or the afferent visual pathways. Nevertheless, persons with idiopathic CN usually have reduced acuity, typically in the range of 20/25 to 20/80.

Visual acuity varies with parameters of the eye movements in CN, most notably the duration of the foveation periods. Foveation periods are brief intervals during the CN wave form when eye velocity is a few deg/s or less and the target of regard is imaged on or very close to the fovea [2]. Better visual acuity is associated with longer foveation periods [3,4]. In addition, a relationship exists between visual acuity and the beat-to-beat variability in eye position during foveation periods [5]. The issue that we address here is whether a sensory deficit exists in the visual system of persons with idiopathic CN, or whether impaired visual functioning is attributable solely to the retinal image motion.

Two approaches can be used to evaluate whether impaired visual functioning is attributable to a sensory deficit in persons with idiopathic CN. The first was adopted by Abadi and King-Smith [6], who showed that contrast sensitivity for a briefly flashed line, particularly when vertical, is worse than normal in persons with idiopathic CN. Because each line was exposed for only a fraction of a ms, CN eye movements produced no appreciable motion or smear of the retinal image, implying that the measured reduction in sensitivity resulted from a sensory deficit. The second approach, used in the studies of letter and Vernier acuity summarized here, is to examine the influence of image motion similar to that in persons with CN on the visual performance of *normal* subjects. This strategy reveals the visual impairment that is directly attributable to image motion. Any additional impairment in persons with idiopathic CN is presumably the result of a sensory abnormality.

Letter acuity

Image motion simulating the amplitude and frequency of that in persons with CN was produced when normal subjects monocularly viewed acuity targets after reflection from an oscillating mirror. Currie et al. [7] verified that visual acuity for projected Landolt Cs depends primarily on the duration of the simulated foveation periods, and not on the

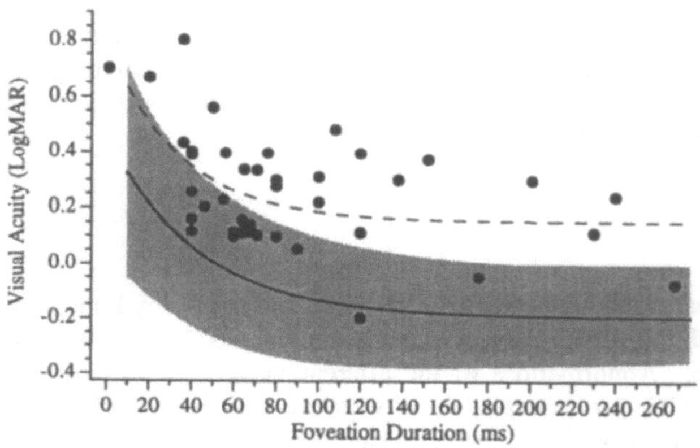

Figure 1. **Visual acuities (log MAR) for 41 subjects with idiopathic CN (filled circles) are compared to the 95% confidence interval for acuity for 16 normal observers (shaded area), measured during image motion simulating that in CN. The solid and dashed lines are exponentials fit to the normal and CN data.**

amplitude or the intensity of the imposed image motion. Position variability of the simulated foveation periods also has a small deleterious effect on visual acuity, especially when the simulated foveation duration is long [7]. Chung and Bedell [8] compiled data for 16 normal subjects across 4 studies that investigated how Landolt C acuity improves with the duration of the simulated foveation period. The average exponential function has a time constant of 42 ms, with a range among studies of 26 to 75 ms. Assuming that optimal acuity is reached after 3 time constants (i.e., about 95% of the way down the exponential curve), these results indicate that letter acuity should be normal if the foveation duration of the CN wave form is about 125 ms or longer.

Letter acuity for normals is compared with those for 41 subjects with idiopathic CN in Figure 1. This comparison reveals that more than half of the individuals with idiopathic CN exhibit worse acuity than expected on the basis of their retinal image motion. Presumably, the vertical distance of each point above the normal region in Figure 1 represents the magnitude of the sensory deficit in that subject with CN.

Vernier acuity

Under optimal conditions, Vernier acuity in normal observers is highly precise. It therefore represents a sensitive indicator of visual loss as demonstrated, for example, in persons with amblyopia [9]. In our study, we used bright, high-contrast, 30-min arc horizontal or vertical lines, presented on an oscilloscope at a frame rate of 240 Hz. The visual field was otherwise dark and viewing duration was unlimited. Vernier thresholds were determined by probit analysis and correspond to a change from 50% to 84% on psychometric functions determined using the method of constant stimuli.

Previous investigators have shown that the threshold for discriminating direction of offset for a stationary Vernier stimulus is lowest when the component lines abut or are

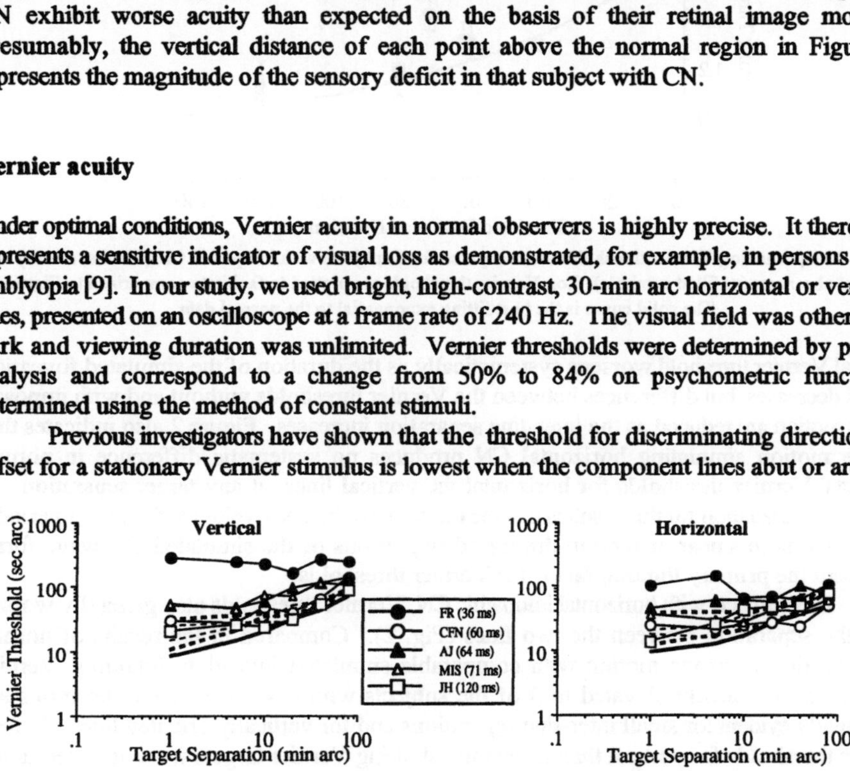

Figure 2. **Vertical and horizontal Vernier thresholds for 5 subjects with CN are compared to the average data for 2 normal observers during imposed image motion. Mean foveation durations for each subject with CN are indicated in the key. Normal data for different simulated foveation durations are shown as thick (20 and 120 ms) and thin (40 and 80 ms) *dashed* lines. The thick *solid* line represents normal thresholds without motion. For all subjects, thresholds for abutting Vernier targets are plotted at an x-axis value of 1 min arc.**

separated by only a few min arc [10, 11]. We confirmed this result for two normal subjects and demonstrated that best Vernier thresholds continue to occur at small inter-line separations in the presence of image motion simulating that in CN (Fig. 2). The

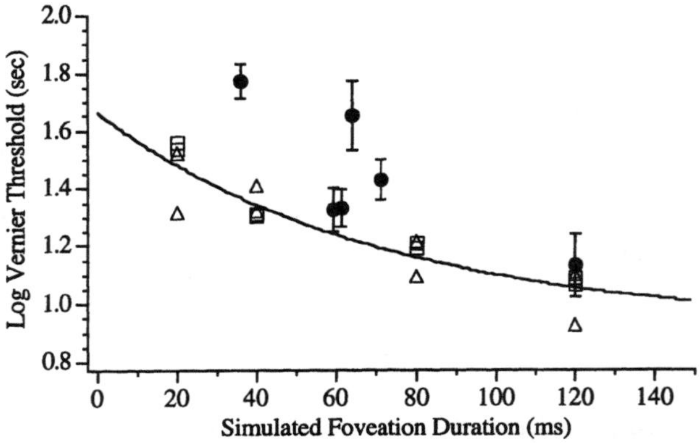

Figure 3. **Optimal log Vernier thresholds are compared for 6 subjects with idiopathic CN (filled symbols) and 2 normal observers (unfilled symbols). Log Vernier thresholds are plotted to facilitate comparison to Figure 1. The solid curve is the best fitting exponential to the normal data.**

optimal Vernier threshold worsens systematically as the duration of the simulated foveation period decreases, but differences between the Vernier thresholds without and with imposed image motion are reduced as the inter-line separation increases. Figure 2 also indicates that image motion simulating horizontal CN produces no systematic difference in normal subjects' Vernier thresholds for horizontal vs. vertical lines, at any target separation. A plausible explanation for this result is that the duration of the zero-velocity foveation periods, and not image smear or motion during other portions of the simulated CN wave form, represent the primary limiting factor for Vernier thresholds.

In 5 subjects with horizontal idiopathic CN, Vernier thresholds also generally worsen with the separation between the two lines (Fig. 2). Compared to the results of normal subjects during image motion with comparable simulated foveation durations, Vernier thresholds are clearly elevated in 3 of the subjects with CN. Threshold elevations are particularly evident for small inter-line separations and for vertically oriented lines. In fact, poorer thresholds for vertical than horizontal abutting Vernier targets were obtained in the 5 CN subjects whose data are plotted in Figure 2, and for another subject who contributed only partial data.

Optimal Vernier thresholds measured during image motion in the normal observers improve with the duration of the foveation period of the simulated CN wave form. The time constant of the best-fitting exponential function is about 71 ms (Fig. 3). Although this time constant is longer than the average value for letter acuity, the difference may not be significant as different normal subjects participated in the two studies. Compared to the normal data, optimal Vernier thresholds are elevated for 3 of the 6 subjects with CN. Of these 3, two also have letter acuities that lie above the normal region in Figure 1. Letter acuities for the other 4 subjects with CN fall within the normal area

Conclusions

Some, but not all, individuals with idiopathic CN have letter and Vernier acuity that are worse than normal subjects during comparable motion of the retinal image. This implies that a sensory deficit contributes to reduced vision in these individuals, along with the retinal image motion that results from the CN. Our Vernier data, along with the earlier results of Abadi and King-Smith [6], indicate that the sensory deficit in CN is at least partially meridional.

Clinically, the importance of a sensory deficit in some individuals with CN is that its contribution to reduced vision is likely to be more difficult to reverse than the reduction of vision that stems directly from excessive retinal image motion. Identification of the separate contributions that a sensory deficit and retinal image motion make to reduced vision is useful for making clinical decisions about the management of individual patients with CN.

Acknowledgment

This research was supported in part by NEI research grant R01 EY05068.

References

1. Cogan DG. Congenital nystagmus. Can J Ophthalmol 1967;2:4-10.
2. Dell'Osso LF, Daroff RB. Congenital nystagmus waveforms and foveation strategy. Doc Ophthalmol 1975;39:155-182.
3. Abadi RV, Worfolk R. Retinal slip velocities in congenital nystagmus. Vision Res 1989;29:195-205.
4. Sheth NV, Dell'Osso LF, Leigh RJ, van Doren CL, Peckham HP. The effects of afferent stimulation on congenital nystagmus foveation periods. Vision Res 1995;35:2371-2382.
5. Bedell HE, White JM, Abplanalp PL. Variability of foveations in congenital nystagmus. Clin Vision Sci 1989;4:247-252.
6. Abadi RV, King-Smith PE. Congenital nystagmus modifies orientational detection. Vision Res 1979;19:1409-1411.
7. Currie DC, Bedell HE, Song S. Visual acuity for optotypes with image motions simulating congenital nystagmus. Clin Vision Sci 1993;8:73-84.
8. Chung STL, Bedell HE. Velocity criteria for "foveation periods" determined for image motions simulating congenital nystagmus. Optom Vision Sci 1996;73:92-103.
9. Levi DM. Spatial vision in amblyopia. In: Regan DM, editor. Spatial Vision. Boca Raton, FL: CRC Press, 1991:212-238.
10. Westheimer G, McKee SP. Spatial configurations for visual hyperacuity. Vision Res 1977;17:941-947.
11. Williams RA, Enoch JM, Essock EA. The resistance of selected hyperacuity configurations to retinal image degradation. Invest Ophthalmol Visual Sci 1984;25:389-399.

OPTICAL TRANSFER FUNCTIONS, POLYPLOPIA, AND SELECTIVE SPATIAL FREQUENCY LOSS IN CONTRAST SENSITIVITY FUNCTIONS

LO BOUR[1] and PATRICIA APKARIAN[2]
[1]*Dept of Neurology, Clinical Neurophysiology, Academic Medical Centre, Amsterdam.*
[2]*Dept of Physiology, Medical Faculty, EUR, THE NETHERLANDS.*

Abstract

Simulations of modulation transfer functions of the eye's optics were performed to demonstrate an optical origin for selective contrast sensitivity (CSF) losses. Wave aberration functions include standard spherical aberration, coma and small amounts of irregular aberrations. Under such conditions, simulation of slight refractive error with also larger pupil sizes optically induces selective decreases in spatial frequency contrast. As a result, selective CSF loss at intermediate and lower (2-15 cpd) spatial frequencies in patients with visual pathway pathology should be attributed to neural factors only with caution and with carefully controlled, well defined optical variables.

Introduction

The quality of spatial vision is determined by various visual system transfer functions, i.e., optical, retinal and/or neural. Optical and retinal transfer functions can be considered as front-end, visual system processing stages. Proper functioning of particularly these early system stages is prerequisite for optimal spatial vision [1,2]. In general, when a transfer function is known, processing of the object, typically sine wave gratings, readily can be defined by Fourier theory for any linear system. That is, linear superposition of sine wave gratings with the appropriate phase and amplitude may define any spatial object. For incoherent light, optical and retinal transfer functions are linear, and therefore, the spatial transfer of the eye's optics can be characterized by modulation transfer functions and/or corresponding point spread functions [3,4]. Sine wave gratings typically have been used to determine subjective contrast thresholds for varying spatial frequencies, thus yielding the classic contrast sensitivity function (CSF) [5]. However, not only do optical and retinal transfer functions determine the CSF but neural transfer functions, that are definitely not linear, also play a major role [6]. Consequently, although determination of the CSF is based on Fourier methodology, the superposition principle cannot be applied. The CSF also cannot be implemented to comprehensively characterize spatial resolution of the visual system. That the CSF is a limited approach to visual spatial processing should be considered particularly as applied to visual function assessment.

Although, historically, selective CSF loss particularly within the intermediate spatial frequency ranges was attributed to visual pathway malfunction, subsequent studies have identified the presence of narrow band, spatial frequency losses as resulting from optical artifact, e.g., monocular polyplopia as based on the cos ^{2} law [7]. Recently, the optical artifact explanation for selective CSF loss has been extended by a more comprehensive model that includes calculations of optical transfer functions of the eye as based on the wave aberration function [8]. For this model, peak selective CSF loss is dependent upon e.g., the degree of irregular aberration, refractive error and pupil size. In the present overview, concomitant theoretical limitations of the CSF in clinical assessment of spatial vision in patients with various vision disorders also is considered [8,9].

Methods

Contrast sensitivity was measured empirically with a computer controlled method of ascending limits as described previously [7]. Theoretical, numerical evaluation of the convolution integrals for computing MTFs of the optical system of the human eye in

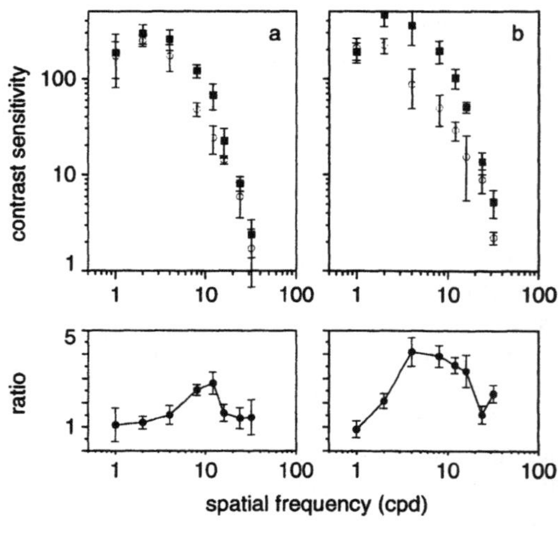

Figure 1. Effects of artificial pupil. a) CSF with optimum correction (closed symbols) and artificial pupil compared to .75 D over correction and artificial pupil (open symbols). b) same as in (a) but with natural pupil. Sensitivity ratios depicted below. Adapted from reference [9].

polychromatic light were performed following the method of Hopkins [10], also as described in more detail previously [3,8]. Simulated aberration coefficients of the wave aberration function were adapted from reference [11]. Chromatic aberration components for various wavelengths were taken from reference [12]. To account for irregular aberration, an extra term to the wave aberration function was added, consisting of a circular segment centered in the middle of the pupil with a slight difference in refractive power from the surround. The refractive increment D_i is given by: $D_i = 0.4\ D$ *if* $x^2 + y^2 < 0.25$ *mm; otherwise* $D_i = 0$.

Results

In Figure 1, the influence of pupil size on selective CSF loss is depicted for a normal control. The CSF measured with (a) a 3 mm artificial pupil (with mydriaticum) and (b) with a natural pupil are compared. Closed squares depict the CSF with optimum correction; open circles the CSF with 0.75 Diopters (D) over correction. Lower pan-els depict sensitivity ratios. The lower, left panel, dem-onstrates substantial select-ive loss, despite an arti-ficial pupil of 3 mm; note also the peak attenuation at 12 cycles/degree. With the larger natural pupil, the optically induced selective loss broadens and enhances; peak sensitivity loss now occurs at about 8 cycles/degree.

Figure 2 (left) depicts a surface plot together with a contour plot of an MTF calculated with a positive irregularity (0.5 mm, 0.4 D) and a 5 mm pupil. Figure 2 (right) shows theoretical sensitivity ratios for various pupil sizes derived from the MTF (depicted at the left) with a negative miscorrection (−0.1 D is compared to −0.8 D). Note that there is a shift in the peak of the sensitivity ratios as a function of pupil diameter. With a positive irregularity, the peak frequency increases with pupil size (13 to 18 cycles/degree); however, with a negative irregularity, (see also e.g., reference [9]), the peak spatial frequency decreases with pupil size (17 to 10 cycles/degree).

Discussion

The experimental data as well as the optical model based on optical transfer functions show that selective spatial frequency losses may occur due to optical factors. For example, Figure 1 demonstrates that selective CSF loss can readily be introduced by a small degree of refractive error and that the magnitude and the spatial frequency peak of selective loss depends also on pupil size. The theoretical model of Figure 2, explains the relationship between monochromatic aberrations and the occurrence of selective loss of spatial frequency contrast. Essential is the presence of small amounts of irregular aberration in combination with slight refractive error. Concurrent with selective loss, polyplopia is present. Experimental data in normal controls as well as the optical model show that for minimizing optical aberrations, optimal pupil sizes range from about 2-3 mm. As described in more detail elsewhere [9], to avoid optically induced selective losses with CSF testing in patients, optical variables such as pupil size and refractive correction require careful attention.

The optical model described herein shows the effect of an irregularity consisting of a circular element centered relative to the pupil plane with a slight refractive increas with respect to the surround. Under normal conditions, these irregularities of the the eye's optics are attributed primarily to the crystalline lens and its corresponding segmented character. Irregularities in refraction may also be located along different loci in the pupil plane [13]. In general, the optical model predicts that minor irregularities lead to an increased depth of focus with an enhancement of the retinal image contrast on flanks of the optimum focus plane. As noted above, optical irregularities may introduce, unexpected selective losses at intermediate and lower spatial frequency ranges (2 - 15 cycles/degree). To obtain a better and more comprehensive understanding of regular and irregular aberrations and how they contribute to image quality of the retinal image, new techniques, such as the double-pass technique, based on a hybrid optical-digital method [4] and the Hartmann-Shack wave-front sensor [14], may be used in the future for routine evaluation.

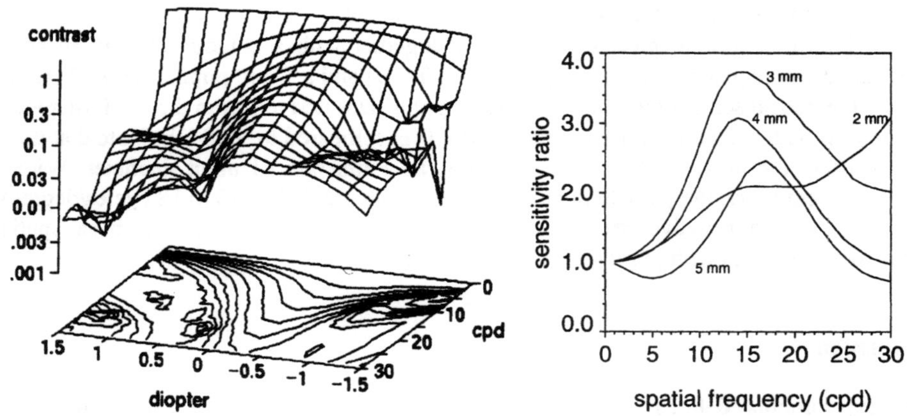

Figure 2. Left: Surface and contour plot of theoretically calculated MTF's in white light at varying degrees of defocus for a 5-mm pupil diameter. The wave aberration function incorporates regular aberrations (mean values), Stiles-Crawford apodization, and also a small positive additional irregularity. Right: Sensitivity ratios derived from theoretical MTF's for various pupil sizes. A focus setting of −0.1 D is compared to a focus setting of −0.8 D. Adapted from references [8,9].

References

1. Campbell FW and Green DG. Optical and retinal factors affecting visual resolution. J.Physiol. 1965;181: 576-593.
2. Ohzu H, Enoch JM, O'Hair J. Optical modulation by the isolated retina and retinal receptors. Vision Res. 1972; 12: 231-244
3. Bour LJ. MTF of the defocused optical system of the human eye for incoherent monochromatic light. J Opt Soc Am. 1980;70:321-328.
4. Artal P, Iglesias I, López-Gil N and Green DG. Double-pass measurements of the retinal image quality with unequal entrance and exit pupil sizes and the reversibility of the eye's optical system. J Opt Soc Am A. 1995;12:2358-2366.
5. Bodis-Wollner I and Diamond SP. The measurement of spatial contrast sensitivity in cases of blurred vision associated with cerebral lesions. Brain. 1976; 99: 695-710.
6. Regan D. Disorders of spatial vision. Human Brain Electrophysiology. Elsevier/New York. 1989; Part 3: 509-515.
7. Apkarian P, Tijssen R, Spekreijse H and Regan D. Origin of Notches in CSF: Optical or Neural? Invest Ophthalmol Vis Sci. 1987;28:607-612.
8. Bour L and Apkarian P. Segmented refraction of the crystalline lens as a prerequisite for the occurrence

of monocular polyplopia, increased depth of focus and contrast sensitivity function notches. J Opt Soc Am A. 1994;11:2769-2776.

9. Bour LJ and Apkarian P. Selective, broad band spatial frequency loss in contrast sensitivity functions: comparison with a model based on optical transfer functions. Invest Ophthalmol Vis Sci. 1996; in press.
10. Hopkins HH. The numerical evaluation of the frequency response of optical systems. Proceedings Physical Society B. 1957; 70: 1002-1005.
11. Howland HC and Howland B. A subjective method for the measurement of monochromatic aberrations of the eye. J Opt Soc Am. 1977; 67:1508-1518.
12. Charman WN and Jennings JAM. Objective measurement of the longitudinal chromatic aberration of the human eye. Vision Res. 1976;16:999-1005.
13. Von Helmholtz H. Southall JPC, editors. Treatise on Physiological Optics Vol I. The Optical Society of America. 1924.
14. Liang J, Grimm B, Goelz S, and Bille JF. Objective measurement of wave aberrations of the human eye with the use of a Hartmann-Shack wave-front sensor. J Opt Soc Am A. 1994;11:1949-1957.

A NEW LOOK AT UTROCULAR DISCRIMINATION

ALEXANDER I. COGAN
The Smith-Kettlewell Eye Research Institute, San Francisco, California 94115

Abstract

Flashes incrementing or decrementing the luminance may differ in perceived direction depending on whether the flash goes to one, the other, or both eyes. This directional bias is sufficient for discrimination between monocular and binocular conditions of stimulation, but it does not ensure correct utrocular discrimination. It is proposed that the bias and 'the feeling in the eye' both arise from unequal stimulation of the two eyes and are related to a primitive and perceptually ambiguous visual orientation response.

Introduction

The question "Which eye saw the stimulus?" is neither an easy, nor a natural question to answer [1]. Yet, *some* observers were capable of utrocular discrimination, even when carefully tested by Enoch et al. [2], who used blurred targets in conditions which eliminated extraneous cues that could arise from interocular differences in image shape, contrast, chromaticity, etc. Blake & Cormack [3], too, found that some observers could tell which eye was stimulated by a grating of low spatial frequency (1 cyc/deg); no observer could identify the eye stimulated with a high-frequency grating (8 cyc/deg). This finding has been recently confirmed by Cormack et al. [4], who achieved utrocular discrimination also with random dot fields of unequal binocular contrast.

The recognized cue for utrocular discrimination is somesthetic, "a feeling" [5, 2, 3, 4]. That 'feeling' is generally assumed to be monocular, but its true origin is unknown, nor has any reason been suggested why only some observers seem to have it.

I propose that the somesthetic cue is part of a vestiginal, primitive *orientation response* that gives an organism equipped with eyes symmetrically placed about the median plane a choice for orientation of the body axis either towards the side of stronger visual stimulation, or away from it. The feeling is thus tied to a *directional* cue which arises from unequal stimulation of the two eyes and is inherently ambiguous, as it can point either towards the more- or the less-strongly stimulated eye.

The directional bias of test flashes

As an observer in many studies concerned with binocular summation at the differential luminance threshold I formed the impression that the sites of stimulation might be discriminable with flashes that were above threshold: while binocular flashes were centered in the field, the right-eye and left-eye flashes seemed biased to the right or left, respectively. [The bias would be unremarkable if the stimuli were not centered on the foveae. In experiments of Ono & Barbeito [6] a local stimulus was flashed to one side of the fixation point, and the observers' responses "right eye" or "left eye" were either always correct—when the monocular stimulus fell on the nasal retina, or always incorrect—when it fell on the temporal retina. Ono & Barbeito concluded that they disproved "utrocular identification", but their results obtained with extrafoveal stimuli were trivially dependent on hemispheric projection and showed, not surprisingly, that visual direction mediated by the local sign mechanism has nothing to do with utrocular discrimination.] The differences in perceived direction of test flashes in my experiments could not be dependent on image position relative to the fovea, because the visual field was always centered on the median plane and the flashes were spatially coextensive with the field, whether they occurred in one, the other, or both eyes. In some experiments the field was uniform; in other experiments it displayed a random dot stereogram (RDS) and the field was stereoscopically three-dimensional. The 3D image remained unaffected by increments and decrements of luminance, which were seen merely as fleeting changes of brightness within the stable field. These brightness 'wiggles' were biased slightly to the right or left with monocular flashes only. Is the bias real? (Expt. 1) Could it provide an unambiguous perceptual cue for utrocular discrimination? (Expt. 2).

General Methods

A field 12 deg in diameter was illumined by white light. The field displayed an RDS and was viewed with a stereoscope providing effortless fusion with near-parallel visual axes. [Our four observers all had normal acuity and stereopsis; fixation disparity was equal to or less than 2 arc min.] Base luminance was 120 cd/m² in Exp. 1 and 30 cd/m² in Exp. 2. The surround was dim (about 2% of field luminance). Flashes, given in a random sequence, incremented or decremented the base luminance in the right eye (RE), the left eye (LE), or both eyes (B); in the 'dichoptic' condition (Bx) the two eyes received flashes with the opposite sign of brightness contrast.

Experiment 1

The observer was to indicate the directional bias of a test flash.

Method: Flash duration was 200 msec, 24 cd/m² amplitude (suprathreshold). The observer pressed one of 3 buttons to indicate the directional bias of a flash as 'Left', 'Center', or 'Right'. In a single session each of the four conditions was presented 40 times and at least 160 responses total was collected from each of the four observers.

Results: All observers showed a directional bias such that flashes going to the right or the left eye appeared to deviate towards the right or the left side of the field, respectively, while binocular flashes were centered in the field. No bias was found in the dichoptic condition (Bx). [The chi-square table had a 4 x 3 design: four conditions versus three responses; df=6. The χ^2 score was significant in all observers (LW: $\chi^2 = 288.7$; $r=0.975$; $P < 0.001$; MK: $\chi^2 = 103.6$; $r=0.805$; $P < 0.001$; AC: $\chi^2 = 146.7$; $r=0.957$; $P < 0.001$; AR: $\chi^2 = 20.4$; $r=0.357$; $P < 0.005$)].

The next question was whether the directional cue would be sufficient for an explicit identification of each condition and provide for correct utrocular discrimination.

Experiment 2

The observer was to name the condition of stimulation.

Method: The conditions were the same as in Exp. 1, but the stimulus was a pulse train: 1-msec flashes separated by a 350-msec interval. Pulse amplitude was set initially at zero. The observer adjusted pulse amplitude until he could just see flicker. (The criterion flash brightness was thus about the same in all conditions.) No time limit was set. 320 responses were collected from each of the two highly experienced observers (AC and AR) while each condition was presented 80 times.

Results: Good discrimination among the conditions of stimulation was shown by both observers. [AC: χ^2=161.9; r=0.71; df=9; $P < 0.001$, and AR: χ^2=270.7; r=0.92; df=9; $P < 0.001$.] However, while conditions RE and LE were mostly named correctly by observer AC, observer AR consistently *misidentified* these monocular conditions: the directional bias found in Exp.1 did not ensure utrocular discrimination in Exp.2. Obviously, discrimination between monocular and binocular stimulation does not imply utrocular discrimination, contrary to the notion of Blake & Cormack [3].

Discussion

With full-field stimulation (involving the monocular segment), perceived direction at the light source is biased temporalwards: the nasal hemiretina is prevalent [7]. The ability to associate 'Left', 'Right', and 'Center' directions with stimulation of the left eye, the right eye, and both eyes, respectively, in Expt. 1 is consistent with the notion that the nasal hemiretina was directionally prevalent whenever the flash was monocular. If hemiretinal prevalence were a sufficient explanation, then the directional bias would have a purely monocular origin.[1] However, the results of observer AR in Exp. 2 are not in agreement with this notion. Was the temporal hemiretina prevalent in that instance? There is no justification for such a switch in hemiretinal prevalence.

Alternatively, the directional bias arises from a difference in the stimulation of the two eyes. This notion was originally suggested by the 'interocular yoke' effect [8] discovered using counterphase modulation of luminance in the two eyes. At frequencies below 3Hz observers experienced 'motion' oscillating across the median plane [9, 10].[2] A striking finding was an ambiguity in the observer's judgment of direction; although the timing of his button press was in precise keeping with the modulation frequency, 'brightest right' was sometimes signaled when the right eye's field was in fact darkest. The ambiguity was apparently due to the *somesthetic* cue, because the motion was *felt*, either at the eyes or inside the head, rather than 'seen'. The 'feeling' thus did not always point to the more strongly stimulated eye, which may explain misidentification of the stimulated eye by observer AR; the directional ambiguity also may be the reason why some observers respond at chance in the task of utrocular discrimination.

Acknowledgment. My thanks go to M. Clarke for programming the computer, to my observers, and to A. Rossi for his help in running the experiments. The author is supported by SKERI grant #2802.

References

1. Helmholtz H von. Handbook of Physiological Optics. Translated from the 3d German Edition, Southall JPC, Editor. New York: Dover, 1962:Vol. III p.458.

2. Enoch J, Goldmann H, Sunga R. The ability to see which eye was stimulated by light. Invest Ophthalmol 1969; 8:317-331

3. Blake R, Cormack RH. On utrocular discrimination. Percept & Psychophys 1979; 26:53-68

4. Cormack LK, Landers DD, Stevenson SB. Correlation detection and utrocular discrimination in displays with unequal monocular contrasts. Invest Ophthalmol Vis Sci (Suppl) 1996; 37:5652

5. Smith S. Utrocular or 'which eye' discrimination. J Exp Psychol 1945; 35:1-14

6. Ono H, Barbeito R. Utrocular discrimination is not sufficient for utrocular identification. Vision Res 1985; 25:289-299
7. Jampolsky A. Unequal visual inputs and strabismus management: a comparison of human and animal strabismus. In Halveston EM, Jampolsky A., Knapp P., McNeer KW, Parks MM, Reinecke RD, Scott WE, von Noorden GK, Editors Symposium on Strabismus. Transactions of the New Orleans Academy of Ophthalmology St. Luis: The C.V. Mosby Company, 1978:374
8. Cogan AI. The interocular luminance yoke: A vestige of phototaxis? Vision Res 1990; 30:181-185
9. Cogan AI, Chan H, Clarke M. 'Utrocular discrimination' as a quasi-cyclopean response. Invest Ophthalmol Vis Sci (Suppl) 1985; 26:186
10. Cavonius CR. Binocular interactions in flicker. Percept & Psychophys 1979; 31:273-280

Notes

[1] My monocular tests with the nontest eye occluded proved inconclusive: although flashes seen with the left eye were biased to the left, the right-eye flashes were centered, and another observer showed no directional bias with flashes going to either eye.

[2] Notably, 'motion', albeit somewhat weaker, was also present if luminance was modulated in *one* eye only, provided that the field was binocular; if the other eye was occluded, then brightness alone was seen to fluctuate in the (monocular) field.

THE EFFECT OF AGE ON THE WESTHEIMER FUNCTION

JAMES COMERFORD, DONNA MALLOY, AMY PRUSZENSKI
FRANK THORN
The New England College of Optometry, Boston, MA

Abstract

The Westheimer function is relatively stable in healthy observers between 20 and 70 years of age. The sensitization portion of the function is unaffected by age and only in the oldest observers does a small but significant decrease in desensitization occur.

Introduction

The Westheimer function, a component of Layer-by-Layer Perimetry [1], is a psychophysical measure of receptive field organization. The results of this test for peripherally viewed stimuli correlate well with single cell recordings of ganglion cell receptive fields in monkeys [2].

In this test, detection thresholds are measured for small test probes as a function of the size of a background disc. Small backgrounds elevate thresholds (desensitization), presumably due to convergent receptor input into bipolar cells; larger background sizes reduce thresholds (sensitization) due to lateral inhibition that shifts the sensitivity of the cell.

We are interested in the clinical application of this test. Since most of the ophthalmic and neurological deficits to be examined occur in old age, we wished to determine the extent to which aging itself could be a confounding factor in our studies.

In a previous study, Yuan, Yager and Davis [3] found both a slight tendency for an increase in sensitization with age and large individual differences in the magnitude of the effect. Benedetto and Armstrong [4] studied the sensitization effect and found that older observers needed increased surround intensity to occlude the perception of an increment in light intensity. They hypothesized that their large effect was due to decreased contrast sensitivity with age rather than interpreting it in terms of sensitization within the Westheimer paradigm. They do not give any information about the variability of their results. Neither study offered a statistical analysis of the effect of aging on their visual tests.

Method

We tested 40 observers aged 20 to 69. There were 4 male and 4 female subjects for each decade of life. All were healthy and were not taking medication for any ophthalmic condition. All observers had visual acuity that was 6/6 (20/20) or better.

An interactive animation program (Macromedia Director) was used to present stimuli on a monochrome high intensity monitor (Image Systems). Two positions were tested at 8° eccentricity in the nasal visual field of the right eye. One position was 45° above and the other 45° below the horizontal meridian. The test probe was a 2 min of arc 500 msec flash. Increment thresholds for the probe were determined against background discs ranging in diameter from 0.3° to 2° of arc. The illuminance of the backgrounds was 0.65 log cd/m^2 and that of the surrounding visual field was 0.46 log cd/m^2. We used a method of limits with 20% catch trials to assess guessing. Eye movements were monitored by observation or by an infrared video system (Eyescan).

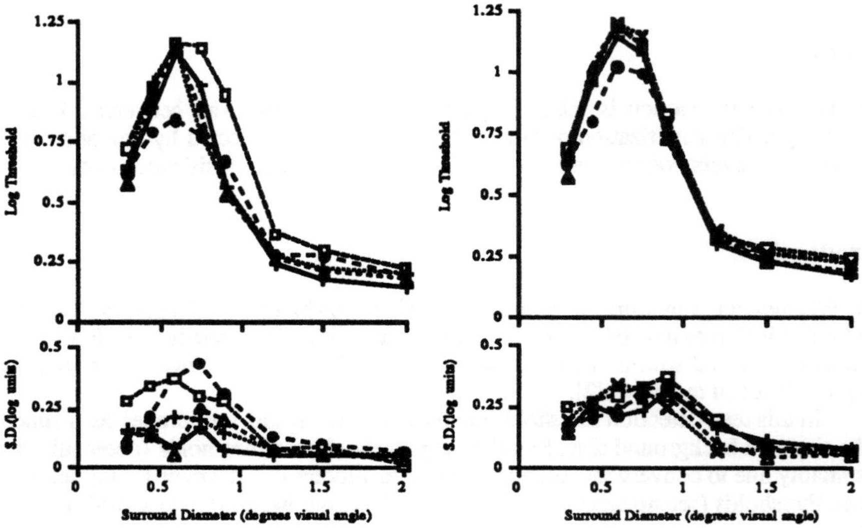

Figure 1. The Westheimer function for 8° eccentricity in the upper (left graph) and lower (right graph) visual field as related to age. Age categories: 20's, +; 30's, ×; 40's, Δ; 50's, □ ; 60's •.Standard deviations are plotted in the lower graph and are small for the sensitization portion of the function.

Results

Our procedures provide large sensitization and desensitization effects (See Fig.1). From the minimum background diameter of 0.3° to a background of 0.6°, a 0.5 log unit desensitization occurs. This is followed by a sensitization of 0.9 log units as the background increases to 2°. As seen in Fig. 2, this sensitization endpoint represents both great sensitivity and great consistency between subjects (s.d.= 0.06 log units for subjects across all ages at each test location).

There is no age, gender, or age x gender effect on the mean increment threshold. But, sensitivity is slightly greater in the lower visual field (0.075 log unit difference) ($F= 11.4;1/30$; $P = 0.002$). The ANOVA does not show a significant effect of age on the Westheimer function ($F = 1.31$; 28/210; $P = 0.150$). Nor is age associated with the difference between the upper and lower visual fields ($F = 1.27$; 28/210; $P =0.174$).

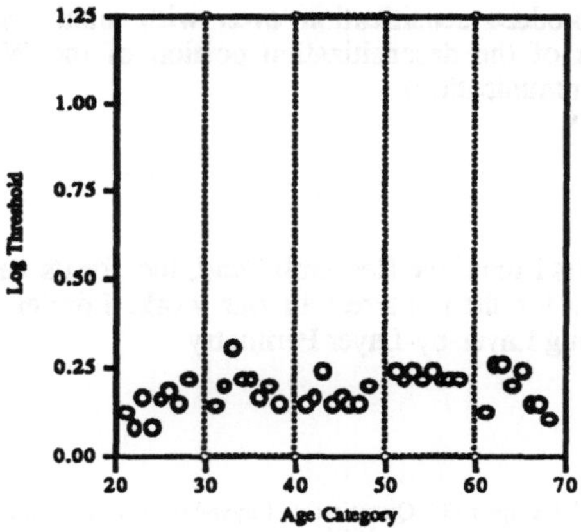

Figure 2. A plot of the increment thresholds for the largest background disc used in determining the Westheimer function. They are quite uniform and do not change with the age of the observer.

While the sensitivity of the Westheimer function is virtually identical for the three younger groups, the functions for the two older groups in figure 1 may differ slightly. By using several younger age groups we may have swamped out the differences for older subjects in the ANOVA. To evaluate this possibility, we combined the three youngest groups into a single young-adult group in a post-hoc ANOVA. The background size x age effect in this case is highly significant (F = 4.35; 7/196; P = .0002) indicating a strong effect of age on the Westheimer function. The Westheimer effect does not differ between any of the four younger groups. However, there are significant differences between 60 year olds and the 20, 30, and 40 year olds (F = 2.14; P = 0.048; F = 2.17; P = 0.045; F = 3.22; P = 0.0045).

Discussion

The Westheimer function is relatively stable for healthy people between 20 and 69 years of age. Between the ages of 20 and 49 there is no change in the shape or amplitude of the function. The only change is a slight decrease in the desensitization effect for the 60 years old.

There may be two reasons that our data differs from the earlier results of Yuan et al [3]. We evaluated perpheral vision where eye movements may cause fewer artifacts than under the foveal conditions they used [5]. In addition, the longer duration of our test increment may optimize the sensitization effect and reduce variability.

Our differences with Benedetto and Armstrong [4] are more difficult ti determine because their procedures are not described in detail. If they used procedures similar to those of Eoch [1], their results suggest a large increase in sensitization with age. Neither our results nor those of Yuan et al [3] support that finding.

Our results suggest that a small change late in liife of a neural component in spatial summation induces small changes in vision [6]. Alternatively, lenticular scatter in aged observers may produce sensitization even with small background stimuli, thereby reducing the peak of the desensitization portion of the Westheimer function (Bruce Drum, personal communication).

Acknowledgements

We thank the Massachusetts Lions Eye Research Fund, Inc. for its support, and Dr. Jay Enoch and Dr. Mark Zorn for their interest in our work. Lorelei DeGalla wrote the computer program for testing Layer-by-Layer Perimetry.

References

1. Enoch JM, Fitzgerald C, Campos EC. Quantitative Layer-by-Layer Perimetry: An Extended Analysis. New York: Grune and Stratton, 1981.

2. Spillman L, Ransom-Hogg A, Oehler R. A comparison of perceptive and receptive fields in man and monkey. Human Neurobiol 1987; 6:51-62.

3. Yuan R, Yager D, Davis ET. Some aspects of spatial sensitization in foveal cone vision: age of subject; psychophysical method; and individual differences. Invest Ophthalmol Vis Sci 1990;31(suppl.):357.

4. Benedetto MD, Armstrong DA. The effect of aging upon psychophysical receptive field properties. In:Armstrong DA, Marmor MF, Ordy JM, editors. The Effects of Aging and the Environment on Vision, New York: Plenum Press, 1991: 35-43.

5. Yuan R, Yager D, Davis ET. Reduction of foveal desensitization with blurred backgrounds. Vis Res 1991; 32:577-582.

6. Latham K, Whitaker D, Wild JM. Spatial summation of the differential light threshold as a function of visual field location and age. Ophthal Physiol Opt 1994;14:71-78.

EXTENSIONS OF THE SUSTAINED-LIKE AND TRANSIENT-LIKE EFFECTS

EDWARD A. ESSOCK[1,2], JASON S. MCCARLEY[1], MICHAEL J. SINAI[1], BYUNG-GEUN KHANG[1], STEPHEN LEHMKUHLE[3], WILLIAM K. KREBS[1] AND CONG YU[1]
[1]*Departments of Psychology and* [2]*Ophthalmology and Visual Sciences, University of Louisville, Louisville KY 40292*
[3]*School of Optometry, University of Missouri - St. Louis, St. Louis, MO 63121*

Abstract

We report physiological and psychophysical studies that further expand and delineate two of the tests of Enoch's Layer-by-Layer Perimetry. In the physiological studies we show that single ganglion cells give responses comparable to human responses. In the human studies we demonstrate that a corresponding sensitization response exists in the OFF-channel, that a "pure" flicker mechanism smaller than the transient-like mechanism exists, and that an orientation bias exists in the cortical properties mapped with a variation of these tests. These results offer extensions of layer-by-layer perimetry for the clinical testing of additional layers of the visual system.

One of Jay Enoch's most important contributions to vision science is Layer-by-Layer Perimetry. In Layer-by-Layer Perimetry, functional status is assessed layer-by-layer through the layers of the visual system as well as perimetrically point-by-point across the retina. At its core are two tests that reflect the functional integrity of the inner retina at the tested visual field locations [1,2]. Both tests involve the detection of a small test probe on a small background. In the sustained-like test, test threshold increases, then decreases as background diameter is increased, with the latter branch taken to reflect intact organization of surround antagonism. In the transient-like test, threshold on a windmill-shaped background is compared for static and rotating conditions. If the motion raises test threshold, intact organization of a particular retinal pathway driven by temporal modulation is presumed [3]. In this paper we report some of our findings that expand and elucidate these phenomena.

To demonstrate that these perceptual phenomena are indeed closely linked to receptive field properties, we tested single cells directly. We recorded from single cells in anesthetized cats while presenting them a small test probe (2 Hz LED) on a bright variable-diameter background, that was either static or temporally modulated (rotating vanes or flickering homogeneous field). Full details of the recording procedure and the test methods are presented elsewhere [3]. We reported previously that cat LGN X-cells show responses comparable to normal humans on these tests: desensitization followed by strong sensitization on the sensitization test and strong suppression on the transient-like test when temporal modulation is introduced. Here we report that identical results were found for ganglion cells recorded presynaptically in the LGN (Figure 1). These results suggest that the responses shown by humans are indeed closely linked to basic receptive field spatiotemporal properties at the retinal level.

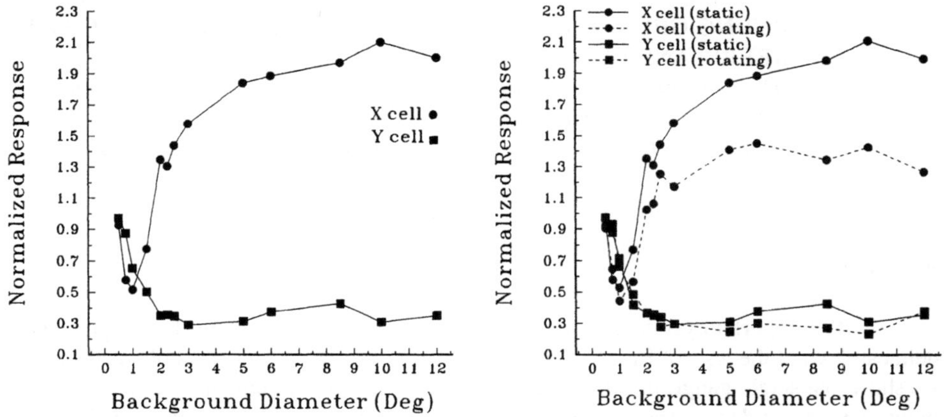

Figure 1. The 2 Hz fundamental response plotted as a function of background diameter. Ganglion X-cells, but not Y-cells, match the normal human response of sensitization (Left) and of strong suppression at the larger background diameters characterizing the human transient-like effect (Right).

In other experiments we investigated whether analogous sensitization and center/surround organization can be demonstrated in humans in the OFF-pathway. Since the OFF-pathway is presumed to detect decrements [4], we measured decrement threshold

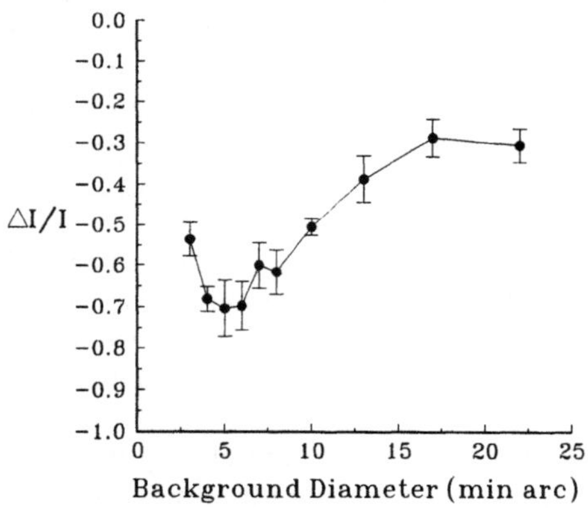

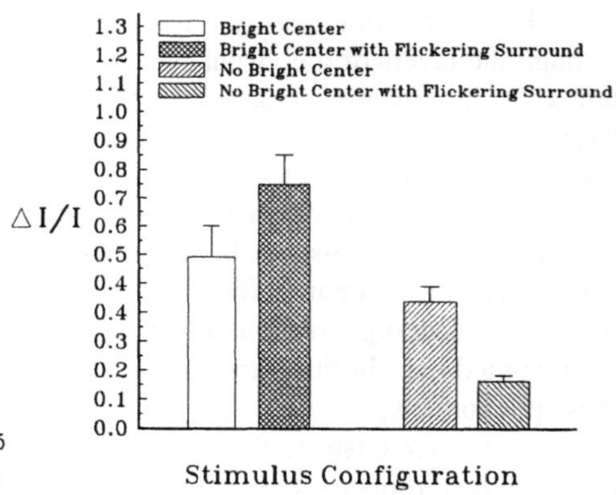

Figure 2. (Left) Decrement threshold for a 1.5' test on a 119 cd/m^2 background on a 189 cd/m^2 monitor screen, 2AFC staircase method. Threshold increases in magnitude (i.e., larger decrements) then decreases as the diameter of the decrement background is increased.

Figure 3. (Right) A local contrast-gain mechanism demonstrated with a flickering annulus (2 Hz, 20% depth, 3' inner diameter, 2AFC staircase). Temporal modulation of the annulus causes suppression when the annulus center is bright (80 cd/m^2), and facilitation when the annulus center equals the screen luminance (16 cd/m^2).

for a decrement test and varied the diameter of a decrement background to map the center/surround organization. Figure 2 shows that decrement threshold increased, then decreased, revealing comparable spatial interactions on this decrement version of the Westheimer paradigm and suggesting a Layer-by-Layer test suitable to assess the center/surround integrity in the OFF-pathway.

In our work investigating the basis of the desensitization induced by temporal modulation, we have discovered that near-by temporal modulation can be either desensitizing or sensitizing. We find that, in addition to the suppressive mechanism demonstrated by Enoch that is maximal for 6' inner diameter vanes, there exists a smaller mechanism that is driven by "pure" flicker (i.e., temporal modulation about the mean screen level) and that this mechanism can be suppressive *or sensitizing*. This new temporal mechanism differs from the transient-like mechanism in that it is a different size (3' inner diameter) and can be sensitizing. Figure 3 shows that whether it suppresses or facilitates probe detection is dependent upon whether the region inside the annulus is bright (as in the transient-like test) or is set at the screen luminance, respectively. This newly demonstrated local temporal mechanism is revealed by temporal modulation *per se* rather than by motion of a bright pattern. Since this process affects sensitivity based on pure temporal modulation, it appears to correspond to the contrast-gain control mechanism reported previously that is distinct from illuminance-based gain control mechanisms [5]. Thus, these data provide the basis for a new perimetric layer-by-layer test that reflects the local organization of a contrast-gain control mechanism.

In another extension of the sensitization paradigm we have used a modified test configuration to assess cortical spatial interactions as proposed originally by Fuld [6]. We used a small line target (1' x 7') on a rectangular background and found that when the width of the background is increased, threshold again increases to a point, then decreases, suggesting a central summation region 6' wide with lateral regions of flank inhibition [7].

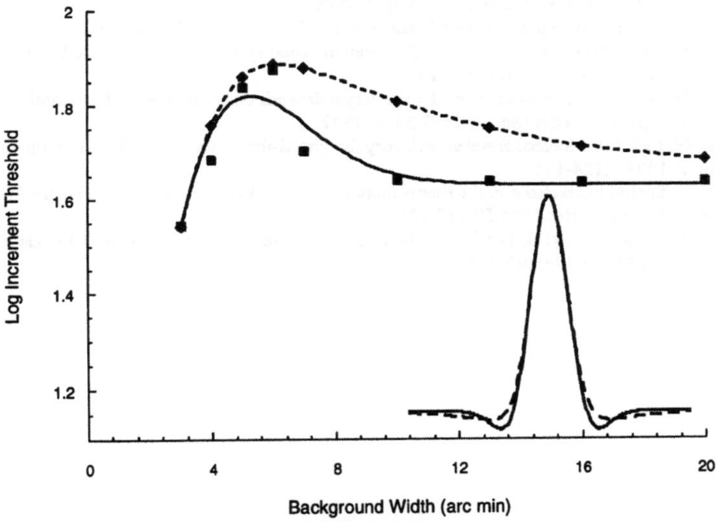

Figure 4. Data, integrated-DOG fit and DOG sensitivity profiles (inset) at vertical (solid lines) and oblique (dashed lines) orientations. Data obtained in Maxwellian-view with 2.4 log troland background on a 2.0 log troland surround and method of adjustment.

Furthermore, like many cortical phenomena, an oblique effect is demonstrated (Figure 4). This test paradigm is described well by an underlying difference-of-Gaussians mechanism over which light is integrated as the background's width is increased. The inset in Figure 4 shows the sensitivity profiles inferred to underlie detection at the two orientations. The steeper sensitization translates into greater inhibition at the 0° orientation. We have suggested [8] that the shape of the mechanism fits with a medium-size psychophysical mechanism (Wilson's 'D' mechanism [9]) and appears to be mediated by M-cells in the retina due to the correspondence to their spatial scale and high sensitivity [10,11].

Together, these various findings extend our understanding of local sensitivity regulation in the visual system and expand the domain of layer-by-layer perimetry. Thus, these findings offer additional tests to be employed clinically (e.g., tests of the OFF-pathway and local contrast-gain control response) and provide new layers to be tested by Layer-by-Layer Perimetry.

Acknowledgement Sigma Xi Grant-in-Aid of Research (JSM).

References

1. Enoch JM. Quantitative Layer-by-Layer Perimetry. Invest Ophth Vis Sci 1978;17:208-257
2. Enoch JM, Essock EA, Williams, RA, Barricks MA. Functional visual effects of lesions located near the optic nerve head. Doc Ophthalmologica 1985;61:137-156.
3. Essock EA, Lehmkuhle S, Frascella J, Enoch JM. Temporal modulation of the background affects the sensitization response of X- and Y-cells in the dLGN of cat. Vis Res 1985:25;1007-1019.
4. Schiller PH, Sandell JH, Maunsell JHR. Functions of the ON and OFF channels of the visual system. Nature 1986;322:824-825.
5. Shapley R, Enroth-Cugell C. Visual adaptation and retinal gain controls. In Osborne N, Chader G, editors. Progress in Retinal Research 1984:3;263-346.
6. Fuld K. A sensitization effect with rectilinear stimuli. Vis Res 1978;18:1045-1051.
7. Essock EA. Stimulus orientation biases of the human visual system: A unifying model [dissertation]. Providence (RI): Brown University, 1981.
8. Essock EA, Krebs WK. Sensitization of a line target depends on orientation and temporal modulation rate. Invest Ophthal Vis Sci (Suppl) 1992;33(4):1349.
9. Wilson HR, Gelb DJ. Modified line-element theory for spatial-frequency and width discrimination. J Opt Soc Am A 1984:1;124-131.
10. Oehler R. Spatial interactions in the rhesus monkey retina: A behavioral study using the Westheimer paradigm. Exp Brain Res 1985;59:217-225.
11. Crook JM, Lange-Malecki B, Lee BB, Valberg A. Visual resolution of macaque retinal ganglion cells. J Physio (Lond) 1988;396:205-224.

FUNCTIONAL AND IMAGING INVESTIGATIONS IN PATIENTS WITH WELL-DEFINED ABNORMALITIES OF THE VISUAL SYSTEM

F.W. FITZKE
Laboratory of Physiological Optics,
Department of Visual Science, Institute of Ophthalmology,
University College London, London EC1V9EL, UK

Abstract

Enoch has led and inspired a school of research activity which aims to further our understanding of the visual consequences of specific and well characterized abnormalities of the visual system. For example, using psychophysical and imaging techniques has led to understanding some of the fundamental mechanisms underlying rod and cone functional abnormalities in some retinal degenerations which can be related to specific mutations in rhodopsin and other photoreceptor specific molecules. Preferential loss of magnocellular function such as motion sensitivity may provide a means for earlier detection of damage and for determining the effects of interventions in conditions like glaucoma. New imaging techniques have revealed structures which have never before been seen in the living human eye to allow direct correlation with the functional measurements. This type of research owes much to the work of Enoch who has been instrumental in promoting this approach to understanding the eye and its function.

Introduction

Investigations of visual function in patients who have specific abnormalities of certain components of the visual system have contributed to the understanding of both normal visual function and underlying mechanisms of pathology. Retinitis pigmentosa (RP), hereditary and acquired macular degenerations and other conditions have recently been reviewed [1,2] and have been the subjects of recent, intense study in our group [3-11]

Methods

Modified Humphrey Visual Field Analysers have been used to make measurements of rod and cone mediated function in scotopic conditions. Following 45 minutes of dark adaptation, perimetric full threshold determinations throughout the visual field of the dilated eye are followed by light adaptation for two minutes and monitoring of recovery of sensitivity in the dark over a period of approximately one hour.

Results

In some patients with retinitis pigmentosa with known mutations in opsin which result in a single amino acid substitution at the binding site for retinal, no measureable rod function is detected even in locations with normal absolute cone sensitivity and normal cone dark adaptation kinetics. In some cases of RP with an opsin mutation leading to regional losses of rod and cone function, final rod and cone sensitivities can be nearly normal in some retinal locations despite severely delayed recovery of sensitivity following light adaptation. Similar, striking delays in the recovery of dark adapted sensitivity despite normal final thresholds have been found in some patients with Sorsby's pseudovitteliform macular dystrophy and some patients with age related macular degeneration.

Discussion

In these and other conditions, characteristic abnormalities of visual function may not be evident using conventional tests. Clues to the mechanisms underlying the abnormalities are given by comparing the spatial distribution of rod and cone losses, the relation to visual pigments levels measured with the technique of reflection densitometry, and imaging the fundus with the scanning laser ophthalmoscope. These are compared for the different mutations and changes over time to determine the degree of similarity at various stages of the evolution of the diseases. With further understanding of the nature of the functional losses, a logical framework can be devised to consider possible therapeutic interventions which would be expected to differ depending on the mechanism of the pathophysiology.

Acknowledgements

The financial support of The Foundation Fighting Blindness (U.S.) and the Medical Research Council (U.K.) and the collaboration of clinical and research colleagues particularly those noted as co-authors in the list of referenced papers is gratefully acknowledged.

References

1.Bird AC. Retinal photoreceptor dystrophies. The Edward Jackson Memorial Lecture. Am J Ophthalmol, in press.

2.Fitzke FW and Kemp CM. Probing Visual Function with Psychophysics and Photochemistry. Eye 1989; 3:84-89.

3.Wells J, Wroblewski J, Keen J, et al. Mutations in the human retinal degeneration slow (RDS) gene can cause either retinitis pigmentosa or macular dystrophy. Nature Genetics 1993; 3:213-217.

4.Moore AT, Fitzke F, Jay M, et al. Autosomal dominant retinitis pigmentosa with apparent incomplete penetrance: a clinical electrophysiological, psychophysical and molecular biological study. Br J Ophthalmol 1993; 77:473-479.

5.Kim RY, Al-Maghtheh M, Fitzke FW, et al. Dominant retinitis pigmentosa associated with two rhodopsin mutations. Arch Ophthalmol 1993; 111:1518-1524.

6.Wroblewski JJ, Wells JA, Eckstein A, et al. Macular dystrophy associated with mutations at codon 172 in the human retinal degeneration slow (RDS) gene. Ophthalmology 1994; 101:12-22.
7.Owens SL, Fitzke FW, Inglehearn CF, et al. Ocular manifestations in autosomal dominant retinitis pigmentosa with a Lys-296-Glu rhodopsin mutation at the retinal binding site. Br J Ophthalmol 1994; 78:153-158.
8.Wroblewski JJ, Wells JA, Eckstein A, et al. Ocular findings associated with a three-base pair deletion in the peripherin-RDS gene in autosomal dominant retinitis pigmentosa. Br J Ophthalmol 1994; 78:831-836.
9.Evans K, Duval-Young J, Fitzke FW, Arden GB, Bird AC. Chromosome 19q cone-rod retinal dystrophy: ocular phenotype. Arch Ophthalmol 1995; 113:195-202.
10.Kim RY, Dollfus H, Keen TJ, et al. Autosomal dominant pattern dystrophy of the retina associatd with a 4 bp insertion at codon 140 in the RDS/peripherin gene. Arch Ophthalmol, in press.
11.Kim RY, Fitzke FW, Moore AT, et al. Autosomal dominant retinitis pigmentosa mapping to chromosome 7p exhibits variable expression. Br J Ophthalmol 1995; 79:23-27.

EVALUATION OF QUANTITATIVE MEASUREMENT OF PRISM INDUCED METAMORPHOPSIA

HIROSHI HIROSE[1], JAY M. ENOCH[2], KUAN MONG TUAN[2]
[1]Nagoya University, School of Medicine, Department of Ophthalmology, 65 Tsuruma-cho, Showa-ku, Nagoya 466, JAPAN
[2] School of Optometry, University of California, Berkeley, CA.

Abstract

We developed a technique to measure metamorphopsia rapidly, finely and quantitatively [1,2]. A model providing constant optical distortions and resultant perceptual metamorphopsia was devised using plane prisms of 15Δ. Three short vertical lines and CRT display were used to assess image distortion in the central retinal area. It is possible to measure accurately prism-induced directional biases using this method and judgements were made with less than ± 3% error.

Introduction

The Amsler grid tests, the classical approach employed for metamorphopsia, while useful, are crude and only can be used qualitatively. However, when observing an Amsler grid pattern with central fixation point, one finds the task of the observer to be either a bisection or a doubling of a distance in some dimension. These visual functions are hyperacuities, which are the finest visual responses. Based on this idea, we reported a model of quantification of prism induced metamorphopsia and usefulness of doubling tasks to eliminate individual bias at '95 ARVO. Here, to obtain more reliable data, We evaluated accumulating data of normals and the factors affecting judgements.

Subjects and method

Subjects are 5 persons from 16 to 34 y.o. Two of them have eyes with high myopia corrected by soft contact lenses(SCL). Other two have eyes with myopia less than 3D corrected by spectacles. One is emmetropia eye.

An instrument with beamsplitter, CRT display, IBM computer and mouse was used. Three short vertical lines, each separated by 128 arcmin at a test distance of 2 m were displayed on the CRT which was seen straight ahead through the beamsplitter cube. A

plano trial 15Δ prism is inserted in the left hand path. Testing is monocular. [Fig.1]

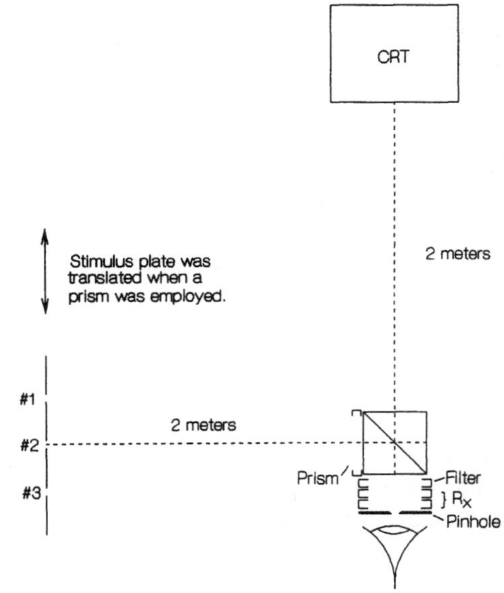

Figure 1. Schematic diagram of the instrument. The prism was removable/interchangeable.

The location of each of the projected lines was measured precisely by using Vernier alignment matches. Projections of 3 slits in the CRT were determined as settings x_1, x_2, and x_3 . From these measurements, the physical extent of a', b', and c' (x_1x_2 = a', x_2x_3 = b', x_1x_3 = c') were determined. This allowed estimation of the optical distortion caused by the prism.[Fig.2A]

Determination of the extent of each half of the display (a' and b') when prisms were used: Because of distortions induced by the prism, a' is not b'. This difference between a' and b' was separated analytically from the observer's internal setting bias. The doubling task where the distance x_1x_2 was matched by third line, $x_{3'}$ (to the right), while the observer fixated x_2.(Fig.2B). Similarly, to assess b' , a moveable line, $x_{1'}$ (to the left), was used to double the separation of x_2x_3 (Fig.2C).

Analysis: 15Δ is an example of a prism used; 0Δ refers to the no prism case. We utilize equalities obtained from the doubling experiments in order to estimate a' and b' for the prism case.

$$(a_{0\Delta})'/\,(x_2x_{3'})_{0\Delta} = (a_{15\Delta})'/\,(x_2x_{3'})15\Delta$$

from Figs.2A, B and rearranging terms and solving for $(a_{15\Delta})'$,

$$(a_{15\Delta})' = [(x_2x_{3'})_{15\Delta}]\,[(a_{0\Delta})'/\,(x_2x_{3'})_{0\Delta}].$$

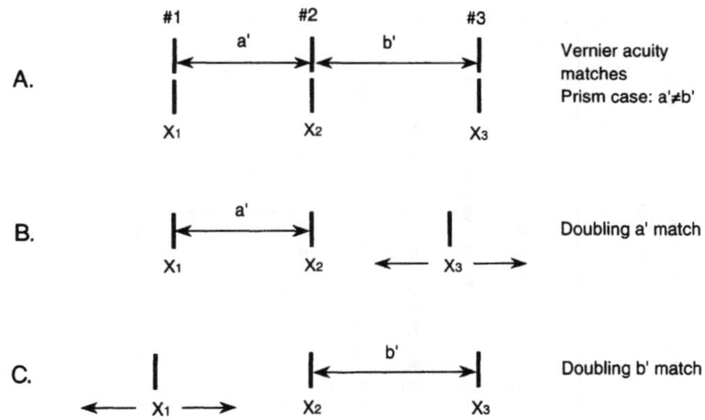

Figure 2. Schematic diagrams of displays utilized: A. The Vernier match with x_1, x_2, x_3 on the CRT. B. The doubling task where the distance x_1x_2 was matched by x_2x_3.. C. The doubling task where $x_1.x_2$ was set equal to the distance x_2x_3.

From Figs.2A,C and then solving for $(b_{15\Delta})'$,

$$(x_1.x_2)_{0\Delta} / (b_{0\Delta})' = (x_1.x_2)_{15\Delta}' / (b_{15\Delta})',$$

$$(b_{15\Delta})' = [(x_1.x_2)_{15\Delta}]\,[(b_{0\Delta})' / (x_1.x_2)_{0\Delta}].$$

The following values are compared for both analytical schemes:

$(a_{15\Delta})' / (b_{15\Delta})'$[Determined] compared to $(a_{15\Delta})' / (b_{15\Delta})'$[Vernier].

Results and discussion

According to the above analysis, errors between Vernier and determined measurements were calculated. Data of high myopic eyes corrected by SCL(Fig.3, case 1,2) showed unstable and inaccurate results in each trial. However, other 3 cases (Fig3, case 3,4,5), two of mild myopic eyes and one emmetropia eye demonstrated stable doubling judgements and have errors within ± 3% (Fig.3). It is possible to factor out the internal bias using this doubling technique and to measure distortions accurately. However, cases with high myopia corrected SCL do not seem to be adequate for performing this test probably because unexpected SCL small movement might affect to make judgements in each session.

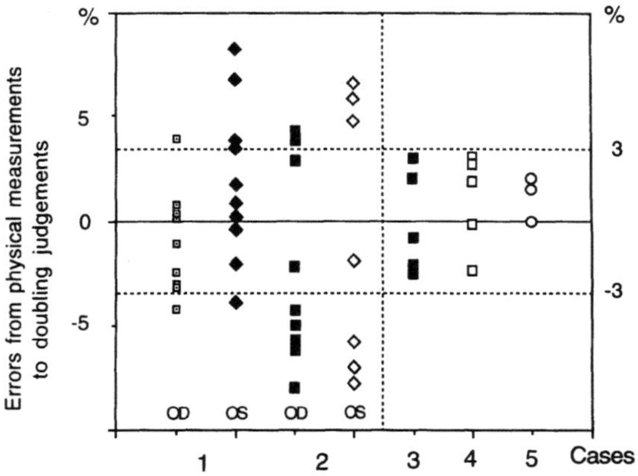

Figure 3. Results of 5 cases. Two of high myopia corrected by SCL (case 1,2) show unstable judgments in each trial compared with other 3 cases (case 3,4,5) demonstrating small errors less than ±3%.

References

1. Enoch JM, Baraldi P, Lakshminarayanan V, Savage GL, Fendick M. Measurement of metamorphosia in the presence of ocular media opacities. Am J Optom Physiol Optics 1988;65:349-53.
2. Lakshminarayanan V, Aziz S, Enoch JM. Quantification of metamorphosia using hyperacuity techniques. Optom Vis Sci 1991; 68:942-45.

AN ANALYSIS OF HUMAN VISUAL RECEPTIVE FIELDS USING THE PERIMETRIC METHOD

KAZUTAKA KANI[1], MISUZU TAKASHIMA[1], SATORU NAGATA[1],OSAMU MIMURA[2], KAZUNORI TAKUBO[2]

[1] *Dept. of Ophthalmology, Shiga University of Medical Science, Seta-tsukinowacho, Ohtsu, 520-21 JAPAN*

[2]*Dept. of Ophthalmology, Hyogo College of Medicine, Mukogawacho, Nishinomiya, 630 JAPAN*

Abstract

We measured the visual thresholds using subjective and pupillographic perimetry of various stimulation sizes, drew diameter-threshold curves and performed computer simulations which showed the shape, area and density of the receptive fields. The visual thresholds were determined using pulse or ramp stimulation. The diameters of the center of the receptive fields obtained using pulse stimulations were 6.2 minutes at the fovea. Those obtained using ramp stimulations were 4.4 minutes at the fovea. The results from the pupillographic perimetry could be simulated by W-cells.

Introduction

In perimetry, the relation between target size, threshold and receptive field of the retinal ganglion cell is generally considered as follows. If the light that falls on the retina is smaller than the on-center of the receptive field, the threshold of the cell depends upon the light energy, i.e. intensity by area (complete spatial summation). When the light is larger than the receptive field center, the threshold depends not upon the energy, but the intensity of the light (non-spatial summation). This idea is simple to understand, but the function of the off-surround area is not considered. Moreover, many receptive fields overlap each other, so it would not be appropriate to discuss their relationship in a single receptive field. In this paper we present measured visual thresholds and examine the results using computer simulation.

Methods

Experiment 1: A Topcon automated projection perimeter was used. The projection perimeter was modified so that smaller targets, two steps smaller than Goldmann No.0, and ramp stimuli were available. The background brightness was set at 31.5 asb. Pulse stimulations of 200 ms in duration were presented and the subject was instructed to press akey if the target was seen, and do nothing if it was not. The increment threshold was determined to 1 dB using a standard threshold program bracketing strategy in the perimeter.

Experiment 2: The same projection perimeter was used. The target intensity was initially set about 15 dB lower than the normal threshold and was gradually increased 30 dB in 15 seconds by means of a rotatory wedge neutral density filter. The subject was asked to press a button the instant he or she saw the target.

Experiment 3: A fundus perimeter, composed of an infrared video fundus camera, pupil monitoring apparatus and a target projection with a Maxwellian view system was used. The background brightness was set at 0.56 Trolands. The target diameters were from 6.8 min. to 125 min. The thresholds for pupillary reaction to light were determined by the up and down method.

Computer Simulation: When light falls on the receptive field of a ganglion cell, it is stimulated as the volume of the lighted part of the receptive field, and the output of the cell then equals the volume beyond the threshold (θ_n). If the total output of all overlapping cells concerned with the target exceeds the psychological threshold (θ_p), the target is detected. A total activity model increment threshold (TAMIT) [1,2] was used. The parameters in this model are: maximum center sensitivity (A), maximum surround sensitivity (AQ), the radius of the receptive field center (σ_e), the radius of the receptive field surround (σ_i), the threshold of one neuron (θ_n), the psychological threshold (θ_p), the receptive field density (Dr) and retinal eccentricity (E). These parameters are described by the following equations [1-7]:

$$G(r) = A\exp\left(\frac{-r^2}{\sigma_e^2}\right) - AQ\exp\left(\frac{-r^2}{\sigma_i^2}\right)$$

$$1/\sqrt{Dr} = 0.0055(1 + 0.59E)$$

$$2\sigma_e = 2.2 + 0.21E \qquad \text{(in X cell)}$$

$$2\sigma_e = 4.15 + 0.55E \qquad \text{(in Y cell)}$$

$$2\sigma_e = 30 + 6.0E \qquad \text{(in W cell)}$$

$$A = 2.13/\sigma_e^{1.23}$$

The results of our computer simulation when the parameter θ_n and Q are changed is shown in Figure 1. When the targets are large, the stronger the inhibition (Q), the lower the total output becomes (Figure 1, top). When the targets are small, the higher the threshold of the neurons (θ_n), the lower the total output becomes (Figure 1, bottom).

Results and Discussion

The solid line in the upper set of curves in Figure 2 shows the diameter-threshold curve measured at the fovea in experiment 1 obtained by pulse stimulation [8]. The best fit curve obtained from the simulation is shown by dotted line. The parameters of the best fit curve of the computer simulation are similar to those of the Y-cells if the radius of the receptive field center is a little larger than that of Y-cells.

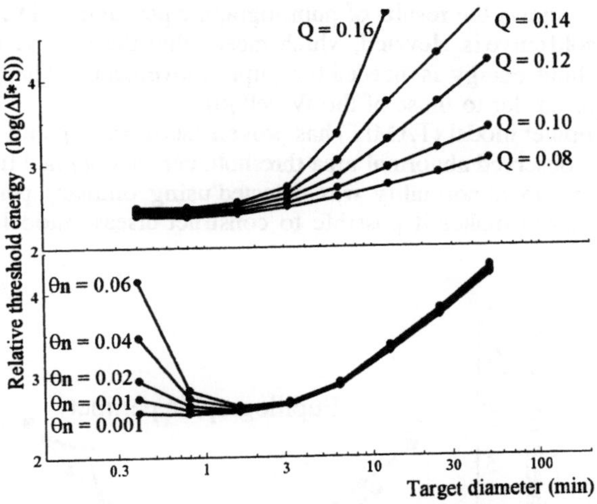

Figure 1. Computer simulation of diameter-threshold curve. The sensitivity ratio of the center to the surround (Q) and the threshold of the neuron (θ_n) are varied.

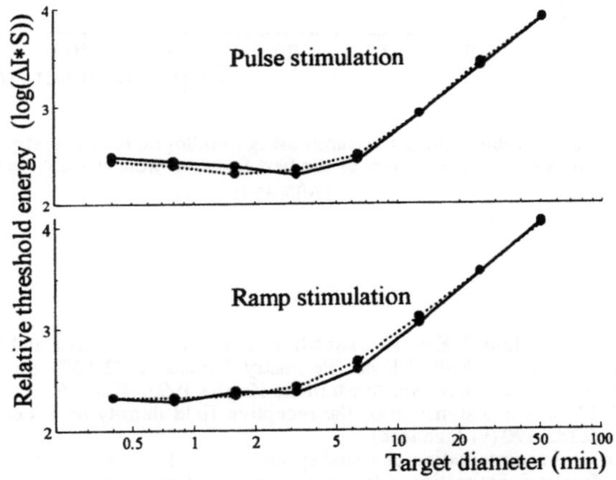

Figure 2. The diameter-threshold curve. The solid line shows the average of 15 normal subjects at the fovea, and the dotted line shows the best fit curve from computer simulation. The upper set of curves are the results measured by pulse stimulation, and the lower, with ramp stimulation. The parameters were σ_e=3.12', Q=0.135, θ_n=0.005 and $1/\sqrt{Dr}$=3.3' by pulse stimulation and σ_e=2.2', Q=0.122, θ_n=0 and $1/\sqrt{Dr}$=0.74' by ramp stimulation, respectively.

The lower set of curves in Figure 2 shows the results of experiment 2 obtained by ramp stimulations [9] and by simulation. The parameters indicate that these responses were different from those obtained using pulse stimulation. In this simulation, the receptive field was smaller than that of the Y-cells but larger than that of the X-cells, and the density was similar to that of the X-cells.

Figure 3 shows the results of pupillographic perimetry. The left of side of the diameter-threshold curve is elevated, which means that the smaller the stimulus size, the more threshold energy is needed for pupil movement. The parameters of the simulation were similar to those of the W-cell [6].

Our computer model (TAMIT) has proven useful in explaining psychophysical data. We have observed abnormal area-threshold curves obtained from patients with glaucoma, where no abnormality was detected using ordinary perimety [8,9]. Our computer simulation makes it possible to construct disease models of the retina or optic nerve.

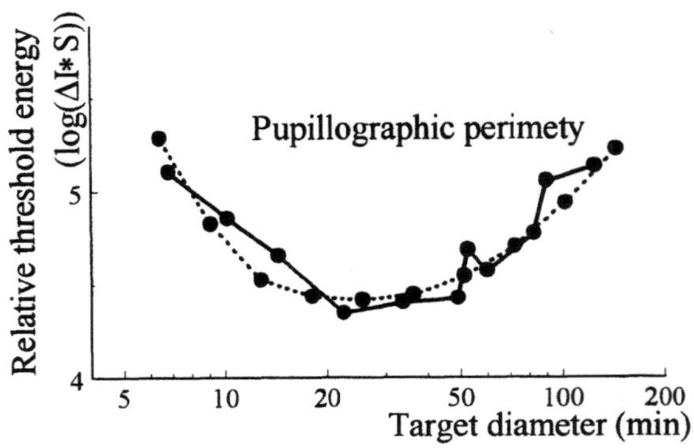

Figure 3. The diameter-threshold curve measured using pupillographic perimetry. The thresholds were measured at the fovea. The parameters of the best fit curve were σ_e=45', Q=0.1, θ_n=0.005 and $1/\sqrt{Dr}$=2.0

References

1. Nagata S, Takashima M, Inui T, Kani K. Estimation of receptive field area and density of human retina using computer simulation. In: Mills RP ed. Perimetry Update 1992/1993 Proceedings of the Xth International Perimetric Society Meeting. Amsterdam: Kugler 1993: 533-535.
2. Inui T, Kani K, Miyake S. Estimation of the receptive field density of Y cells in the human retina. Shinkeiganka 1989;6:383-390 (in Japanese).
3. Drasdo N. The neural representation of visual space. Nature 1977;266:554-556.
4. Inui T, Kani K, Miyake S. Estimation of the receptive field density of X cells in the human retina and visual acuity. Shinkeiganka 1989; 6:391-395 (in Japanese).
5. Inui T, Mimura O, Kani K. Retinal sensitivity and spatial summation in the foveal and parafoveal regions. J Opt Soc Am 1981;71:151-154.
6. Stone J, Fukuda Y. Properties of cat retinal ganglion cells: A comparison of W-cells with X- and Y-cells. J Neurophysiol 1973;36:551-567.
7. Linsenmeier RA, Frishman LJ, Jakiela HG, Enroth-Cugell C. Receptive field properties of X and Y cells in the cat retina derived from contrast sensitivity measurement. Vision Res 1982;22:1173-1183.
8. Takashima M, Nagata S, Kani K. Estimation of receptive fields using an automatic perimeter. In: Mills RP ed. Perimetry Update 1992/1993 Proceeding of the Xth International Perimetric Society Meeting. Amsterdam: Kugler, 1993: 537-541.
9. Takashima M, Nagata S, Tsukada H, Obata N, Kani K. Ramp stimulation perimetry in testing the X-system. In: Mills RP, Wall M editors. Perimetry Update 1994/1995 Proceedings of the XIth International Perimetric Society Meeting. Amsterdam: Kugler, 1995:149-157.

REACTION TIMES FOR RECOGNITION OF DEGRADED FACIAL IMAGES

VASUDEVAN LAKSHMINARAYANAN[1], SANJIV K. BHATIA[2], ASHOK SAMAL[3], and GRANT V. WELLAND[2]
[1]*School of Optometry and Department of Physics & Astronomy,*
[2]*Department of Mathematics & Computer Science*
University of Missouri - St. Louis, St. Louis, MO
[3]*Department of Computer Science & Engineering*
University of Nebraska - Lincoln, Lincoln, NE

Abstract

We report data from experiments measuring reaction times necessary to discriminate human faces from non-faces. The study is a continuation of our previous work [1] to establish a benchmark in human face recognition using degraded images. A two-alternative forced-choice (2AFC) experiment is used. Both stimulus images (face/non-face) are uniformly degraded in terms of the number of pixels (using a modification of the Haar wavelet) and the number of gray scales.

Introduction

Human face identification begins with the recognition that the stimulus is a human face as opposed to an alternative such as an inanimate object or an animal. There is a considerable body of literature on various aspects of face recognition by machines and humans [2, 3]. For example, it is well known that the ability of an observer to recognize a human face is influenced by the distinctiveness of the face, the orientation in which it is seen, and the race of the face. Often, the human system is presented a scene containing faces for a brief period of time during which he/she must pick out the faces. In many applications of human face recognition using automatic methods, undue delays in processing may be unacceptable, *e.g.*, authentication in routine environments. Automated face recognition systems have many practical applications [4].

As part of an ongoing study aimed towards elucidation of human face recognition, we conducted extensive psychophysical experiments. The aim was to establish a benchmark criteria for automated face recognition. The present experiments were specifically designed to measure the reaction time required by humans in recognizing face patterns. The aim is that these researches will provide insight into the design of an automated system that will match the performance level of human vision system. Such studies can be used as bench-marks to evaluate automatic face recognition systems. In developing an intelligent system to match human level performance, the computation requirements will be guided by the time required to perform the task. We present our experimental results in this article.

Methods

Four sets of images were used in the experiment – human faces (target images), mammalian faces (including primates), scrambled human faces, and inanimate objects. The images were presented to the subjects on a CRT using a SPARCstation 2 computer. Each image occupied an area of 3.62 × 3.62 cm^2 on the screen and was viewed at a distance of 58.1 cm from the screen (visual angle of 3.56° at the eye). All images were presented in a 128 × 128 pixel array with an aspect ratio of 1:1 as mug shots. Additionally, each facial image was devoid of any background noise and was unobstructed.

A total of 92 facial images, 92 mammalian faces (including 41 primates), and 85 inanimate objects (natural and man-made objects, including landscapes and non-mammalian animals) were used. Scrambled faces were developed from the original facial images by an algorithmic manipulation of the image pixels. Ninety facial images were scrambled for this experiment. A modified Haar wavelet formulation for the degradation of stimulus images using fractional pixels [1], was used. This procedure is equivalent to block averaging and removal of detail in an image. Additionally, images were degraded by reducing the number of gray scales.

The experiments were performed using ten adult subjects. They used a view tunnel to minimize the stray light noise etc., and wore appropriate correction to the test distance. Each subject was presented a sequence of panels each comprising of a pair of images (a target and a non-target). The subject's task was to decide whether the human face (the target) appeared on the left panel or the right. Each panel was presented for 500 msec and the subject *had* to make a decision. A new panel was presented to the subject after they had made a response or after four seconds had elapsed. The response time was automatically measured by the computer. The subject pressed either the left or the right mouse button corresponding to whether he/she saw the target in the left or the right panel. Each subject was given approximately 5000 to 6000 panels, selected at random at different degradation levels.

Results

We collected a total of 69,302 responses. The number of correct responses was 56,347. The psychometric results have been reported separately [1]. The mean of the reaction time for all stimuli was 0.846 seconds with a variance of 0.168 seconds. For correct responses, the mean reaction time was 0.855 seconds with a variance of 0.149 seconds. The corresponding data for incorrect responses are 0.806 seconds (mean) and 0.248 seconds(variance). The data were also subdivided into categories and are displayed in Table 1. Table 2 gives a detailed distribution of the responses as a function of reaction time.

Table 1: Reaction time from Experiment. (the variances are within parentheses)

Category	Number of Responses	Overall time (seconds)	Correct Responses		Incorrect Responses	
			Number	Time	Number	Time
Primate	9256	0.868 (0.175)	7047	0.878 (0.157)	2210	0.837 (0.230)
Scrambled	28533	0.835 (0.162)	23386	0.843 (0.143)	5148	0.800 (0.246)
Objects	19866	0.845 (0.169)	16525	0.858 (0.150)	3342	0.782 (0.252)
Mammals	20889	0.862 (0.175)	16435	0.870 (0.155)	4445	0.830 (0.245)

Table 2: Distribution of reaction times

Response time	Overall	Correct	Incorrect
0.0-0.5	12	10	22
0.5-1.0	62	65	50
1.0-1.5	20	20	20
>1.5	6	5	8

In Figures 1 and 2, we have plotted times for different levels of image degradation (spatial and gray scale resolution levels). The data indicate that there is little or no effect of spatial and gray scale resolution on response time.

Statistical test were performed to verify the null hypothesis on both the means and variances of the data sets. With the sole exception of scrambled faces *vs* object categories, the null hypothesis was verified for all comparisons at $P = 0.01$ level (2 tailed t-test). Here, the statistical tests were inconclusive probably since the means and variances are approximately equal. This is being investigated. It should also be noted that even though the subjects were allowed up to four seconds to respond, almost all the responses were made within 1.5 seconds with approximately 75% of the responses being made within 1.0 seconds. Common observation dictates that as the amount of detail in a scene/picture increases, the sooner we will be able to detect/identify it. This situation is replicated in

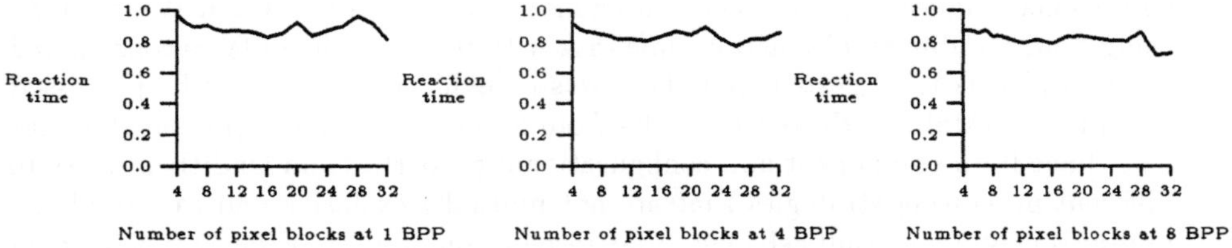

Figure 1: Plot of average reaction times as a function of pixel block size. Independent parameter is gray scale.

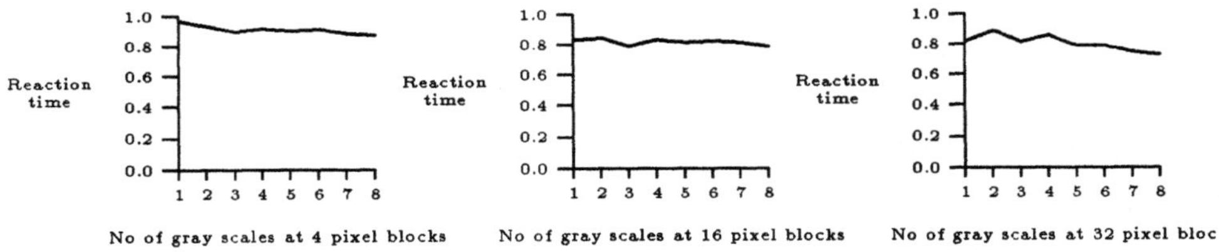

Figure 2: Plot of average reaction times as a function of gray scale degradation. Independent parameter is pixel block size.

our experiments by increasing the number of pixel blocks (greater resolution). However, our results indicate that reaction time is practically constant for all definition levels used in the experiment.

Discussion

Reaction times have been studied extensively in face recognition tasks. Valentine and Bruce [5, 6] measured reaction times and showed that distinctive faces were recognized more quickly than typical faces. Shepherd et al., [7] have studied the effects of distinctiveness and presentation time on face recognition. It has been shown that reaction times for inverted faces was affected much more than for nonface stimuli . A more interesting phenomenon in face perception is the "Margaret Thatcher Illusion" [9]. Reaction times were measured for both rotated normal and "Thatcher" faces and it was concluded that the orientation effect was essentially the same for both type of faces suggesting that processing of faces is qualitatively not different from the processing of other types of stimuli [10].

Galton [11] has suggested that relationship among features of a face may be a more critical factor to its recognition than the contribution of any particular facial feature. Using this Gestaltan approach it is concluded that a face is processed as a whole unit [12]. In the Gestaltan approach, the importance of configurational relationships between features is stressed. Bradshaw and Wallace [13], using "same"-"different" reaction time task with tests of pairs of faces constructed from an identikit, suggested that there was no evidence for faces to be processed as unitary Gestaltan. However, results from a paper by Sergent [14] suggest that faces have both component and configurational properties and lend themselves to different processing strategies that are not mutually exclusive and can unfold simultaneously. Our results showing that recognition of a face is fairly independent of level of degradation suggest that the face processing system is at a more global level (at least at the initial stages of the process), thus suggesting a Gestaltan approach. We emphasize that the task in our experiments was *not* what the face is (an identification problem) but rather, of the two images, which is the human face (a recognition problem).

Individual components of a face are not indispensible for recognizing faces. The fact that we can recognize and identify a face 30 or 40 meters away suggests that we are not doing a feature or piecewise analysis. At those distances small features of a face are not visible and only the relationship amongst them are useful. Harmon [15], for example, has shown that even under severe blur conditions, we are successful in recognizing faces. He also showed that a face made of a 16 $\times$ 16 matrix of a quantized pixel blocks can be accurately identified (*e.g.*, the famous Lincoln Photo). At this resolution level, only the configuration resulting from coarse quantification allows recognition. Ginsburg [16] has shown that only low spatial frequency information (about 2 cycles/degree) carries basic portrait frequency information. Since a higher level of spatial frequency information would be required for resolution of individual features it can be hypothesized that face recognition may not rely exclusively on a feature analysis [17]. Milner [18] has suggested that the process of recognizing wholes necessitates descending or attenuating component parts. The relationship among features, in addition to particular shape of each feature, may thus represent a source of information for face identification.

Size of a face seems to play an important in its recognition [19]. Here, the size of all our targets and non-targets images were approximately constant throughout the set of experiments and therefore can be factored out. There has been much interest recently in studies of recognition of human faces degraded by spatial quantization [20, 21]. In particular, it has been shown that if facial images are degraded by spatial quantization or block averaging, there is a non-linear acceleration of the decline in accuracy of recognition as block size increases, leading to a suggestion that recognition requires a critical minimum range of object spatial frequencies, namely 8–16 cycles/face of information. In this study, we have not addressed this aspect. To the best of our knowledge, we are not aware of published reaction time studies on degraded/quantized facial images. The other curious aspect of the reaction times measured here is the relatively long response times. In this paradigm, subjects are assumed to look at one of the pair and see that it is either a face or not and make that decision. The long time might represent this longer decision making process. This has to be investigated in future research. Another factor which has been left out in our experiment is the memory parameter. Sergent [14] has hypothesized that since memory of a face cannot be completely faithful, relying on component parts of a face for recognition tasks might not be an effective strategy and therefore configural properties might have a more determinant role, and make the processing of these properties necessary for face recognition.

We performed two sets of two-alternative forced-choice (2AFC) experiments to measure the reaction time for the face detection task, *i.e.*, recognizing a pattern to be a face, without identifying it. The first set of experiments was used primarily to determine the role of spatial and grayscale resolution in human face perception [1]. We recorded the response times from this experiment even though the experiment was not designed to measure the reaction time *per se*. The second set of experiments was designed primarily for accurate measurement of the reaction times. The main difference between the two was the way the subjects recorded their response. In the first, there is some amount of motor movement to position the mouse, while in the second there is practically none.

The results show that motor movement does not seem to affect the overall response time for recognition. Furthermore, it appears that neither spatial resolution nor gray scale resolution plays a significant role in the overall recognition time. The subjects roughly take a little under a second to recognize a pattern as a face irrespective of its resolution. Previous studies have shown that as the spatial resolution improves, so does the performance of the subjects in terms of percentage of patterns correctly identified as a face [1]. The current study indicates that the visual system does not take any more time to process the lower resolution image.

By showing the invariance of reaction times to different levels of degradation (both resolution and gray scale) we have further extended the earlier results of Harmon on degraded (blurred) faces. The present results were obtained in a 2-AFC discrimination task in which both stimuli were simultaneously presented with no verbal cues and no memorization was involved. In this sense, caution should be exercised in comparing results to those of other researchers since different experimental conditions (*e.g.*, identikit images) and tasks (*e.g.*, "same"–"different" reaction time measurements) were utilized.

Acknowledgements

This study was partially supported by NSF grants CDA-9022445 and USE-9152764 (AS) and Air Force Grant 90-0307 (GVW).

References

1. Bhatia SK, Lakshminarayanan V, Samal A, Welland GV. Human face perception in degraded images. J Visual Comm Image Rep 1995;6:280–295.

2. Bruce V, Cowey A, Ellis AW, Perrett DL. Processing the Facial Image. Oxford, UK: Clarendon Press, 1992.

3. Bruce V, Burton M. Processing Images of Faces. Norwood, NJ: Ablex Publishing Corp., 1992.

4. Samal A, Iyengar PA. Automatic recognition and analysis of human faces and facial expressions: A survey. Pat Recog 1992;25:65–77.

5. Valentine T, Bruce V. The effects of distinctiveness in recognising and classifying faces. Perception 1986;15:525–536.

6. Valentine T. A unified account of the effects of distinctiveness, inversion and race in face recognition. Quart J Exp Psychol 1991;43A:161–204.

7. Shepherd JW, Gibling F, Ellis HD. The effect of distinctiveness, presentation time, and delay on face recognition. In:Bruce V, editor. Face Recognition. Hillsdale, NJ: Lawrence Earlbaum Associates, 1991:137–145.

8. Diamond R, Carey S. Why faces are not special: An effect of expertise. J Exp Psychol:Gen 1986;115:107–117.

9. Thompson P. Margaret Thatcher – A new illusion. Perception 1980;9:483–484.

10. Sjoberg W, Windes J. Recognition times for rotated normal and "Thatcher" faces. Percept Motor Skills 1992;75:1176–1178.

11. Galton F. Component portraits made by combining those of many different persons in to single resultant figure. J Anthropological Institute 1879;8:132–144.

12. Ellis HD. Recognising faces. Brit J Psychol 1975;66:409–426.

13. Bradshaw JL, Wallace G. Models for the processing and identification of faces. Percept Psychophys 1971;9:443–448.

14. Sergent J. An investigation into component and configural processes underlying face perception. Brit J Psychol 1984;75:221–242.

15. Harmon LD. The recognition of faces. Scientific American, November 1973;70–82.

16. Ginsburg A. Visual Information Processing Based on Spatial Filters Constrained by Biological Data [dissertation]. Cambridge:University of Cambridge, 1978.

17. Tieger T, Galz L. Recognition of faces in the presence of two-dimensional sinusoidal masks. Percept Psychophys 1979;26:163–167.

18. Milner PM. A model for visual shape recognition. Psychol Rev 1974;81:521–535.

19. Kolers PA, Duchnicky RL, Sundstroem G. Size in the visual processing of faces and words. J Exp Psychol 1985;11:726–751.

20. Bachmann T. Identification of spatially quantized tachistoscopic images of faces: How many pixels does it take to carry identity? Eur J Cog Psychol 1991;31:87–103.

21. Costen NP, Parker DM, Craw I. Spatial content and spatial quantization effects in face recognition. Perception 1994;23:123–146.

FUNCTIONAL DIVISION OF HUMAN RETINA

LEI LIU[1], CLIFTON M. SCHOR[2]
[1] *The Arlene Gordon Research Institute, The Lighthouse Inc., NY.,*
[2] *School of Optometry, University of California, Berkeley, CA.*

Abstract

The retina can be functionally divided according to apparent horizontal (isoelevation) and vertical (isoazimuth) contours. Monocular apparent horizontal positions across the visual field were measured at different elevations in a psychophysical experiment. Our data suggests that the isoelevation divisions of the human retina provide a relatively stable perceptual reference framework.

Introduction

The discrepancies between the perceptual-visual world and the physical world provide vision scientists an opportunity to investigate the mystery of visual-spatial information processing. While many of these perceptual discrepancies are small in magnitude some of them become pronounced in large fields of view. One such constant error is the apparent curvature of long horizontal and vertical lines.

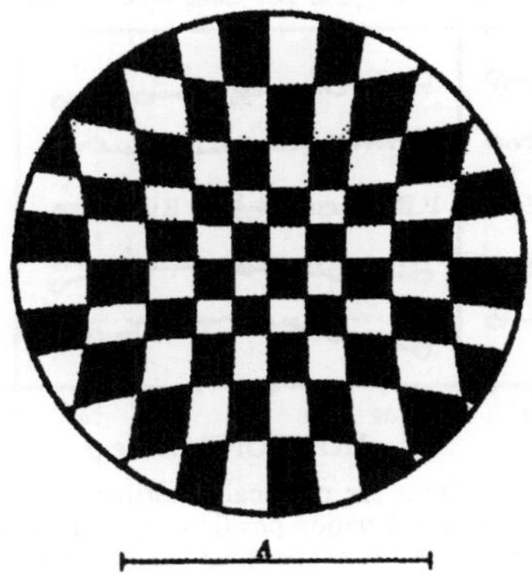

Figure 1. Helmholtz's checkerboard. The pincushion distortion was meant to compensate for the apparent curvature of long horizontal lines. When this checkerboard is positioned in front of one eye, at a distance of *A*, it appears rectilinear.

It is well established that the horizontal meridian of the retina mediates the sense of horizontal [1,3]. The question is, what retinal elements mediate the sense of horizontal above and bleow the horizontal meridian of the retina? Dividing the retina according to apparent horizontal and verticality is referred to as functional division of the retina [3]. A horizontal retinal division line is the collection of retinal units which, when stimulated, give rise to the sense of a horizontal line. Interestingly, these lines do not always coincide with physically straight lines.

When a horizontal line is fixated upon, it appears horizontal and straight to the observer. However, long horizontal lines above and below this line appear concave toward the fixation point. In order to perceive a line as straight, this perceptual barrel distortion has to be nulled with the opposite pincushion distortion in which hroizotnal lines are convex toward the fixation point. This is demonstrated by the famous Helmholtz checkerboard [1] shown in Figure 1. Helmholtz claimed that when this checkerboard with a pincushion distortion was viewed at a distance indicated by *A*, it would appear rectilinear.

Although this phenomenon is well known, it has not been quantitatively studied because spatial localization is very poor in the peripheral [2,3], making curvature judgments difficult. We have developed a equal height judgment criterion to quantify this perceptual error. Our study of the retinal division started with measuring the spatial loci of apparent horizontal above and below the level of fixation. The data was then used to derive the retinal loci which mediated the sense of horizontal.

Methods

We measured position along apparent horizontal contours, or isoelevation positions at two close viewing distances (15 and 27 cm). A set of binocular fixation targets and nonius lines were always present at the center of the display. A reference dot (8 arcmin in diameter) was presented to one eye above the binocular fixation target. A test dot of the same size was presented at a given horizontal eccentricity (ranging from 13-25 deg) to the same eye. Polarioid filters isolated targets for one eye. The isoelevation curves in the

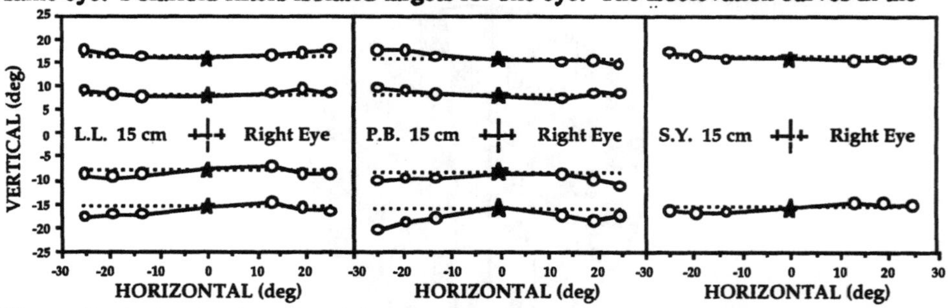

Figure 2. Isoelevation data. Dotted lines are physically horizontal in space. Stars are the reference dot position and the data points are apparent isoelevation positions as a function of retinal eccentricity. Each data point is the mean of 10-30 adjustments. Error bars are about the size of the symbols.

two eyes were measured separately. In each stimulus presentation, both the reference dot and the test dot were flashed for 200 msec. The observer, while keeping his fixation at the center of the display, adjusted the vertical position of the test dot until it appeared to be at the same height as the reference dot. This criterion demanded that the observer made judgment based on his innate sense of horizontal. 10 to 30 adjustments were taken at each test location. The tests were conducted on a 6-by-4 matrix, covering 50-by-30 degrees of visual field. The stimulus was generated by a Mac II computer. All the experiments were done in a dark room. Chin rest and head rest were used to stabilize head position. One of the authors and two undergraduate students who were naive about the purpose of this study participated in the experiments. LL and SY were emmetropic. PB had mild myopia and did not wear her refractive correction during the experiment.

Results

The isoelevation positions for the right eyes of 3 observers are shown in Fig.2. As expected, the apparent horizontal contours deviate from physical horizontal lines in space such that isoelevation curves were convex toward the fixation point. There was also a trapezoidal vertical expansion in the nasal (left) side of visual field because the fronto-parallel screen viewed in symmetrical convergence was not perpendicular to either visual axis at the finite viewing distance.

In order to infer functional division of retina from the isoelevation data in space, we assumed that the retina was a perfect sphere. Its center coincides with the origin of the coordinate system. The optics of the eye are simplified as a projection through the mean nodal point of eye (5.7 mm in front of the origin). A horizontal retina division line is defined as the intersection of a plane and the retinal sphere. This retinal division plane is parallel to the x-axis and it intersects the z-axis at the *retinal division point* which is z_p mm in front of the origin. A family of retinal division lines are the intersections of the retina sphere with all the planes which are parallel to the x-axis and which intersect the z-axis at the same retinal division point z_p.

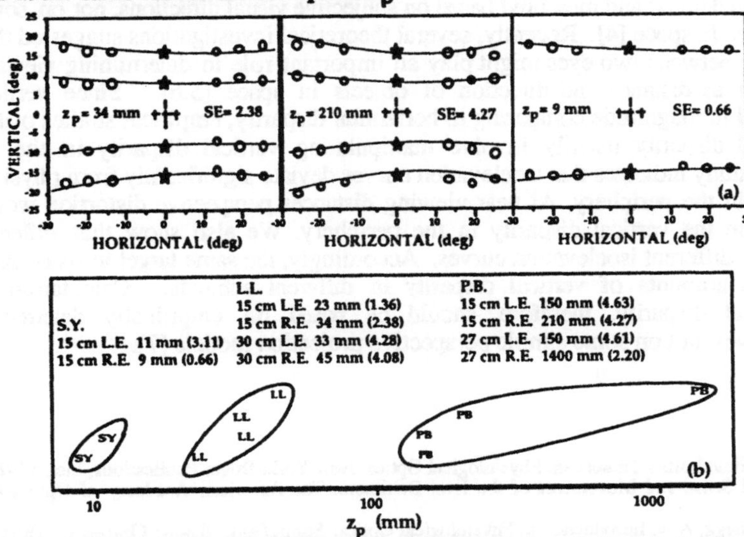

Figure 3. Estimates of isoelevation curves. (a) Best zp fit of the data shown in Figure 2. Best fit zp values and square errors are shown in the middle of each graph. (b) Summary of best fitting zp values for both eyes of each observerand at two viewing distainces.

Different schemes of functional retinal division can be distinguished by different retinal division points. The projection of a retinal division line through the nodal point onto a planer screen in space is always a conic curve. When such a curve is displayed on a tangent screen, it is perceived as a horizontal line. This curve, therefore, is the theoretical isoelevation curve under this given retinal division scheme.

The single parameter z_p of the projection curve was manipulated to fit our isoelevation data. Fig.3a shows the best fitting curves for the right eye isoelevation data of three observers. For LL, the best fitting z_p was 34 mm and for PB it was 210 mm. The isoelevation lines for these two observers were much more curved than that suggested by Helmholtz and the z_p values were much larger than the physical dimension of the eyeball. For SY, z_p was 9 mm.

Fig.3b summarizes the best fitting z_p values for all the data. Although the positions of the retinal division points for different observers differ significantly, the z_p values for the two eyes of the same observer are very similar. Observer LL and PB also conducted the same experiment at a longer viewing distance (27 cm). The best fitting z_p values obtained for the two distances are also very similar, indicating that the retinal division specified by the z_p value may represent a constant perceptual reference framework.

Discussion

This study provides a means of summarizing the barrel distortion of the eye with a single parameter (z_p). It also provides important information about binocular vision. Binocular correspondence is defined and measured based on subjective visual directions, not on some physical measures in space [4]. Recently, several theoretical investigations suggested that vertical disparity between two eyes might play an important role in determining viewing parameters, such as distance and direction of objects in space [5,6]. Since vertical disparity is small in magnitude comparing to horizontal disparity, empirical studies of the effect of vertical disparity usually involve manipulating vertical disparity in the far periphery. Our study indicates that isoelevation curves deviate significantly from physical horizontal lines in the periphery. At near viewing distances perspective distortion would further exaggerate the vertical disparity in the periphery. We also show that different people may have different isoelevation curves. Accordingly, the same target in space may subtend different amounts of vertical disparity in different subjects. Calculation of binocular vertical disparity, therefore, should be based on empirically determined isoelevation curves, not on some simple perspective projection models [7].

References

1. Helmholtz, H. v. Helmholtz's Treatise on Physiological Optics New York: Dover Publications, Inc., 1962.
2. Hering, E. Spatial Sense and Movements of the Eye. Baltimore: The American Academy of Optometry, 1942.
3. Tschermak-Seysenegg, A. v. Introduction to Physiological Optics. Springfield, Illinois: Charles C. Thomas, 1952.
4. Ogle, K. N. Researches in Binocular Vision. New York: Hafner, 1950.
5. Mayhew, J. The interpretation of stereo-disparity information: the computation of surface orientation and depth. Perception 1982;11:387-403.
6. Gillam, B. and Lawergren, B. The induced effect, vertical disparity, and stereoscopic theory. Perception & Psychophysics 1983;34:121-130.
7. Rogers, B. J. and Bradshaw, M. F. Vertical disparities, differential perspective and binocular stereopsis. Nature 1993;361:253-255.

GRATING VISUAL ACUITY WITH SHORT EXPOSURE DURATION

SHINICHI YAMADE and MOMOYO KONO
Dept. of Ophthalmology, Shiga University of Medical Science, Shiga, JAPAN

Abstract

Previously we reported that the critical duration of Landolt 'C' visual acuity was significantly prolonged in eyes with central serous retinochoroidopathy and macular edema, but that the critical duration for the increment threshold was not prolonged in these diseased eyes. To clarify the mechanisms behind this phenomenon, we measured the critical duration of grating visual acuity using grating charts generated on a monitor. The mean critical duration of 3 trials for a normal subject was 73.0 msec and 140 msec under two different conditions. These values were rather close to that of the threshold testing. The mechanisms behind critical durations in Landolt 'C' visual acuity and grating acuity are suspected to be different. The time dependency of grating acuity is rather similar to that of the increment threshold.

Introduction

During visual acuity testing patients occasionally require longer stimulus duration for proper reading of the targets, although they demonstrate relatively high levels of visual acuity using the conventional method. In our previous study [1], we reported that the critical duration of Landolt 'C' visual acuity was significantly prolonged in eyes with central serous retinochoroidopathy (CSR) and macular edema (ME). The mean critical durations of the CSR and ME groups were 3.25 ± 0.60 log msec (1.78 sec., n=13) and 3.43 ± 0.22 log msec (2.69 sec., n=6) respectively. These values were significantly longer than that of the normal group (2.79 ± 0.19 log msec or 0.62 sec., n=17). But the critical duration for the increment threshold was not prolonged in these diseased eyes. Figure 1 shows the calculated threshold-time curves of 4 eyes with CSR and 4 eyes with macular edema. Although the mean relative threshold energy of the diseased groups was significantly ($p<0.02$) higher than that of the control group, the mean critical durations were 1.77 ± 0.17 log msec (58.9 msec) for the normal group, 1.74 ± 0.04 log msec (55.0 msec) for the CSR group, and 1.86 ± 0.04 log msec (72.4 msec) for the ME group. These values were not significantly different from each other.

To clarify the mechanisms behind these phenomenon, we measured the critical duration of grating visual acuity in a normal eye.

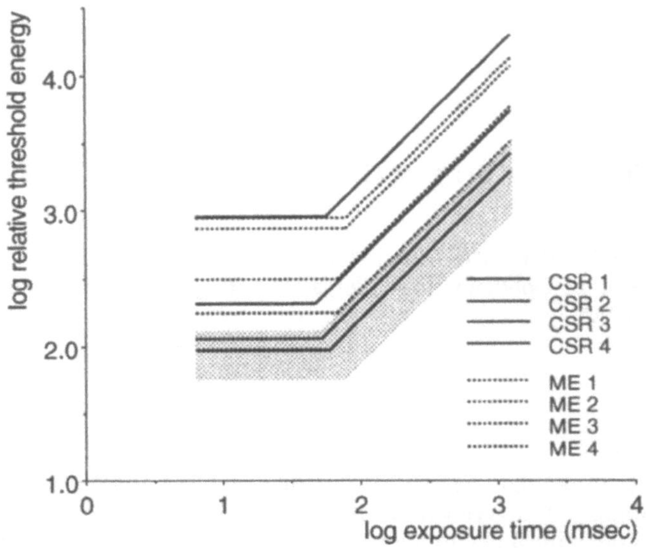

Figure 1. The threshold-time curves of CSR (solid lines, n=4) and ME (dotted lines, n=4). The shaded area indicates the approximate normal range taken from 10 normal eyes. The critical durations are not significantly different from each other.

Methods

Grating targets of 8 different spatial frequencies of 3 different grating directions were generated on a monitor. The target was a 10 cm circle, which subtended 1.43 degrees at testing distance (4 m). The spatial frequencies were 4.28, 6.41, 9.62, 12.1, 16.4, 20.0, 25.7, and 35.6 cycles/degree. Directions of the grating were vertical, tilted to the right or tilted to the left by 15 degrees. The visual acuity of each exposure time was determined by showing these charts in a random sequence. The same target appeared four times, so 96 charts were displayed per session. To indicate the exposure timing, a gray circle of 500 msec duration was displayed three times with a 500 msec interval, and the grating test chart was shown after the last interval. The exposure duration was 10,20,30,50,100,200,300,500 or 1000 msec. The observer was required to indicate the direction of the grating or 'could not see' , by pushing a button. The observer was not allowed to guess the direction when he could not see it.

The rates of correct answers for each target were plotted against its spatial frequency and the most acceptable function, and so the visual acuity (to be at the 50% correct level) for that exposure time, was calculated as shown in Figure 2. The function was assumed as $p(x) = \exp(-x)/(\exp(x)+\exp(-x))$, where $x = 2s$(target size-observer's visual acuity) (in log c/d) and $s=-p'(0)$. The least squares algorithm was used.

The calculated visual acuity in log spatial frequencies for 9 exposure times (10 to 1000 msec) were plotted and the critical duration was determined, assuming that the function was composed of two straight lines. We assumed that the function had a gradient for the shorter exposure time, where a kind of temporal summation occurred, and that it had no gradient (constant) for the longer exposure time, where no temporal summation occurred. The least squares method was used here again.

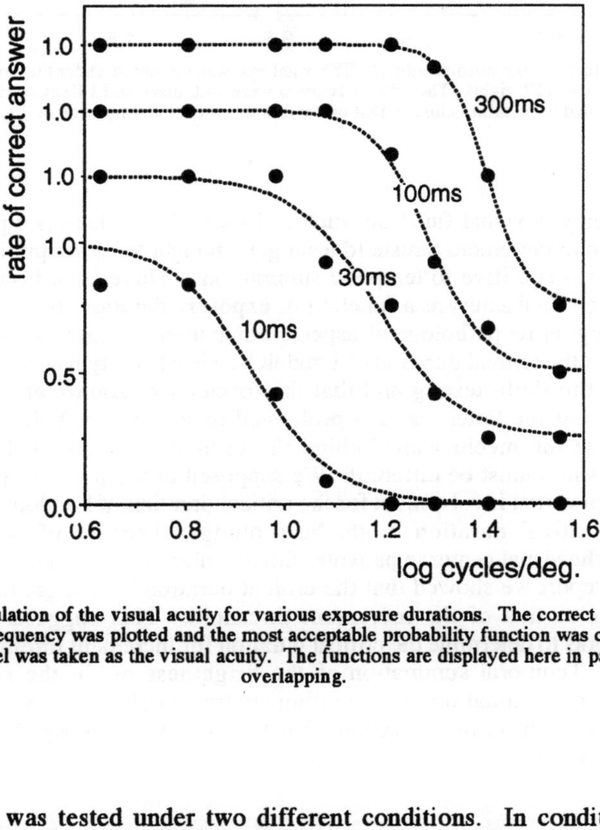

Figure 2. Calculation of the visual acuity for various exposure durations. The correct rates for each target's spatial frequency was plotted and the most acceptable probability function was calculated. The 50% correct level was taken as the visual acuity. The functions are displayed here in parallel to avoid overlapping.

Results

A normal eye was tested under two different conditions. In condition 255, the brightness of white background was 92.9 cd/sqm and the grating constant was 92.5%. In the other condition (127), the background brightness was 23.2 cd/sqm and the contrast was 73.1%. The mean critical duration of the 3 trials for the normal subject SY's right eye were 73.0 msec for condition 255 (Fig. 3 left) and 140 msec for the condition 127 (Fig. 3 right). These values were rather close to that of the threshold test (58.9 msec as shown in Fig. 1).

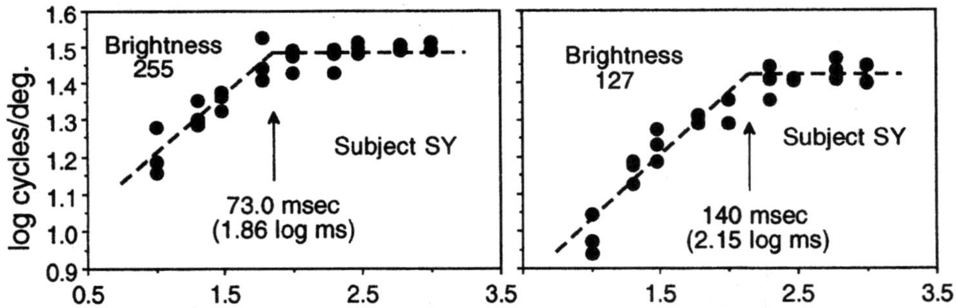

Figure 3. The results from the normal subject. SY's right eye was measured under the bright (255, left) and less bright conditions (127, right). The critical duration were 73.0 msec and 140 msec respectively, which seemed to be rather close to that of the threshold test (58.9 msec as in Fig. 1).

Discussion

Time-dependency in visual function, such as Bloch's law, which is a phenomenon of critical duration in increment threshold testing, is thought to be as applicable to visual acuity as it also is sensitive to temporal summation. There have been a few reports [2-6] addressing visual acuity as a function of exposure duration, but we could find no papers reporting on its pathological aspects other than our previous paper [1]. We reported [1] that the critical duration of Landolt 'C' visual acuity was longer than that of the increment threshold testing and that the former was significantly prolonged in diseased eyes, but the latter was not prolonged under such pathological conditions. This means that the mechanisms behind the critical durations of Landolt 'C' and increment threshold must be different. We supposed in our previous paper that there might be central neural involvement for the critical duration of Landolt 'C' visual acuity and that the critical duration might be prolonged because of poor information transmitted to the visual center in patients with macular involvement.

In this report we showed that the critical duration for the grating visual acuity was very close to that of the increment threshold. This suggests that a similar mechanism works to determine the critical duration for increment threshold and grating visual acuity. Temporal summation of the brightness or, in the case of grating patterns, temporal summation of the grating contrast might occur when the exposure time is shorter than the critical duration. Whether it will be prolonged in diseased eyes or not is our next task.

References

1. Kono M, Yamade S. Temporal integration in diseased eyes, Int Opthalmol 1996 submitted.

2.Graham CH, Cook C. Visual acuity as a function of intensity and exposure time. Am J Psychol 1937;49:654-661.

3 Kahneman D. Temporal summation in an acuity task at different energy levels - A study of the determination of summation. Vision Res 1964;4:557-566.

4.Kahneman D. Time-intensity reciprocity in acuity as a function of luminance and figure ground contrast. Vision Res 1966;6:207-215.

5.Kahneman D, Norman J, Kubovy M. Critical duration for the resolution of form: centrally or peripherally determined? J Exp Psychol 1967;73:323-327.

6. Baron WS, Westheimer G. Visual acuity as a function of exposure duration. J Opt Soc Am 1973;63:212-219.

DOUBLE FLASH RESOLUTION ALTERED IN AGING AND EARLY GLAUCOMA

TETSUSHI YASUMA[1], NORIKO MIYAKAWA[1], JUN YAMAZAKI[2], NORIAKI YAMAMOTO[3], HIROSHI HIROSE[4]
[1]*Yasuma Eye Hospital, Nagoya,* [2]*Toyohashi City Hospital,* [3]*Gamagouri City Hospital,* [4]*Nagoya University School of Med, Nagoya, JAPAN*

ABSTRACT

Double flash resolution (DFR) and critical flicker fusion frequency (CFF) were measured in 30 patients with glaucoma. These patients had no abnormality in any isopter evaluated using the Goldmann perimeter or any elevation of thresholds using the Tubinger perimeter at parafoveal field locations. These two tests, DFR and CFF, were also performed in 24 normal subjects divided into 3 age groups. Ten out of the 30 patients with glaucoma showed a significant deterioration of DFR in the temporal visual field without any abnormality in CFF. In the normal subject group, however, functional abnormalities with aging were observed in the upper visual field. Therefore, the deterioration of time-dependent sensitivity in the temporal visual field in the cases with glaucoma was judged as early glaucomatous changes. The DFR is thought to be a more sensitive method for detecting early glaucomatous functional changes than flicker or static perimetry, and seems to be a promising test for the understanding of pathophysiologic process underlying retinal or optic nerve diseases.

Materials and Methods

The methods of measurement were reported in detail(1). Three red circular light-emitting diodes (LED), with dominant wavelength of 700 nm, mean luminance of 210 nit, and visual angle of 34 minutes, are set on the Foerster perimeter. In the DFR test, the fusion thresholds (msec) of double flashes, with exposure duration of each flash being 10 msec, are measured by controlling the intervals of these two flashes generated by one LED. These two tests were performed after 10 minutes of adaptation to 80 lux background.

Central and paracentral field locations, 10 (degree) away from the center on every 30 (degree) meridian were selected for test points in a glaucoma study. In a study, on the other hand, central and paracentral field locations on every 90(degree) meridian were selected. This is because, the results in the previous studies on DFR and CFF in the normal subjects displayed significantly great individual variations in the superior and inferior visual fields(1).

Subjects

In the glaucoma study, 30 patients with glaucoma were examined. They had a high intraocular pressure of 21 mmHg or higher for over 2 months in the past, and had no visual field defect using the Goldmann perimeter or elevation of thresholds using the Tubinger perimeter.

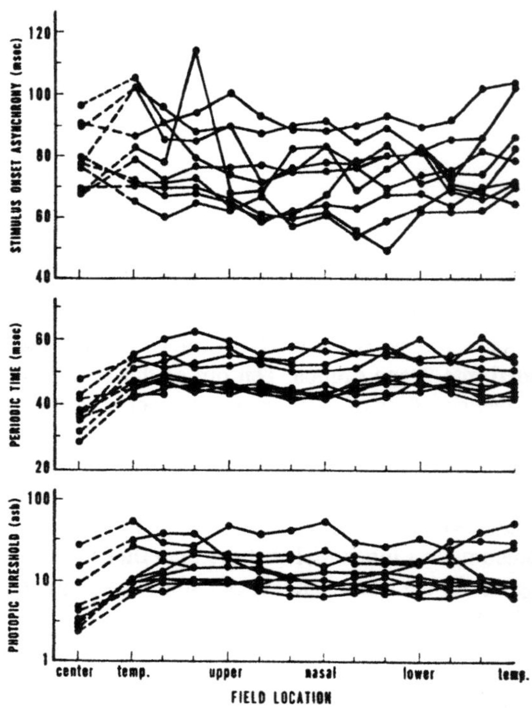

Figure 1. Results of 3 tests. Top: DFR test. Middle: CFF test. Bottom: Static Perimetry. Results from group with early glaucoma having abnormal DFR and normal CFF.

On the other hand, 24 normal persons aged from 11 to 75 years participated in the study. These normal subjects were classified into three groups; ie, 8 subjects in children group aged from 11 to 13 years, 8 subjects in adults group aged from 20 to 41 years, and 8 subjects in aged group aged from 60 to 75 years.

Results & discussion

Sixteen out of the 30 patients with glaucoma not having field defect using a Goldmann perimeter or a Tubinger perimeter showed functional abnormalities in the DFR; 10 patients showed abnormal DFR with normal CFF and 6 atients exhibited abnormalities both in DFR and CFF(Fig.1). None of these patients disclosed abnormality only in CFF without any abnormality in DFR.

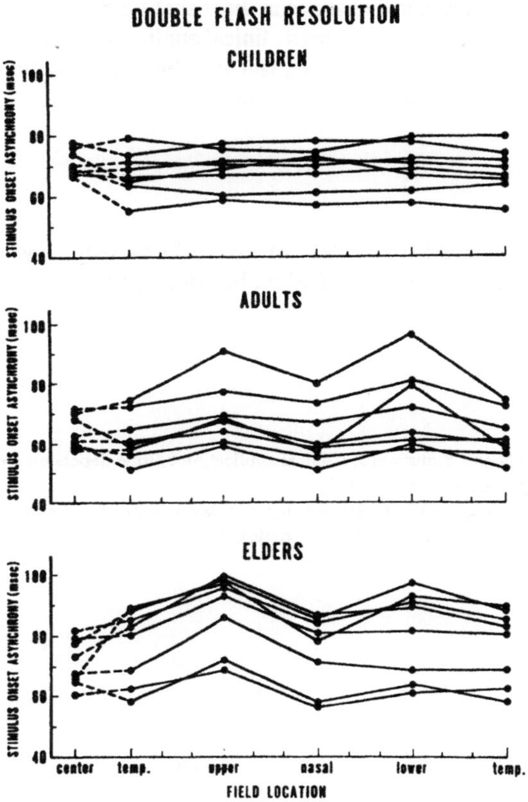

Figure 2. The thresholds of DFR for children, adults and aged groups.

Significant differences in DFR were found between the thresholds at the temporal quadrant and those at the nasal quadrant in group B(Student t-tests). Furthermore, significant differences in CFF and perimetric thresholds were found between the center and the nasal quadrant in all three groups.

The results of DFR in normal observers are shown in Figure 2. The top, middle and bottom data illustrate results in a) children, b) adults and c) aged group, respectively. Abnormal DFR was found at the upper and lower visual fields in adults and aged group, but there was no such abnormality in children group. On the other hand, the values of CFF among various visual fields were nearly the same in all age groups.

Significant differences in DFR at the upper and lower visual field were found between the children and adults group, and between the children and aged group. At the upper visual field, significant difference in DFR was also found between the adults and aged group. On the other hand, no significant difference among the three age groups was found in the case of CFF.

The essence of the DFR test resides in its simplicity with use of two pulsed-lights which are not so intense as to stabilize the neural interactions in the visual pathway, and in enabling one to evaluate functional changes in the visual system that may not be detected by other tests. The present study indicates a clinical applicability of this test not only as a diagnostic aid for the early detection of glaucoma but also for the understanding of pathophysiologic processes of retinal or optic nerve diseases.

Acknowledgments

The authors thank Saiichi Mishima, MD of Tokyo University, Jay M Enoch, PhD of University of California at Berkeley, and Shinobu Awaya, MD of Nagoya University for kind discussion.

References

1. Yasuma T, Miyakawa N and Yamazaki J: Clinical application of time-dependent perimetry: 1. Results in normal subjects. Jpn J Ophthalmol 1986; 30:330.
2. Enoch JM, Fitzgerald CR, Campos EC. Quantitative layer-by-layer perimetry. An extended analysis. Current Ophthalmology Monographs. New York: Grune & Stratton, 1981.

DESCARTES' CONTACT TUBE:

A CONTRIBUTION TO CONTACT LENS HISTORY

ROBERT F. HEITZ
Dpt. Ophthalmology, Central Hospital, F-67504 Haguenau,FRANCE.

Abstract

In his Discours de la Méthode, La Dioptrique, VII (1637), René Descartes proposed various methods to improve vision, in particular a water-filled tube in contact with the eye. This contact-tube used unintentionally a principle of contact lenses: the elimination of corneal power by a fluid and the substitution of this negated corneal surface by a new optical surface. Descartes did not intend to fit a corrective device in contact with the cornea, but he was attempting to improve the properties of the Galilean telescope for illustration of his new rules for simple and easy reasoning.

Introduction

In his fundamental work "Discourse on the Method of rightly conducting one's reason and seeking the truth in the sciences" *(Discours de la Méthode pour bien conduire sa raison et chercher la vérité dans les sciences*), the french philosopher René Descartes, born 400 years ago in 1596, discussed a number of controversial scientific issues in areas ranging from cosmology to physiology. The first edition of the Discourse also included three specific essays illustrating Descartes' method, namely the Optics *(La Dioptrique),* the Meteorology *(Les Meteores)* and the Geometry *(La Geométrique).* Descartes had begun work on the Optics in the late 1620s, and its publication in 1637 aroused considerable scientific interest. The work provides a good example of Descartes' application of mathematical techniques to problems in the physical sciences.

The Discourse seven of the Optics, under the title "Means for perfecting vision" (*Des moyens de perfectionner la vision*), take into consideration three factors to improve vision, --1-- the interior organs which receive the action emanating from the objects, --2-- the exterior organs by which these actions are disposed to produce the best effects and finally --3-- the object themselves. We can do nothing to improve the interior organs: the nerves and the brain. A near object produces a larger image upon the retina than a distant object of the same size, but bringing a distant object near to the eye is not always possible. The only effective action to have an enlarged retinal image is to act on the exterior organs, which include all the transparent parts of the eye as well the appliances we can interpose between the eye and the object being viewed [1,2]

Method

In his explanation of the perception of a bigger image, Descartes explains that "the greatness of the images depend only on three things: the distance which is between the object and the place where the rays cross...;then, on the one between this same place and the background of the eye; and finally on the refraction of these rays" *(Pour la grandeur des images, il est à remarquer qu'elle dépend seulement de trois choses, à savoir, de la distance qui est entre l'objet et le lieu où se croisent les rayons ...; puis, de celle qui est entre ce même lieu et le fond de l'oeil ; et enfin, de la réfraction de ces rayons.)*

"There remain only one other means of increasing the greatness of images, which is to cause the rays which come from various points of the object, to cross as far as possible from the backgound of the eye; but it is certainly, without comparison, the most important and the most considerable of all." *(Il ne reste plus qu'un autre moyen pour augmenter la grandeur des images, qui est de faire que les rayons qui viennent de divers points de l'objet, se croisent le plus loin qu'il se pourra du fond de l'oeil; mais il est bien, sans comparaison, le plus important et le plus considérable de tous.).*

In order to obtain elongation of the eye, Descartes suggested applying to the eye devices in which the rays coming from different objects in the visual field cross as far as possible from the retina. These devices are often interpreted as contact lens systems.

To construct these devices, Descartes proposed the following reasoning: "How, for example, the first of the three liquids with which the eye is filled has nearly the same refraction as common water, if we apply directly against a tube full of water, like EF, and the end of which there is a glass GHI, whose figure is similar to that of the skin BCD which covers this liquid and has the same relation to the distance from background of the eye, there will not be any refraction at the entry of this eye; but that which took place formerly there, will take place at the entry of the tube GI: so that these rays crossing there, form an image RST much larger than if they only crossed on the surface BCD; and they will form it more and more larger according to the increasing length of the tube. And thus the water EF performing the function of the humor K; the glass GHI, that of the skin BCD; and the entry of the tube GI, that of the pupil; the vision will be made same so as if the Nature had made the eye longer than it is, over the whole lenght of this tube". *(Comme par exemple, d'autant que la première des trois liqueurs dont l'oeil est rempli cause à peu près même réfraction que l'eau commune, si on applique tout contre un tuyau plein d'eau, comme EFF, au bout duquel il y ait un verre GHI, dont la figure soit semblable à celle de la peau BCD qui couvre cette liqueur, et ait même rapport à la distance du fond de l'oeil, il ne se fera plus aucune réfraction à l'entrée de cet oeil; mais celle qui s'y faisait auparavant se fera dès l'entrée du tuyau GI: si bien que ces rayons, se croisant dès la, formeront une image RST beaucoup plus grande que s'il ne se croisoient que sur la superficie BCD; et ils la formeront de plus en plus grande selon que ce tuyau sera plus long. Et ainsi l'eau EF faisant l'ofice de l'humeur K; le verre GHI, celui de la peau BCD; et l'entrée du tuyau GI, celui de la prunelle; la vision se fera en même façon que si la*

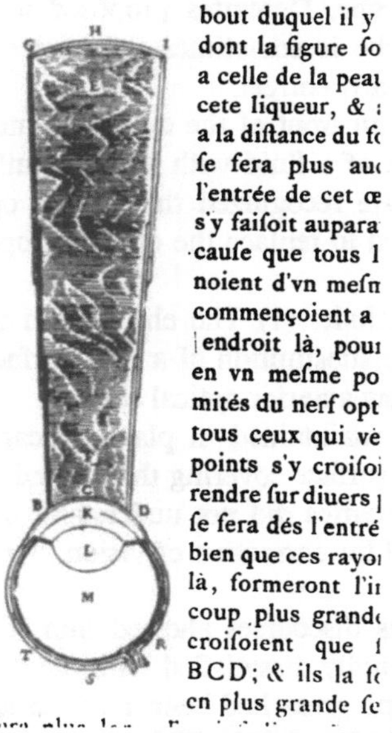

Fig.1. Descartes' water-filled tube placed against the eye, as step one of his demonstration.
EF: water filled tube - K: anterior humor of the eye
BCD: anterior skin of the eye (cornea)
GHI: distal glass, "similar to the skin BCD".

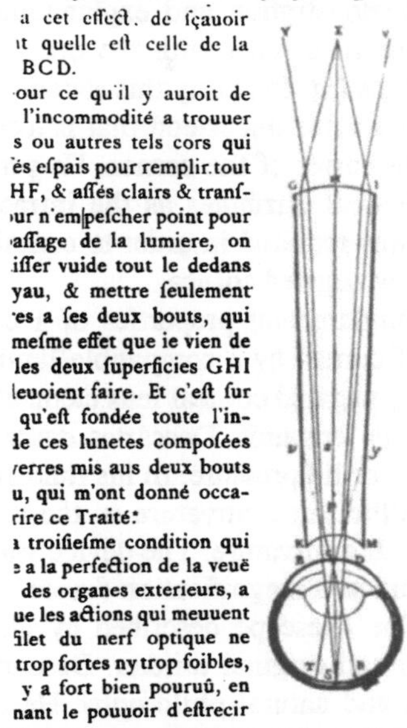

Fig.2. Step two of Decartes' demonstration: the water-filled contact-tube is replaced by a tube filled with water, or by a glass rod, but not applied to the eye.

Nature aurait fait l'oeil plus long qu'il n'est, de toute la longueur de ce tuyau.)

"But, the more that it would be much discomfort to apply water to the eye, so as I have explaind; and likewise, it is impossible to know exactly the figure of the skin BGD which covers him; it would be impossible to determine exactly this of the glass GHI , for to substitute him. *(Or, d'autant qu'il y aurait beaucoup d'incommodité à joindre de l'eau contre notre oeil, en la façon que je viens d'expliquer; et même que, ne pouvant savoir précisément quelle est la figure de la peau BCD qui le couvre, on en saurait déterminer exactement celle du verre GHI, pour le substituer à sa place).*

Descartes proposes therefore in the second step to employ another appliance consisting of a tube filled with water with a glass at each end and not applied to the eye and in a third step to replace the water-tube with a solid piece of glass" Finally he proposes, to leave the inside of the tube empty and apply a lens to each end, which will produce the same effect.

"This is the principle of the device formed by a lens at each end of a tube, named a telescope, which is the object of this treatise." *(C'est sur ceci seul qu'est fondée toute l'invention de ces lunettes composées de deux verres mis aux deux bouts d'un tuyau, qui m'ont donné occasion d'écrire ce traité).*

Discussion

In his demonstration and explanation of the telescope, Descartes proposed a water filled tube in contact with the eye. This contact tube is sometimes interpreted as a contact lens [3]. In reality this statement is only partially correct.

Descartes undestood that placement of water in front of the eye eliminates the refractive power of the cornea. He proposed the use of a fluid with approximatly the same physical attributes as the intraocular fluids. He recognized that a new optical surface was required in order to contain the fluid and to replace the optical properties of the now negated cornea.

Fundamental properties of a contact lens include: (1) The elimination of the power of cornea by a compatible liquid, and (2) the substitution of a new surface for the (now) negated corneal lens element by using a new anterior optical surface.

The lens-unit, Descartes described, was not maintained in place by capillary attraction or lid pressure. In his fluid-filled tube, the surface covering the far end of the tube has the same curvature as the cornea, and Descartes did not understand how to measure this curvature. The device was not intended for correction of vision, per se. It was meant as a magnification device.

The telescope described by Descartes in this discourses showed him to be a powerful and original thinker. Descartes was profoundly dissatisfied with the state of learning and natural philosophy. He felt that little progress had been made since the time of Aristotle. Descartes enunciated new rules for simple and easy reasoning particularly, ".to divide difficulties into as many parts as possible for better solution" and "to conduct his thoughts in order and to proceed by step from the simplest and easiest to know to more complex knowledge".

The analysis of a Galilean telescope, begining with a water-filled contact tube for effective eye elongation, to the final Galilean telescope, is a remarkable demonstration of this new approach to reasoning which Descartes introduced in the 17th century.

It is particularly interesting that he recognized a need to employ the principle of corneal neutralization as the first step of his demonstration, but he did not recognize that corneal neutralization can be used in the correction of refraction.

References:

1. Adam Ch,Tannery P. Oeuvres de Descartes. rev ed. Paris: Vrin/CNRS, 1964-1976
2. Cottingham J.,Stoothoff R.,Murdoch D. The philosophical writings of Descartes. Cambridge: University Press, 1988
3. Enoch JM. Descartes' contact lens Am J Optom Physiol Opt & Arch Am Acad Optom 1956; 33: 77-85
4. Heitz RF. History of contact lenses. In:Dabezies OH., editor.:Contact lenses. The CLAO guide to basic science and clinical practice. Orlando: Grune & Straton, 1984:1.1-1.19

MACH BANDS AND ART

MICHAEL F. MARMOR,
Dept. of Ophthalmology, Stanford University, Stanford, CA.

Abstract

Some illusions depend on cultural experiences or expectations, but Mach bands are innate to everyone. Ernst Mach postulated that the perceptual enhancement of contrast at border derived from physiologic interactions with the retina. This insight explained phenomena tht had been used consciously or unconsciously by artists for millennia. This is discussed with examples in this article.

The recognition of contrast is at the core of vision, and vision is at the core of art. The phenomena of Mach bands are one manifestation of cellular organization in our retina and brain that favors contrast sensitivity, and it is instructive physiologically and aesthetically to see how these effects have been used intentionally or inadvertently in art.

This topic has special meaning for me with respect to Jay Enoch. Some years back, in evaluating contrast sensitivity in retinal disease, I struggled to separate the effects of reduced acuity from those of disease pathology . We made some simple measurements of contrast sensitivity after optical blur from plus lenses [1], but of course, the interpretation was not so simple. We needed advice from an expert -- and I called on my friend Jay. In characteristic fashion, he suggested that the science would be improved by good food: we arranged to meet halfway between Stanford and Berkeley and he patiently tutored me on the fine points of contrast sensitivity over an excellent Chinese lunch.

The Czech scientist, Ernst Mach (1838-1916) was a Renaissance man who made major contributions in physics, psychology and philosophy. His name is best known today with respect to supersonic speeds (e.g., Mach 1), and his advocacy of "positivism" in science led to increased experimental and theoretical rigor in physics. Early in his career Mach had studied perception, and he analyzed the bands of light and dark that appear at the margins of shadows.

These phenomena were not new, but Mach had the insight to recognize that the enhancement of contrast at borders might derive from physiological processes within the eye rather than the brain [2]. His concept was based on anatomic studies of his day which showed that there were more photoreceptors than ganglion cells, so that convergence had to occur within the retina. He realized that convergence might incorporate different types of excitation, and thus favor the perception of contrast: "It appears to me that the phenomena discussed can only be explained on the basis of a reciprocal action of neighboring areas of the retina." This was quite a remarkable insight, considering that the relevant circuitry for inhibitory action, center-surround organization, and contrast perception within the retina, would not be clearly delineated for nearly 100 years.

The exquisite contrast sensitivity of the retina and brain leads to many well-known visual illusions. For example, the same patch of gray will appear quite light on a black background, and quite dark on a white background, because our eye is more influenced by contrast than by the absolute brightness of the gray itself. Mach bands represent a related type of illusory phenomenon. Broadly speaking, two aspects of Mach bands can be described. The first are perceptual Mach bands which represent the

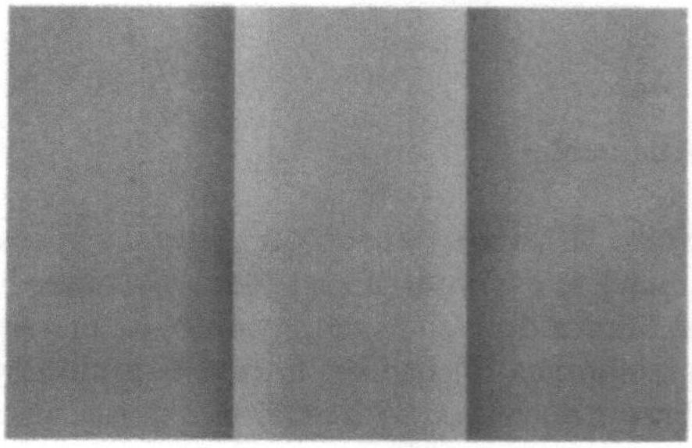

Figure 1: (Left) Perceptual Mach bands. Each grey rectangle is evenly colored (i.e., has the same brightness throughout), but we perceive an illusory darkening or lightening near the junctions.

Figure 2: (Right) Illusory brightness effects created by Mach bands. All three parts of this figure are an identical grey, but the light-dark junctions (Mach bands) between each zone fool the eye into thinking that the entire zone is light or dark.

illusory appearance of darkening or lightening at the edge of a light-dark boundary (Figure 1). The second type of Mach band phenomenon is the use of Mach bands to produce an illusion of lightness or darkness where it doesn't exist (Figure 2). Both of these phenomena -- perceptual Mach bands, and Mach bands that create illusory contrast -- have been used in art [3].

I have not rigorously sought the origins of Mach bands in art, but they are drawn at the edges of shadows in Greco-Roman art from the walls of homes in Pompeii and Herculaneum. These are depictions of perceptual Mach bands, and they show that ancient painters were careful observers of natural phenomena. Since much of the Roman art in this period copied the styles of earlier Greek artists whose work has been lost, we don't know the actual dates at which these techniques were first practiced.

Mach bands are also a mainstay of Asian art, perhaps in part because brush paintings lack color and the artist must use every trick of contrast and texture to convey the nature of the scenery. A frequent use of Mach bands in Asian art is to create the illusion of darkness or lightness in different areas of a painting (Figure 3). For example, the top of a mountain will get darker near its edge, making the whole mountain appear to loom dark in the distance. These techniques can be traced back at least to the Tang Dynasty (618 to 907). These artists could not have been aware of the concept of retinal integration, but they clearly understood the illusory power of contrast upon perception.

The use of Mach bands, and indeed also the use of shadows, perspective, and other components of realism in art, largely disappeared during the Middle Ages. Most art of that period was produced under the aegis of the church, and its purpose was no longer to decorate but solely to inspire and spread the doctrines of the church. The spirit of scientific inquiry returned during the Renaissance, along with artistic devices that portrayed a more realistic perceptual world. Brunelleschi and Alberti popularized perspective at the beginning of the 15th century, and the portrayal of shadows reappeared. Mach bands were soon to follow. Painters like Montegna and Leonardo drew light bands at the edge of dark borders and vice versa, showing awareness of both

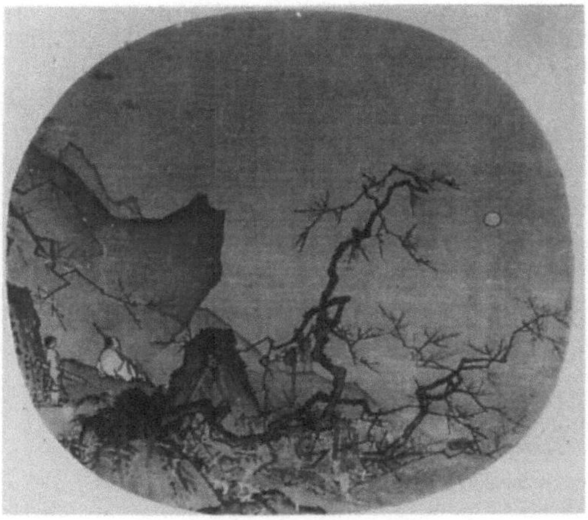

Figure 3: Ma Yüan (active 1180-1230). Plum Blossoms by Moonlight. Copyright 1986 by the Metropolitan Museum of Art, all rights reserved; gift of John H. Crawford, 1986. The mountains appear dark relative to the sky, but the difference disappears if one covers the edges (which represent a Mach band).

the perceptual phenomena of Mach bands and the ability of contrast to heighten the recognition of edges and space [4]. Later in the 19th century, Blanc would write, "Leonardo da Vinci says we should place a light background in contrast to a shadow and a dark background to a mass of light, and it is a general principle, a precept not to be attacked." [5]

This precept was followed by many artists. For example, the French pointillist, Georges Seurat, owned Blanc's book and apparently took Leonardo's advice very seriously [6]. In his sketches as well as his paintings, he exaggerated the contrast between subject and background no matter whether a figure stood against a lawn, a wall or a distant body of water. Sometimes this technique made for rather odd effects: in The Bathers at Asnières and A Sunday on La Grande Jatte there is so much alternation from light to dark around figures that the water is very strange-looking.

Twentieth century artists have also embraced Mach bands, both perceptual and illusory. The American painter, Arthur Dove, liked to paint bands and concentric circles of graded intensity (Figure 4), calling them "power bands". These designs, much like the pattern in Figure 1, create powerful Mach bands which perhaps were a part of Dove's fascination with them. Georgia O'Keeffe used Mach bands more in the style of the Asian brush painters, to create an enhanced sense of lightness or darkness in space. She was a master of shading, and Mach band effects are evident in many of her works.

Mach band effects have been incorporated into paintings and prints by "Op artists" such as Vasarely. In these works, the perceived bands and illusory effects intrigue and confuse us, and become intrinsic parts of the image. Some critics have argued that such Op art is merely design or a pleasing presentation of psychology experiments. I argue strongly to the contrary, since the use of Mach bands in art is no more or less justified than the use of other visual substrates such as color, perspective, or a particular image such as the Rouen Cathedral. The measure of art is whether the visual tools have been used to challenge and engage the viewer -- not which tools were used [7].

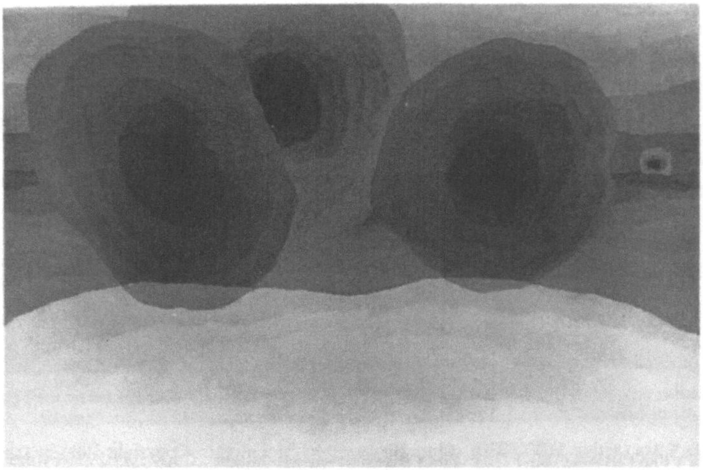

Figure 4: Arthur Dove. Fog Horns, oil, 1929. Colorado Springs Fine Arts Center. The stepwise shading creates perceptual Mach bands at the junctions between steps.

Some artists have produced visual effects by the conscious avoidance of Mach bands. An example is Renoir whose figures, particularly women, have a misty and soft appearance, much like the heroine in an old movie. A close inspection of these canvases show that Renoir carefully blurred the border of his subjects with a band of paint having a color and brightness intermediate between the flesh and background. By eliminating edge effects, including Mach bands, he removed cues of contrast and gave his figures an ill-defined and hazy boundary.

Ernst Mach did not "invent" the bands that bear his name, since their perception resides within the retinal circuitry of us all. He was also not the first to observe these phenomena, which have been portrayed or used by artists for millennia. However, Mach had the insight to recognize that the bands are derived from excitatory and inhibitory signals within the retina. Mach bands are found in the art of many ages, but Mach first told us why.

References:

1. Marmor MF and Gawande A. Effect of visual blur on contrast sensitivity. Invest Ophthalmol Vis Sci 1988;95:139-143.
2. Ratliff F. Mach Bands: Quantitative studies on neural networks in the retina. San Francisco, Holden-Day, 1965.
3. Marmor MF. The bands of Ernst Mach: Edge effects in art. In: Marmor MF and Ravin JG, eds. The Eye of the Artist. Philadelphia, Mosby-Year Book, Inc., 1996.
4. Weale RA. Discoverer of Mach-bands. Invest Ophthalmol Vis Sci 1979;18:652-654.
5. Homer WI. Seurat and the Science of Painting. Cambridge, MIT Press, pp 85-6, 1964.
6. Ratliff FA. Paul Signac and Color in Neo-Impressionism. New York, Rockefeller University Press, 1992.
7. Marmor MF. Illusion and optical art. In: Marmor MF and Ravin JG, eds. The Eye of the Artist. Philadelphia, Mosby-Year Book, Inc., 1996.

AUTHOR INDEX

Documenta Ophthalmologica Proceedings Series

1. J. François (eds.): *Symposium on Light-Coagulation.* Argon Laser and Xenon Arc (Ghent, Belgium, 1972). 1973 ISBN 90-6193-141-X
2. J.T. Pearlman (ed.): *10th ISCERG Symposium* (Los Angeles, Calif., USA, 1972). 1973 ISBN 90-6193-142-8
3. H.E. Henkes (ed.): *Photography, Electro-Ophthalmology and Echo-Ophthalmology in Ophthalmic Practice.* 1973 ISBN 90-6193-143-6
4. E. Dodt & J.T. Pearlman (eds.): *11th ISCERG Symposium* (Bad Nauheim, Germany, 1973). 1974 ISBN 90-6193-144-4
5. W.J. Holmes (ed.): *Public Health Ophthalmology.* Papers Presented at the Conference on the Prevention of Impaired Vision and Blindness (Paris, France, 1974). 1975 ISBN 90-6193-145-2
6. A. Th. M. van Balen (ed.): *First International Symposium on Artificial Lensimplantation* (Utrecht, The Netherlands, 1974). 1975 ISBN 90-6193-146-0
7. A.F. Deutman (ed.): [Symposium on] *New Developments in Ophthalmology.* (Nijmegen, The Netherlands, 1975) 1976 ISBN 90-6193-147-9
8. O. Hockwin (ed.): *Progress of Lens Biochemistry Research.* In Honour of Prof. Dr. med. J. Nordmann. 1976 ISBN 90-6193-148-7
9. J.J. de Laey (ed.): *International Symposium on Fluorescein Angiography* (Ghent, Belgium, 1976). 1976 ISBN 90-6193-149-5
10. R. Alfieri & P. Solé (eds.): *12th ISCERG Symposium* (Clermont-Ferrand, France, 1974). 1976 ISBN 90-6193-150-9
11. E. Auerbach (ed.): *Experimental and Clinical Amblyopia. 13th ISCERG Symposium* (Kibbutz Ginossar, Israel, 1975). 1977 ISBN 90-6193-151-7
12. E.L. Greve (ed.): *Symposium on Medical Therapy in Glaucoma* (Amsterdam, The Netherlands, 1976) 1977 ISBN 90-6193-152-5
13. T. Lawwill (ed.): *ERG, VER and Psychophysics. 14th ISCERG Symposium* (Louisville, USA, 1976). 1977 ISBN 90-6193-153-3
14. E.L. Greve (ed.): *2nd International Visual Field Symposium* (Tübingen, Germany, 1976). 1977 ISBN 90-6391-154-1
15. J. François & A. De Rouck (eds.), J.T. Pearlman and J. Kelsey (co-eds.): *Electrodiagnosis, Toxic Agents and Vision. 15th ISCEV Symposium* (Ghent, Belgium, 1977). 1978 ISBN 90-6193-155-X
16. H.-J Merté (ed.): *Genesis of Glaucoma.* Contributions of the Wessely Symposium in Munich (October 1974) with final Considerations by H. Goldmann. 1978 ISBN 90-6193-156-8
17. A.F. Deutmann & J.R.M. Cruysberg (eds.): *5th International Congress on Neurogenetics and Neuro- Ophthalmology* (Nijmegen, The Netherlands, 1977). 1978 ISBN 90-6193-159-2
18. O. Hockwin & W.B. Rathbun (eds.): *Progress in Anterior Eye Segment. Research and Practice.* In Honour of Prof. J.E. Harris. 1979 ISBN 90-6193-158-4
19. E.L. Greve (ed.): *3rd International Visual Field Symposium* (Tokyo, Japan, 1978). 1979 ISBN 90-6193-160-6
20. J. François, S.I. Brown & M. Itoi (eds.): *Proceedings of the Symposium of the International Society for Corneal Research* (Kyoto, Japan, 1978). 1979 ISBN 90-6193-157-6

Documenta Ophthalmologica Proceedings Series

21. J. François, E. Maumenee & I. Esente (eds.): *First International Congress on Cataract Surgery* (Florence, Italy, 1978). 1979 ISBN 90-6193-162-2
22. E.L. Greve (ed.): *Glaucoma Symposium.* Diagnosis and Therapy (Amsterdam, The Netherlands, 1979). 1980 ISBN 90-6193-164-9
23. E. Schmöger & J.H. Kelsey (eds.): *Visual Electrodiagnosis in Systemic Diseases.* Proceedings of the 17th ISCEV Symposium (Erfurt, GDR, 1979) 1980 ISBN 90-6193-163-0
24. A. Hamburg (ed.): *Symposium on Uveal Melanomas.* On the Occasion of the Snellen Medal Presentation to Dr W.A. Manschot (Utrecht, The Netherlands, 1979). 1980 ISBN 90-6193-722-1
25. H. Zauberman (ed.): *Proceedings of the Conference on Subretinal Space* (Jerusalem, Israel, 1979). 1981 ISBN 90-6193-721-3
26. E.L. Greve & G. Verriest (eds.): *4th International Visual Field Symposium* (Bristol, UK, 1980). 1981 ISBN 90-6193-165-7
27. H. Spekreijse & P.A. Apkarian: *Visual Pathways: Electrophysiology and Pathology.* 18th ISCEV Symposium (Amsterdam, The Netherlands, 1980). 1981 ISBN 90-6193-723-X
28. H.C. Fledelius, P.H. Alsbirk & E. Goldschmidt (eds.): *3rd International Conference on Myopia* (Copenhagen, Denmark, 1980). 1981 ISBN 90-6193-725-6
29. J.M. Thijssen & A.M. Verbeek (eds.): *Ultrasonography in Ophthalmology.* Proceedings of the 8th SIDUO Congress (Nijmegen, The Netherlands). 1981 ISBN 90-6193-724-8
30. L. Maffei (ed.): *Pathophysiology of the Visual System.* Proceedings of a Workshop (Pisa, Italy 1980). 1981 ISBN 90-6193-726-4
31. G. Niemeyer & Ch. Huber (eds.): *Techniques in Clinical Electrophysiology of Vision.* 19th ISCEV Symposium (Horgen-Zürich, Switzerland, 1981). 1982 ISBN 90-6193-727-7
32. A.Th.M. van Balen & W.A. Houtman (eds.): *Strabismus Symposium* (Amsterdam, The Netherlands, 1981). 1982 ISBN 90-6193-728-0
33. G. Verriest (ed.): *Colour Vision Deficiencies VI.* Proceedings of the 6th Symposium of the International Research Group on Colour Vision Deficiencies (Berlin- Steglitz, Germany, 1981). 1982 ISBN 90-6193-729-9
34. A. Roucoux & M. Crommelinck (eds.): *Physiological and Pathological Aspects of Eye Movements.* Proceedings of a Workshop (Pont d'Oye Castle, Habay-la-Neuve, Belgium, 1982). 1982 ISBN 90-6193-730-2
35. E.L. Greve & A. Heijl (eds.): *5th International Visual Field Symposium* (Sacramento, Calif., USA, 1982). 1983 ISBN 90-6193-731-0
36. R. Birngruber & V.-P. Gabel (eds.): *Laser Treatment and Photocoagulation of the Eye.* Proceedings of an International Symposium (Munich, Germany, 1982). 1984 ISBN 90-6193-732-9
37. H.E.J.W. Kolder (ed.): *Slow Potentials and Microprocessor Applications.* 20th ISCEV Symposium (Iowa City, USA, 1982). 1983 ISBN 90-6193-733-7

Documenta Ophthalmologica Proceedings Series

38. J.S. Hillman & M.M. Le May (eds.): *Ophthalmic Ultrasonography.* Proceedings of the 9th SIDUO Congress (Leeds, UK, 1982). 1984 ISBN 90-6193-734-5
39. G. Verriest (ed.): *Colour Vision Deficiencies VII.* Proceedings of the 7th Symposium of the International Research Group on Colour Vision Deficiencies (Geneva, Switzerland, 1983). 1984 ISBN 90-6193-735-3
40. J.R. Heckenlively (ed.), G.H.M. van Lith & T.Lawwill (ass. eds): *Pattern Electroretinogram, Circulatory Disturbances of the Visual System and Pattern-Evoked Responses.* 21st ISCEV Symposium (Budapest, Hungary, 1983). 1984 ISBN 90-6193-503-2
41. E.C. Campos (ed.): *Sensory Evaluation of Strabismus and Amblyopia in a Natural Environment.* In Honour of Prof. Bruno Bagolini. 1984 ISBN 90-6193-508-3
42. A. Heijl & E.L. Greve (eds.): *6th International Visual Field Symposium* (Santa Margherita Ligure, Italy, 1984). 1985 ISBN 90-6193-524-5
43. E.L. Greve, W. Leydhecker & C. Raitta (eds.): *2nd European Glaucoma Symposium* (Hyvinkää, Finland, 1984). 1985 ISBN 90-6193-526-1
44. P.C. Maudgal & L. Missotten (eds.): *Herpetic Eye Diseases.* Proceedings of an International Symposium (Leuven, Belgium, 1984). 1985 ISBN 90-6193-527-X
45. B. Jay (ed.): *Detection and Measurement of Visual Impairment in Pre-Verbal Children.* Proceedings of a Workshop (London, UK, 1985). 1986 ISBN 0-89838-789-2
46. G. Verriest (ed.): *Colour Vision Deficiencies VIII.* Proceedings of the 8th Symposium of the International Research Group on Colour Vision Deficiencies (Avignon, France, 1985). 1987 ISBN 0-89838-801-5
47. P.L. Emiliani (ed.): *Development of Electronic Aids for the Visually Impaired.* Proceedings of a Workshop on the Rehabilitation of the Visually Impaired (Florence, Italy, 1984). 1986 ISBN 0-89838-805-8
48. K.C. Ossoinig (ed.): *Ophthalmic Echography.* Proceedings of the 10th SIDUO Congress (St. Petersburg Beach, Florida, USA, 1984). 1987 ISBN 0-89838-873-2
49. E.L. Greve & A. Heijl (eds.): *7th International Visual Field Symposium* (Amsterdam, The Netherlands, 1986). 1987 ISBN 0-89838-882-1
50. D. BenEzra, S.J. Ryan, B.M. Glaser & R.P. Murphy (eds.): *Ocular Circulation and Neovascularization.* Proceedings of the First International Symposium (Jeruzalem, Israel, 1986). 1987 ISBN 0-89838-892-9
51. J.M. Thijssen, J.S. Hillman, P.E. Gallenga & G. Cennamo (eds.): *Ultrasonography in Ophthalmology 11.* Proceedings of the 11th SIDUO Congress (Capri, Italy, 1986). 1988 ISBN 0-89838-378-1
52. B. Drum & G. Verriest (eds.): *Colour Vision Deficiencies IX.* Proceedings of the 9th Symposium of the International Research Group on Colour Vision Deficiencies (Annapolis, Md., USA, 1987). 1989 ISBN 0-89838-403-6

Documenta Ophthalmologica Proceedings Series

53. R. Sampaolesi (ed.): *Ultrasonography in Ophthalmology 12.* Proceedings of the 12th SIDUO Congress (Iguazú Falls, Argentina, 1988). 1990 ISBN 0-7923-0765-8
54. B. Drum, J.D. Moreland & A. Serra (eds.): *Colour Vision Deficiencies X.* Proceedings of the 10th Symposium of the International Research Group on Colour Vision Deficiencies (Cagliari, Italy, 1989). 1991 ISBN 0-7923-0948-0
55. P. Till (ed.): *Ophthalmic Echography 13.* Proceedings of the 13th SIDUO Congress (Vienna, Austria, 1990). 1993 ISBN 0-7923-1808-0
56. B. Drum (ed.): *Colour Vision Deficiencies XI.* Proceedings of the 11th Symposium of the International Research Group on Colour Vision Deficiencies (Sydney, Australia, 1991). 1993 ISBN 0-7923-1864-1
57. B. Drum (ed.): *Colour Vision Deficiencies XII.* Proceedings of the 12th Symposium of the International Research Group on Colour Vision Deficiencies (Tübingen, Germany, 1993). 1995 ISBN 0-7923-2889-2
58. J.M. Thijssen, H.C. Fledelius & S. Tane (eds.): *Ultrasonography in Ophthalmology 14.* Proceedings of the 14th SIDUO Congress (Tokyo, Japan, 1992). 1995 ISBN 0-7923-3475-2

KLUWER ACADEMIC PUBLISHERS – DORDRECHT / BOSTON / LONDON

MIX
Papier aus verantwortungsvollen Quellen
Paper from responsible sources
FSC® C105338

If you have any concerns about our products,
you can contact us on
ProductSafety@springernature.com

In case Publisher is established outside the EU,
the EU authorized representative is:
Springer Nature Customer Service Center GmbH
Europaplatz 3, 69115 Heidelberg, Germany

Printed by Libri Plureos GmbH
in Hamburg, Germany